# FRONTIERS OF PRIMARY CARE

Series Editor: Mack Lipkin, Jr.

# FRONTIERS OF PRIMARY CARE

## Series Editor: Mack Lipkin, Jr.

Henk G. Schmidt   Mack Lipkin, Jr.
Marten W. de Vries   Jacobus M. Greep   Editors

# New Directions
# for Medical Education

Problem-based Learning
and Community-oriented
Medical Education

Foreword by H. Mahler

With Contributions by O.K. Alausa, D.E. Benor, D. Bok, U. Bollag,
P.A.J. Boujuijs, A.A.M. Crijnen, T. Fryers, E. de Graaff, J.M. Greep,
S.E. Hobfoll, T. Imbos, T. Khattab, H.F. Kraan, J. Lawani,
Y. van Leeuwen, M. Lipkin, Jr., S. van Luyk, D. Maddison, S. Mahler,
F. Makladi, J.H.C. Moust, R.L.B. Neame, V. Neufeld, D. Newble,
Z.M. Nooman, M. Pollemans, M. Prywes, H.G. Schmidt, J.C. Sibley,
H. Snellen, M. Sprooten, B. Stalenhoef, M. Verwijnen,
C. van der Vleuten, M.W. de Vries, J. Zuidweg

With 30 Illustrations

Springer-Verlag
New York Berlin Heidelberg
London Paris Tokyo

Henk G. Schmidt, Ph.D.
Professor of Health Professions
  Education,
University of Limburg,
The Netherlands

Mack Lipkin, Jr., M.D.
Director, Primary Care;
Associate Professor of Medicine,
New York University Medical Center,
  School of Medicine,
New York, NY 10016, USA

Marten W. de Vries, M.D.
Professor of Social Psychiatry,
University of Limburg,
The Netherlands

Jacobus M. Greep, M.D.
Former Dean, Professor of Surgery,
University of Limburg,
The Netherlands

*Series Editor*

Mack Lipkin, Jr., M.D.
Director, Primary Care;
Associate Professor of Medicine,
New York University Medical Center,
  School of Medicine
New York, NY 10016, USA

Library of Congress Cataloging-in-Publication-Data
New directions for medical education.
    (Frontiers of primary care)
    Includes bibliographies and index.
    1. Medical education—Psychological aspects.
2. Humanistic psychology—Study and teaching.
3. Medical logic—Study and teaching.  4. Community
health services.  I. Schmidt, Henk G.  II. Alausa,
O.K. (Ola K.)  III. Series. [DNLM: 1. Community
Health Services—trends.  2. Education, Medical.
W 18 N5315]
R737.N47           362.1′042           86-29859
ISBN 0-387-96390-1

Printed on acid-free paper

Typeset by Publishers Service, Bozeman, Montana.
Printed and bound by Edwards Brothers, Ann Arbor, Michigan.
Printed in the United States of America.

9 8 7 6 5 4 3 2 1

ISBN 0-387-96390-1 Springer-Verlag New York Berlin Heidelberg
ISBN 3-540-96390-1 Springer-Verlag Berlin Heidelberg New York

# Series Preface

Primary care medicine is the new frontier in medicine. Every nation in the world has recognized the necessity to deliver personal and primary care to its people. This includes first-contact care, care based in a positive and caring personal relationship, care by a single healthcare provider for the majority of the patient's problems, coordination of all care by the patient's personal provider, advocacy for the patient by the provider, the provision of preventive care and psychosocial care, as well as care for episodes of acute and chronic illness. These facets of care work most effectively when they are embedded in a coherent integrated approach.

The support for primary care derives from several significant trends. First, technologically based care costs have rocketed beyond reason or availability, occurring in the face of exploding populations and diminishing real resources in many parts of the world, even in the wealthier nations. Simultaneously, the primary care disciplines—general internal medicine and pediatrics and family medicine—have matured significantly. They have become viable alternatives to the specialty approach to care with its potential dehumanization, coordination problems, and increased cost. The primary care disciplines have begun to create new sets of intellectual tools and new educational approaches to support their new paradigm of biopsychosocial care, including clinical epidemiology that examines the efficacy, effectiveness, and efficiency of everyday real-world care; clinical decision making that is beginning to find ways to improve the rational basis for common clinical choice; the medical interview, which is now coming under critical study as the major medium of care; problem-based learning and community-oriented medical education that enable efficient learning of the greatest relevance and with increased satisfaction for learner and teacher; and the philosophic and empiric study of ethical aspects of care.

Several major questions have emerged in the new disciplines. Who is to do primary care? What do these practitioners need to know? How can the needed content, skills, and attitudes be best taught? Who is to teach these new practitioners and what skills do the practitioners need? Persons interested in these questions include primary care professionals, teachers, and researchers in primary medicine.

Frontiers of Primary Care plans to help meet the needs of these overlapping groups, reporting fundamental and applied research findings in clinically relevant, readable ways. It will also provide information to teachers of primary medicine both about necessary content areas such as alcoholism or the medical interview. It will teach teachers about new teaching approaches and methods and include some books teachers may choose to use as texts. Finally, it will publish new conceptual work about the basis of the field and the shifting paradigm of care.

This volume is the latter type of contribution to the series. It is an important introduction for health care teachers, practitioners, and those preparing for such roles concerning two leading innovations in the teaching of person-centered, population-based medicine. It demonstrates the exciting potential for educational innovation. Such major experiments give us hope for the future humanism and relevance of health care.

Mack Lipkin, Jr., M.D.
Series Editor

# Foreword

The development and organization of health systems based on the Primary Health Care Approach is the cornerstone of all national strategies for "Health for All by the Year 2000." These health systems depend, for their effectiveness, on people and particularly on the existence of the right sort of health personnel to deliver health care to whole populations. This means that the basic training and continuing education of health personnel must be adapted to the real needs of communities.

The traditional medical school curriculum is centered on the hospital rather than on the environment in which individuals and communities live. This approach is not conducive to the development of the sort of health staff we need to cope with most people's health problems most of the time.

Educational programs should, therefore, be planned to motivate graduates toward meeting the health needs of the communities they will serve. This implies understanding what technical, social, and behavioural measures are appropriate in the sense of being sound, acceptable to those who use them and those on whom they are used, and applicable at a cost people can really afford. The training of students in direct contact with the community will help the students understand the environment in which people live, and the problems people face in their daily lives. If we try to solve these problems as a basis for learning, it will help to develop health staff sufficiently flexible to solve the problems of tomorrow.

It is vital that more efforts be made to prepare teachers of health workers to promote and implement such ideas. In this way, we can ensure that educational institutions make effective contributions to their country's long-range strategies for health and socioeconomic development.

I firmly believe that this book, which describes the two concepts of community-oriented education and problem-based learning, is particularly timely and valuable. Moreover, I consider it an essential stone that will help pave the difficult way to "Health for All."

H. Mahler, M.D.
Director-General
World Health Organization

# Preface

As Director-General of the World Health Organization, H. Mahler has written, "The development of health personnel able and willing to serve the community by providing health care, promoting health, preventing disease and caring for those in need is a major and formidable task for educators."[1] In his economical way, Mahler has summarized several of the most important challenges for medical education and care in the second half of the twentieth century. Medical education has had to take its share of the blame for the problems perceived in health care systems and the inadequacies perceived in the care of individual patients in this era.

Medicine in the era of genetic engineering, of organ transplantation and artificial hearts, and of the eradication of smallpox, represents one of the highest triumphs of human achievement. Not only does the most advanced care repetitively amaze even seasoned medical scientists, but simple basic care has also become a source of profound wonder and relief. Take, for example, the recent application of elementary physiology to infant diarrhea, a major international killer in tropical and temperate climates, that can carry off an infant in a few hours. Recognition that the cause of death in these children was fluid and electrolyte depletion led to direct treatment. The simple restoration of fluid and electrolytes in these cases has resulted in the saving of thousands of precious lives.

Yet there also exists a harsher side of modern medicine. In many places, it is evident that there are not enough doctors and health care personnel to go around. Health care resources are often misdirected towards glittering new technologies while the life-and-death needs of the poor or remote are denied. Practitioners trained in traditional schools are specialty oriented and sometimes incapable of caring for common problems efficiently and definitively. The traditionalists fail often to apply preventive measures prospectively despite 100 years of demonstration that prevention is much more efficient and causes much less suffering than expenditure of comparable effort and resources for curative care. Similarly, the problems facing citizens in all parts of the world have major psychosocial components—as determinants, precipitants, and reactions to disease and illness. Yet few medical education systems adequately train practitioners to analyze—let alone treat—psychosocial problems that may be more important to the patient's recovery or adjustment than the physical manifestations of the problem.

In parallel to such critiques of medical *systems* are critiques of medical education that are cited as better than ever, yet woefully deficient.[2] These systems are said to be dehumanizing, to stultify creativity, to fail to prepare practitioners for lifetimes of learning at a time when new knowledge doubles in less than five years. It is evident that problem-solving skills are dulled by traditional medical education with the result that practitioners fall back on routine and habit and fail to maintain the active curiosity and alertness needed for the complex tasks of medical practice.

The first half of the twentieth century saw the development of a disease centered approach to medicine exemplified by the growth of medical centers as the home of medical education. This reflected the special needs of medical research and of high-tech approaches to diagnosis and treatment. The medical goals of prevention, of psychosocial integration of care, and of creation of responsible medical-professional citizens who could lead the profession in the direction of service to the population as a whole, were lost. For some, these tasks lay in the hands of schools of public health. But these schools rapidly became specialty ivory towers of their own and lost their ability to communicate with or influence mainstream medicine.[3]

World War II brought home to many the recognition that most medical needs need not be served by specialists, that the common occurs commonly and the unusual rarely so that most practitioners should be equipped to handle the everyday event. General practice was revived and professionalized. National health systems developed in most of Europe. It became increasingly clear that the medical schools, dominated by scholars of great accomplishment but narrow vision, were increasingly remote from the major needs of the people who supported them and depended on them for care. The model institutions and the leading institutions came to be more and more alike in fostering specialty knowledge and in creating physicians increasingly alienated from their surroundings. These schools taught about patients found in referral centers, about extreme and rare cases, and about the newest in preference to the most basic methods. Yet White, Williams, and Greenberg showed that of 1000 illness episodes in the community, only 10 ended up in the university hospital.[4] Yet these 10 formed the experimental basis of the medical approaches of graduates.

In reaction to these and many more problems, a group of medical educational pioneers began to attempt new approaches that would preserve the best of technologically oriented, science-based medicine but include the needs of the entire population and create the needed skills and attitudes in graduates to serve the needs of the people more effectively and efficiently. This book describes two of the most exciting and major educational innovations: community-oriented medical education and problem-based learning.

The work on this book began at the meeting of the Network of Community Oriented Educational Institutions for Health Sciences held at the Rockefeller Foundation's Study Center in Bellagio, Italy, in 1981. This was the second meeting of the Network, an organization begun through the offices of the Health Manpower Development Division of the World Health Organization in 1979. The Network exists to foster cooperation and mutual assistance of the innovative health sciences institutions using community-oriented medical education and problem-based learning. (For a full description of the Network's objectives and a list of member institutions, see Appendices A and B at the end of the book.) Papers from the 1981 meeting became the basis for organization of a volume highlighting recent developments in these fields and building on the prior literature, especially the volumes on *Personnel for Health Care* published by the World Health Organization.

There are three features that make this book a benchmark that will help pave the difficult road toward health for all as Mahler said. First, the volume marks the entry into the exciting world of educational innovation of major traditional institutions such as Harvard University, which, as President Bok's report, "Needed: A New Way to Train Doctors" (Chapter 2), documents, has accepted the argument that major changes are necessary if modern medical education is to meet the demands facing it.

Second, the process of problem-based learning has made major advances in the last few years. Pioneered at McMaster University, in Hamilton, Ontario, Canada, problem-based learning has seen several complementary approaches described and assessed. Here, we report major outcome data about the method. The cognitive and affective effects of problem-based learning have been studied in a unique, experimental way by the faculty of the University of Limburg at Maastricht, The Netherlands. They and others now have detailed knowledge on faculty development and on how to assess student learning.

Finally, the volume illustrates the increasing sophistication of the scholars involved in community-oriented medical education. The chapters presented here include a succinct, profound overview of the conceptual base of community-oriented medical education (Benor et al., Chapter 4), problems arising when implementing it in a developing country (Nooman, Chapter 5), and student experience with it in several entertaining and instructive concrete examples (e.g., Chapter 6 by Bollag and his collaborators and Chapter 7 by Alausa).

We are grateful to many for their help and support in the production of this volume. Kerr White and the Health Sciences Division of the Rockefeller Foundation, led with wisdom and vision by Kenneth S. Warren, provided the wonderful surroundings that stimulated the project. The Foundation of Higher Education in Limburg (SWOL) in The Netherlands has generously supported Dr. Lipkin and Dr. Schmidt and the University of Limburg supported Dr. de Vries, enabling them to collaborate on the book. Debra Kittay, Ine Kuppen, Désirée Bronckers, Petry Thiemann, Tonny deVries, Pauline Schoenmakers, Kay Williams, and Theodore Lester II provided invaluable assistance. Finally, the members of the Network and each of the authors have been most helpful in producing a coherent whole.

The work presented here has been the product of men and women who are truly great medical pioneers. Three of the most noble were with us in Bellagio but have died since. Fred Katz, Jack Sibley, and David Maddison each were dearly loved by us, personally and professionally, for all they have given us. This book is dedicated to them with love, gratitude, and, most of all, the deep respect due to courageous, and brilliant, and human pioneers.

## References

1. Katz FM, Fulöp T (eds). *Personnel for Health Care*. Geneva, World Health Organization, 1978, p 7.
2. de Vries M, Berg R, Lipkin M, Jr. *The Use and Abuse of Medicine*. New York, Praeger, 1982.
3. Evans J. Measurement and management in medicine and health services: training needs and opportunities, in Lipkin M Jr, Lybrand WA (eds). *Population Based Medicine*. New York, Praeger, 1982, pp 3–41.
4. White UL, Williams TF, Greenberg BG. The ecology of medical care. *New Engl J Med*, 1961;265:885–892.

The Editors

# Contents

Series Preface . . . . . . . . . . . . . . . . . . . . . . . . . . . . . . . . . . . . . . . . . . . . . .     v

Foreword . . . . . . . . . . . . . . . . . . . . . . . . . . . . . . . . . . . . . . . . . . . . . . . . .    vii

Preface . . . . . . . . . . . . . . . . . . . . . . . . . . . . . . . . . . . . . . . . . . . . . . . . . . .     ix

Contributors . . . . . . . . . . . . . . . . . . . . . . . . . . . . . . . . . . . . . . . . . . . . . . .    xvii

Part I   The Need: New Ways to Train Doctors

Chapter 1
Towards the Education of Doctors Who Care for the Needs
of the People: Innovative Approaches in Medical Education
*Mack Lipkin, Jr.* . . . . . . . . . . . . . . . . . . . . . . . . . . . . . . . . . . . . . . . . . . .      3

Chapter 2
Needed: A New Way to Train Doctors
*Derek Bok* . . . . . . . . . . . . . . . . . . . . . . . . . . . . . . . . . . . . . . . . . . . . . . . .     17

Chapter 3
A Medical School for the Future
*David Maddison* . . . . . . . . . . . . . . . . . . . . . . . . . . . . . . . . . . . . . . . . . . . .     39

Part II   Community-oriented Medical Education Today
*Mack Lipkin, Jr.*

Chapter 4
Important Issues in Community-oriented Medical Education
*Dan E. Benor, Steven E. Hobfoll, and Moshe Prywes* . . . . . . . . . . . . . . . .     51

Chapter 5
Implementation of a Community-oriented Curriculum:
The Task and the Problems
*Zohair M. Nooman* . . . . . . . . . . . . . . . . . . . . . . . . . . . . . . . . . . . . . . . . . .     66

Chapter 6
Medical Education in Action: Community-based Experience
and Service in Nigeria
*Ulli Bollag, Henk G. Schmidt, Tom Fryers, and John Lawani* . . . . . . . . . .    78

Chapter 7
Community-based Medical Education in Nigeria:
The Case of Bayero University
*Ola K. Alausa* . . . . . . . . . . . . . . . . . . . . . . . . . . . . . . . . . . . . . . . . . . . .    93


Part III   Problem-based Learning: Rationale and Examples
*Henk G. Schmidt*

Chapter 8
The Rationale Behind Problem-based Learning
*Henk G. Schmidt* . . . . . . . . . . . . . . . . . . . . . . . . . . . . . . . . . . . . . . . . . .    105

Chapter 9
Problem-based Medical Education: The Newcastle Approach
*Roderick L.B. Neame* . . . . . . . . . . . . . . . . . . . . . . . . . . . . . . . . . . . . .    112

Chapter 10
Toward an Emphasis on Problem Solving in Teaching and Learning:
The McMaster Experience
*John C. Sibley* . . . . . . . . . . . . . . . . . . . . . . . . . . . . . . . . . . . . . . . . . . .    147


Part IV   Evaluation in Innovative Medical Education
*Marten W. de Vries*

Chapter 11
Evaluation of Health Sciences Education Programs: Program
and Student Assessment at McMaster University
*Victor Neufeld and John C. Sibley* . . . . . . . . . . . . . . . . . . . . . . . . . . . . .    165

Chapter 12
The Evaluation System at the Maastricht Medical School
*Maarten Verwijnen, Tjaart Imbos, Hetty Snellen-Balendong,*
*Betsy Stalenhoef-Halling, Marjan Gruyters Pollemans, Scheltus van Luyk,*
*Mirjam Sprooten, Yvonne van Leeuwen and Cees van der Vleuten* . . . . . .    180

Chapter 13
Issues and Guidelines for Student and Program Evaluation
*Victor Neufeld* . . . . . . . . . . . . . . . . . . . . . . . . . . . . . . . . . . . . . . . . . . .    196

Chapter 14
Teaching and Measuring Interviewing Skills in the
Maastricht Medical Curriculum
*Herro F. Kraan, Alfons A.M. Crijnen, Jaap Zuidweg,*
*Cees van der Vleuten and Tjaart Imbos* . . . . . . . . . . . . . . . . . . . . . . . . .    206

Chapter 15
How Effective Are Problem-based, Community-oriented Curricula:
Experienced Evidence
*Henk G. Schmidt* . . . . . . . . . . . . . . . . . . . . . . . . . . . . . . . . . . . . . . . . .  220

Chapter 16
Dutch Comparisons: Cognitive and Motivational Effects
of Problem-based Learning on Medical Students
*Marten W. de Vries, Henk G. Schmidt, and Erik de Graaf* . . . . . . . . . . . . .  230

Part V    Faculty Development
*Henk G. Schmidt*

Chapter 17
Attitude Change Among Medical Teachers: Effects of a
Workshop on Tutorials
*Henk G. Schmidt, Peter A.J. Bouhuijs, Tymoor Khattab,
and Fathi Makladi* . . . . . . . . . . . . . . . . . . . . . . . . . . . . . . . . . . . . . . . . . .  243

Chapter 18
Training Medical Teachers: Rationale and Outcomes
*Dan E. Benor and Sophia Mahler* . . . . . . . . . . . . . . . . . . . . . . . . . . . . . .  248

Chapter 19
Preparing Faculty and Students for Problem-based Learning
*Jos H.C. Moust and Henk G. Schmidt* . . . . . . . . . . . . . . . . . . . . . . . . . . .  260

Chapter 20
Introducing Problem-based Learning into a Conventional Curriculum
*David Newble* . . . . . . . . . . . . . . . . . . . . . . . . . . . . . . . . . . . . . . . . . . . . .  271

Conclusions . . . . . . . . . . . . . . . . . . . . . . . . . . . . . . . . . . . . . . . . . . . . . . . .  275

Appendix A
The Network
*Jacobus M. Greep and Henk G. Schmidt* . . . . . . . . . . . . . . . . . . . . . . . . .  279

Appendix B
List of Members of the Network of Community-oriented
Educational Institutions for Health Sciences . . . . . . . . . . . . . . . . . . . . . . .  283

Index . . . . . . . . . . . . . . . . . . . . . . . . . . . . . . . . . . . . . . . . . . . . . . . . . . . . .  294

# Contributors

Ola K. Alausa, M.D.
Faculty Coordinator, Faculty of Medicine, Bayero University, Kano, Nigeria

Dan E. Benor, M.D.
Associate Professor of Medical Education, Vice Dean for Curriculum Development and Director, Recanti School for Community Health Professions, University Center for Health Sciences, Ben-Gurion University of the Negev, Beersheva, Israel

Derek Bok, M.D.
President, Harvard University, Cambridge, MA, USA

Ulli Bollag, M.D.
Senior Lecturer in Paediatrics, Faculty of Health Sciences, University of Ilorin, Ilorin, Nigeria

Peter A.J. Bouhuijs, M.D.
Associate Professor of Medical Education, Faculty of Medicine, University of Limburg, Maastricht, The Netherlands

Alfons A.M. Crijnen, M.D.
Assistant Professor of Social Psychiatry, Faculty of Medicine, University of Limburg, Maastricht, The Netherlands

Erik de Graaf
Assistant Professor of Medical Education, Faculty of Medicine, University of Limburg, Maastricht, The Netherlands

Tom Fryers
Professor of Epidemiology, Faculty of Health Sciences, University of Ilorin, Ilorin, Nigeria

Jacobus M. Greep, M.D.
Professor of Surgery, Faculty of Medicine, University of Limburg, Maastricht,
The Netherlands

Steven E. Hobfoll, Ph.D.
Senior Lecturer in Psychology, Faculty of Psychology, Tel Aviv University, Tel
Aviv, Israel

Tjaart Imbos, Ph.D.
Assistant Professor of Medical Informatics and Statistics, Faculty of Medicine,
University of Limburg, Maastricht, The Netherlands

Tymoor Khattab, M.D.
Associate Professor in Gynaecology and Obstetrics, Faculty of Medicine, Suez
Canal University, Ismailia, Egypt

Herro F. Kraan, M.D., Ph.D.
Associate Professor of Social Psychiatry, Faculty of Medicine, University of Limburg, Maastricht, The Netherlands

John Lawani, M.D.
Senior Lecturer in Community Medicine, Faculty of Health Sciences, University
of Ilorin, Ilorin, Nigeria

Mack Lipkin, Jr., M.D.
Director, Primary Care; Associate Professor of Medicine; New York University
Medical Center, School of Medicine, New York, NY, USA

David Maddison, M.D.*
Founding Dean, Faculty of Medicine, University of Newcastle, New South
Wales, Australia

H. Mahler, M.D.
Director-General, World Health Organization, Geneva, Switzerland

Sophia Mahler, Ph.D.
Assistant Professor of Medical Education, Faculty of Health Sciences, Ben
Gurion University, Beersheva, Israel

Fathi Makladi, M.D.
Associate Professor of Family Medicine, Faculty of Medicine, Suez Canal
University, Ismailia, Egypt

---

*Deceased.

Joseph H.C. Moust, M.A.
Assistant Professor of Medical Education, Faculty of Medicine, University of Limburg, Maastricht, The Netherlands

Roderick L.B. Neame, M.A., M.D., Ph.D., M.B.B., Chir.
Senior Lecturer in Physiology, Faculty of Medicine, University of Newcastle, New South Wales, Australia

Victor Neufeld, M.D.
Professor of Internal Medicine, Faculty of Health Sciences, MacMaster University, Hamilton, Ontario, Canada

David Newble, Ph.D.
Associate Professor in Physiology, University of Adelaide, South Australia, Australia

Zohair M. Nooman, M.D.
Founding Dean, Faculty of Medicine, Suez Canal University, Ismailia, Egypt

Marjan Gruyters-Pollemans, M.D.
Assistant Professor of Medical Education, Faculty of Medicine, University of Limburg, Maastricht, The Netherlands

Moshe Prywes, M.D.
Professor of Medical Education, Faculty of Health Sciences, Ben Gurion University, Beer Sheva, Israel

Henk G. Schmidt, Ph.D.
Professor of Medical Education, Faculty of Medicine, University of Limburg, Maastricht, The Netherlands

John C. Sibley, M.D.*
Faculty of Health Sciences, Dean for Educational Affairs, MacMaster University, Hamilton, Ontario, Canada

Hetty Snellen-Balendong, M.D.
Assistant Professor of Medical Education, Faculty of Medicine, University of Limburg, Maastricht, The Netherlands

Mirjam Sprooten-Van Hoof, M.D.
Assistant Professor of Medical Education, Faculty of Medicine, University of Limburg, Maastricht, The Netherlands

Betsy Stalenhoef-Halling, M.D.
Assistant Professor of Medical Education, Faculty of Medicine, University of Limburg, Maastricht, The Netherlands

Cees P.M. van der Vleuten, M.A.
Assistant Professor of Medical Education, Faculty of Medicine, University of Limburg, Maastricht, The Netherlands

Marten W. de Vries, M.D.
Professor of Social Psychiatry, University of Limburg, Maastricht, The Netherlands

Yvonne D. van Leeuwen, M.D.
Assistant Professor of Family Medicine, Faculty of Medicine, University of Limburg, Maastricht, The Netherlands

Scheltus J. van Luyk, M.D.
Assistant Professor of Family Medicine, Faculty of Medicine, University of Limburg, Maastricht, The Netherlands

G. Maarten Verwijnen, M.D.
Assistant Professor of Family Medicine, Faculty of Medicine, University of Limburg, Maastricht, The Netherlands

Jaap Zuidweg
Assistant Professor of Family Medicine, Faculty of Medicine, University of Limburg, Maastricht, The Netherlands

# Part I
# The Need: New Ways to Train Doctors

# 1
# Toward the Education of Doctors Who Care for the Needs of the People: Innovative Approaches in Medical Education

MACK LIPKIN, JR.

This book documents the early, that is, present, stages of one of the most dramatic changes in medical education since Abraham Flexner reported to the Carnegie Foundation in 1910.[1] At that time, medical schools were proliferating without adequate controls or standards. Flexner documented the many deficiencies of these proprietary institutions, including their lack of adequate curriculum and the production of graduates with little knowledge of science or medicine. He wrote of the necessity for a scientific basis of medical education rooted in a scientifically active faculty who would organize a curriculum of basic sciences followed by applied clinical studies. He modeled his recommendations on Johns Hopkins Medical School, which in turn was heavily influenced by the leading German schools of the prior 50 years. Flexner's views, propagated by Carnegie and taken up by leading foundations and philanthropists, led to restructuring of medical education first in the United States and later elsewhere.

In response to pressing problems of modern medicine worldwide, many of them products of the Flexner revolution, a new form of medical education and organization has become the subject of multiple, vigorous experiments involving large institutional commitments. More than 20 medical schools (the number depends on the criteria), spanning the globe and on many portions of the spectrum of global political and social systems, have undertaken varied forms of a common experiment. These schools are attempting to provide community-oriented health education using problem-based learning as the major means of instruction.

These important experiments have two basic roots. First, there is growing recognition that the products of yesterday's medical education—today's medical systems—have systematic and major deficiencies.[2] Second, the last 20 years have seen a qualitative shift in the degree of scholarship and professionalism among teachers of medicine as educators. Using the work of psychologists and educators, they have produced new approaches to thinking and learning about medical teaching. In addition to creative and scholarly bases for new educational approaches is the recognition, increasingly documented during the past two decades, that the process of becoming a doctor or other health worker can be onerous and intellectually diminishing. Some have feared that this process itself contributes to a trend toward dehumanization in medical care.[3] It also is sometimes related to negative effects of the profession on its members: high rates of suicide, addiction, and divorce, and premature morbidity and mortality relative to peers.[4]

The founding of new medical schools has presented the principal opportunity for a small group of innovators to attempt novel forms of organization of school, curriculum, and practice arrangements and methods. These are the subject of this book. This introduction briefly describes the reasons for and the principles of problem-based learning and of community-oriented medical education. The sections that follow elaborate on each in greater detail, followed by studies on the evaluation of these new approaches and by work on the development of the new faculty necessary to implement new approaches. The volume closes with an overview highlighting some of the problems that remain to be solved and future directions for research and development. An Appendix is included to assist those readers who wish to pursue further learning about these institutions and the theories and experiments that underlie their practices.

## Why Community-oriented Medical Education?

On first inspection of the literature, the reasons for undertaking community-oriented medical education seem to vary as a function of locale. However, thoughtful reading shows that the core reasons remain the same regardless of the setting, be it the Sudan or Manhattan. Community-oriented medical education stems foremost from a person-centered model of health care in which the health of the population provides the balance between individual concerns. This view—person-centered and population-based—is seen as balancing the elite care of select individuals coupled with a focus on disease and the advancement of the profession emphasized in traditional, Flexner model, medical-center-based medical schools. This approach does not have an exclusive focus on public health issues as in schools of public health. That approach has led to separation of public health faculties from the mainstream of clinical medicine.[5] Rather, it is a reform movement centered in a rational approach to the care of individual patients *in the context* of a health system that attempts to meet to the fullest extent possible the health and medical needs of the entire population. It is the logical confluence of several streams of thought.

One of these areas is the series of broad criticisms of modern medicine popular in the lay press. Some of these critiques, such as those of Szasz,[6] Illich,[7] and Carlson,[8] emphasize that medicine has created a series of negative practices along with its progress. Iatrogenesis, the creation of illness or disease through medical practice itself, is the most prominent.[9] Although iatrogenic damage to patients is inevitable, the so-called diseases of medical progress have led some to call for the abolition of medicine (see a fuller discussion of these issues in de Vries et al.[10]

A second and more substantial critique argues that modern medicine has a relatively small role in the statistical improvement of the health of populations of people. McKeown argued that control of the great epidemic and endemic infectious diseases happened through social, not medical, progress. For example, the major drop in tuberculosis rates occurred well in advance of Koch's great discovery of the cause and decades before the advent of specific antibiotic therapies.[11] Because modern medicine seemed to have had little effect on gross vital statistics, McKeown viewed it as an amenity.

Many lesser data sets seem to suggest that something is not as it should be. In the United States, for example, surgical rates are two to four times those of Europe without demonstrably meaningful differences in resultant morbidity and mortality. Regional statistical variations in medical practice can be as much as ninefold without rational bases for the differences. Doctors' strikes in Los Angeles and in Israel, for example, lowered the death rates temporarily! (Of course, it is difficult to know if this was a temporary effect that would have been balanced by even greater death rates later.) Fuchs and others have documented the odd Western phenomenon that adding doctors to an area seems to add to the costs of medical care (recently at an annual rate of more than $450,000/doctor/year in the United States) without detectable differences in morbidity and mortality.[12]

Coupled to these basic attacks has been a series of less severe but telling criticisms. First, medicine has been attacked as expansionistic. It is argued that in a time of diminishing real resources medicine must be more selective in its targets and more rational or more democratic in its choice of priorities. Clearly, there have been frequent routine abuses of resource allocation in the direction of high technological solutions to statistically unimportant problems. For example, in the early days of computed tomography (CT), head scanners were widely purchased and justified as a better way to detect early or tiny brain tumors. Yet, as White demonstrated, the number in which early detection made a difference was negligible.[13]

The importance of resource allocation decisions is proportional to the scarcity of resources. When resources for health and illness care are severely limited, as in many countries where annual per capita expenditure for all health care is less than $10, misallocation is lethal. When a decision is made to buy some costly high-tech piece of equipment, other options are eliminated. Too often, health systems in poor nations have elected to buy cardiac surgical units, obstetrical intensive care units, or CT scanners instead of spending funds in less dramatic but more useful ways that might benefit more people, save more (but different) lives,[14] and contribute more to the health of the population served.[2,15,16]

Added to these fundamental critiques of modern medicine are more personal ones having to do with the alienation of doctors and patients. There is a pervasive sense that medicine increasingly is dehumanized as it has become more biological and more technically sophisticated. It is argued that this leads to errors of commission and omission that deprive both doctor and patient of satisfaction and of good care. As well, the disease orientation of modern health systems reflects a too narrow paradigm of health that is directed solely at the biochemical abnormality in what may be a complex etiological process that also includes psychological and social factors. When such factors are omitted, healing through their control is also omitted, with loss of potential healing and benefit.[17] These features of present medical care are reflected not only in the training processes but more basically in the language of medicine. The dominant classifications of medicine give short shrift to psychological and social problems and factors whereas they include exhaustive lists of hair-splitting pathological distinctions.[18]

Finally, expectations of the public for health care have changed dramatically. Whereas even 30 years ago most people did not expect to have health care readily available, it is now seen as a right by some and as a desirable and achievable goal by most. "Health for all by the year 2000," the courageous and ambitious goal of the World Health Organization (WHO), has become a rallying point that characterizes the hopes of people everywhere. It also has become the basis of organization and action for WHO. It means both health and health care, preventive and curative, for all. Few nations can afford all that has been identified as necessary. However, few can afford to ignore the health needs of its populations, as health is tied to productivity of the work force and to political satisfaction. That this is so is illustrated by the large proportion of gross national product spent on health care by populations whose spending is determined by market mechanisms. It is also seen by the practices of some of those nations that are attempting to export their political systems by direct action or by example. Cuba, for example, uses the gift of health care as a vector for its political beliefs.

The intellectual response to these forms of criticism has been to call for *population-based medicine* in some form or other.[2] This approach means medicine that begins with an assessment of the needs of the population, undertakes scientific assessment of the options available to meet the priority problems, and allocates personnel and resources accordingly.

Parallel with the call for population-based medicine is the notion that medical systems and medical education should be population based through a *community orientation*. It is widely believed that the ability of health providers and planners to know and respond to the needs of the population depends on their working and living among the people. This relationship is critical for several reasons. It permits smooth and effective interpersonal relations between health workers and others. It is necessary to understand the complexities of the interaction between the health of an individual or of a population and the environment—physical, biological, social—within which disease is determined or health persists. It is necessary to understand how illness, the human experience of disease,[19] manifests differently in varied settings. It is also necessary to understand how to intervene in ways that are acceptable and efficient.

Moreover, community orientation to medical education and health planning is important because the distribution of health problems varies with the setting. Physicians who have studied disease and illness only in tertiary medical centers are seeing only the rare or extreme case, a tiny fraction of the spectrum of health problems or episodes of illness.[20] Thus their view of the nature of disease is skewed to the acute care of the extreme and diagnosis of the rare. They inevitably omit preventive and social approaches because they have not experienced them as important or useful. They also favor cure over prevention because the cases they see in their training are too late for preventive intervention, and the professors and other role models they work with know, mainly, cure. This approach

TABLE 1.1. Approach to medical care and role of health personnel

| Present | Community-oriented |
|---|---|
| Momentary disease intervention | Concern with antecedents and postintervention as well as intervention in diseases |
| Individual patient | Individual, family, community |
| Organ or suborgan orientation | Totality of man as a system |
| Man isolated from his environment | Man interacting with his environment |
| Hospital-oriented | Home- and workplace-oriented |
| Dependence expected of patients | Supportive role to patients |
| Expert role | Helper role |
| Costs irrelevant | Balanced concern with costs |
| "Technology imperative" | "Appropriate technology" |
| Diagnostic orientation | Functional-outcome orientation |

affects the future shape of health care, as in the kingdom of health care yesterday's graduates are today's rulers. Thus is perpetuated an insulated system that is ineffective, costly, and scientifically invalid because of its focus on a distorted sample.

Katz succinctly summarized some of the differences that characterize the present orientation of medical systems and educational institutions and the community orientation. As the chief scientist for education evaluation of the Division of Health Manpower Development of WHO, Fred Katz played a pivotal role in supporting and advancing the first group of experiments in community-oriented medical education.[21] His analysis is seen in Table 1.1.

In summary, community orientation is a response to the prevailing critiques of modern medicine that attempts to reorient care toward the needs of individuals within populations using a more comprehensive model of care and more extensive diagnostic and therapeutic categories deriving from the life of the patient in his or her own context. As such, it is not put forward as a replacement for what is excellent in present biotechnical medicine. Rather, it is an attempt to place the efforts of medicine in a more complete and appropriate context and thereby extend its value to the people who pay for it and whom it serves. As well, community orientation represents a scientific advance because it corrects the prevalent omission of relevant factors in consideration of disease: the patient as a person, the physical and social environment, and the family and community. The study of these factors, left out of much of the sample of modern medicine's scientific efforts, is the study of epidemiology, the fundamental science of community orientation, and the behavioral and social sciences.[22]

## Why Problem-based Learning?

At the same time that modern medical systems and, by implication, medical education were under fire for distortions and omissions, medical instructional methods were coming increasingly into question. One aspect was the value of the models taught and the relevance and validity of the knowledge communicated.

These issues were touched on above. A second line of criticism had to do with instruction. This analysis focused on issues of relevance, efficiency, and effect on the learning and intellectual traits inculcated in medical graduates. *The Boys in White*[23] showed the devastating effects of a short dose of medical education on creative, idealistic, and highly motivated college graduates (i.e., a typical group) entering medical school. Within a few months of entering, they had changed into passive, unquestioning, authority-oriented followers who no longer engaged the material actively or creatively but, rather, focused on those aspects of their curriculum thought to correlate with success on examinations. Similarly, at a later stage it has frequently been noted that practitioners do not engage in serious continuing education despite the 5-year or less half-life of valid knowledge taught in medical school. Rather, as Charap et al. have shown, practitioners tend to do what they learned in their training.[24] In general, creative problem-solving and lateral thinking were thought to be stifled. Humanistic concerns were lost or diminished. Interpersonal skills lagged, and rigidity and authoritarianism increased. Medical students were taught a language that, although (perhaps) professionally necessary, made them incomprehensible to their patients. Skills in interviewing, the *core* clinical skill that is critical to the gathering of valid data about patients and their problems, were feeble in most curricula.[25]

In parallel with these complaints, a positive series of trends emerged. Socratic teaching methods, known from classical times, found new forms and theoretical bases. As Schmidt describes in detail in a later chapter, cognitive psychologists such as Bruner showed the exciting effects derived from learning methods (note that these are described as learning rather than teaching methods) in which the student-learner discovered knowledge for himself or herself through analysis of practical problems.

There were many antecedents to this trend of the late 1950s. There was the Socratic method itself. Dewey and his school emphasized the importance of self-discovery to enhance motivation for learning and incorporation of what is learned in the student. The Harvard Business School and the Harvard Law School adopted case methods of teaching by which students began with a case study of a problem and then discovered or sought out the knowledge and skills necessary to analyze or understand those aspects of the case they or their teachers had chosen as important. These teachers recognized that problem-oriented learning experiences both increased the efficiency and heightened the relevance of knowledge. It also meant that knowledge learned was incorporated into a *usable* portion of the students' knowledge. This finding is in marked contrast to the discipline-based teaching in most medical schools, which uses lectures on anatomy, biochemistry, pathology, and so forth. Medical students learn factual material organized inversely from the mode in which they will use it. For example, pathology is taught in sections, e.g., "the liver" or "the kidney," in which they learn of the pathological lesions and then reason "down" to symptoms. In contrast, patients experience symptoms so that a physician must think about symptoms first and then follow branching logic or pattern recognition to consider a variety of separate pathological possibilities, each of which has been separately taught.

Several authors contributed to a quickening of the pace of learning about learning. Bruner and others coupled study of infant and child development with concepts about lifelong learning.[26] These reports illustrated the power of student involvement in learning, including both student participation in the setting of problems and student discovery of approaches and new concepts. Rogers, in *Freedom to Learn*[27] documented the utility of problem-based approaches in learning at many levels from child to therapist. Influenced by Bruner, Zacharias at the Massachusetts Institute of Technology (MIT) and top physicists and physics teachers from across the United States developed a totally new approach to teaching physics in high school in which a much more sophisticated curriculum than previously thought possible was taught to students through their own discovery of physical principles facilitated by provision of simple experimental equipment that any school could afford or make. A comparable innovation was made in mathematics in which algebra, geometry, and calculus were discovered by students using basic set theory. Not surprisingly, the results of the physics and mathematics experiments were mixed. Whereas student satisfaction was high among bright students with good teachers, it was less so among dull students with less engaging teachers.

The case method, of course, has long been a part of medicine in clinical teaching. In preclinical teaching, it has been used as raisins in the porridge, to add texture and sweetness to homogeneous mounds of facts. Use of cases has varied, from the case as an opportunity to reason clinically and pathophysiologically, to the case as an example to start a passive lecture. Such exercises, even in a single institution, span a spectrum from highly active independent learning on the part of the student to totally passive observation as the instructor drones on.

Case Western Reserve University introduced an important curricular innovation when it switched from discipline-based teaching, e.g., anatomy, physiology, or immunology, to organ-based teaching in which each discipline contributed material concerning its particular interest in the organ in question. The organ blocks included both normal and pathological features of the organ system. Instructionally, however, they continued to use the usual mix of lectures, illustrative cases, and laboratory exercises. The impact of this sophisticated shuffling of the educational cards was carefully monitored. Although no differences in learning were documented, morale improved. Although some regard this result as a Hawthorne effect, others note that morale has remained high at Case Western Reserve. Following their lead, many other educational leaders undertook to introduce "organ blocks" and other conceptually "integrated" curricula.

McMaster University (Hamilton, Ontario) was one of the first medical schools to introduce *problem-based learning* as the means of instruction from the first day to the last. After an introduction (problem based, naturally) to how to work on problems, students in small groups learn through the analysis of cases and problems. The reasons McMaster tried this approach were several. First, it was thought that it would increase motivation as the relevance of the subject matter would always be evident in the case itself. Second, it was believed that this method would improve students' ability to analyze problems and thereby increase the probability that the graduates would be more effective clinically and as scholars. It was similarly hoped it would increase creativity and the ability to self-educate.

An additional feature of the McMaster curriculum was their attempt to select cases so that the assortment of knowledge accumulated would reflect what is necessary and relevant for the practitioner of medicine in modern Canada. Although not rigidly formalized, this attitude reflects the high visibility in the institution of clinical epidemiology. Finally, the McMaster teachers hoped that the students would learn, from their work in small groups, attitudes and techniques of teamwork, mutual supportiveness, and systems approaches to problem-solving. As discussed below, they anticipated outcomes of improved learner satisfaction, more relevant and better organized learning, and thereby improved and better sustained clinical performance.[28]

The McMaster approach to problem-based learning has been variously adopted and adapted. One significant advance has been the combination of problem-based learning with a laboratory for the learning of skills. The clinical skills laboratory of the Medical Education Department of the State University of Limburg in Maastricht, Holland is a site where students can at any time initiate self-instruction in more than 300 skills, using models, manikins, videotapes, and simulated patients to learn subjects from venipuncture to interviewing. Moreover, the Maastricht faculty has attempted to base some of the curriculum on a epidemiological view of the priority problems.[29]

A similar approach was adopted by the new medical school of the province of New South Wales in Newcastle, Australia. The founding (in his terminology, "foundation") dean of the school in Newcastle was David Maddison. Their initial thought processes and assumptions are included as Chapter 3 in this volume, a description of the "inherent challenge in the development of a new medical school: it provides an unusual opportunity to influence the shaping of medical education so as to prepare practitioners for effective performance of the tasks that will confront the doctor of the future." It will become apparent to the reader that Maddison represented the best sort of innovator: clear-headed, succinct, conservative in values and daring in methods, making changes because of their necessity.

## How Do Community-oriented Medical Education and Problem-based Learning Interrelate?

It is clear from their histories that these two sets of innovations need not be done together. Neither is necessary nor sufficient for the other. Yet they do have a natural connection. On the one hand, problem-based learning that uses common and priority problems inevitably leads the student to recognize the extent to which factors outside the medical center are relevant to the understanding of cases and their care. It happens anyway until such perceptions are trained out of students owing to lack of reward or to actual discouragement. Similarly, if problem-based learning is occurring in a community-oriented faculty, the selection of cases and the patient-centered community-based role models reinforce a comprehensive model of medicine. Each reinforces the effects of the other with respect to relevance, the presence of untraditional considerations such as psychosocial issues, population-centered issues, and the learning of analytical approaches and skills. Moreover, because each of these concerns derives from a combination of scientific concern for proper sampling and humanistic concern for the needs of individuals and populations, they share a world view to some extent (although not necessarily). As innovations, they are similar in style and energy.

## Evaluating Problem-based Learning and Community-oriented Medical Education

Attempts to evaluate these innovations have been integral parts of their development. Because they are $n = 1$ situations, are large institutional efforts, and those doing the innovating are also doing the evaluating, most of the initial evaluations were descriptive. However, some evaluations have been quasi-experimental or have derived a complex view of the innovations through integration of a large variety of objective outcomes. Thus if nothing else, these programs have made noteworthy contributions to the science of curriculum evaluation. As each situation is unique and complex, only highlights are mentioned here. Further details are found in Part IV of this book.

A primary goal of community-oriented schools is to create students capable and motivated to go into primary care community practice—a major goal of the University of the Negev in Beer Sheva, Israel. During the early 1970s Israel faced a problem of medical overspecialization with an inadequate number of primary care physicians to serve remote communities. More than 90% of Israeli medical school graduates at the time of planning of Beer Sheva were going into specialties. In contrast, more than 70% of their first graduating class have elected primary care. McMaster has reported results similar to those of Beer Sheva. Of their graduating classes, 50% of the physicians consistently have gone into primary care.

A second dimension of evaluation is to compare, through standardized testing, graduates in an innovative program to otherwise comparable students who are taking a traditional program. McMaster's students have an annual mean pass rate on the Medical Council of Canada examination of 92%, a superior result. Their graduates rate as good or better than their peers on clinical competence.

Extensive evaluations from Maastricht, The Netherlands, are presented in Chapter 16. Because students in Holland are assigned to medical schools at random or on the basis of geographic rather than merit considerations, and students are neither self nor faculty selected, comparisons among Dutch schools are especially meaningful. In brief, the Maastricht students have higher *satisfaction* ratings than do students at another Dutch medical school, while Maastricht students score at the same level as students at two other schools on quarterly summative examinations consisting of 300 multiple choice questions.

One of the most interesting areas of interest in evaluation has been the attempt of several schools to relate preadmission criteria to how students perform clinically. In Beer Sheva, for instance, preclinical grades and psychometric tests did not predict clinical or grade performances. McMaster University reported similar results. They found that an admission grade point average above 2.5 does not predict student in-course performance or success rates on the Medical Council of Canada licensing examinations. Interestingly, when corrected for age, non-science undergraduate students do as well as science students.

Many of the most interesting studies are still in process. Newcastle University has undertaken a courageous experiment in which they admitted two groups of students. One group was admitted solely on the basis of academic criteria. The second group was admitted on the basis of criteria set by the "Admissions Policy Committee" composed of medical personnel and persons from the community. The criteria were those required for "effective practice of medicine" (see Maddison, this volume) which were reliably measurable. These were "(1) higher mental abilities considered to be specifically related to the problem-solving approach to medicine; (2) creativity; (3) capacity for empathy; (4) capacity to provide supportive/encouraging behavior; (5) perseverance; (6) flexibility of views and attitudes; and (7) ability to deal with ethically difficult situations in an informed and thoughtful manner."[30] They collected identical data sets on both groups so it will be possible to compare their results on both academic and clinical performance criteria.

Overall, then, the innovative nature of these schools has included new approaches to selection of site and subject matter, to the manner of creating learning, and to scientifically sound assessment of the processes undertaken.

# Network of Community-oriented Educational Institutions for Health Sciences

In June 1979 the WHO's Health Manpower Division, directed by Fülöp, brought together representatives of 18 health sciences institutions that were using community-oriented medical education or problem-based learning. They did so because[30]:

... with its member states, WHO has since its inception attempted to ensure that health manpower is available in the quantity needed and of the quality required to service community health needs. In its Health Manpower Development programme (HMD), WHO has actively promoted a closer and more effective linkage between education of health personnel and health services. The importance of educational programmes focussing on community health needs and on total health care rather than curative services only has been stressed. Yet unfortunately such educational programmes are still the exception rather than the rule. There are all too few educational institutions which provide students with adequate learning experiences of community health care and at the same time prepare their students for life-long learning using a problem-solving approach to learning.

Those institutions which are dedicated to provide their students with orientation to community health care and use teaching/learning methods which are problem-based rather than discipline-centered encounter considerable opposition that in their very existence challenges the status quo. At the same time, difficulties are experienced because the experimental nature of the programme makes heavy demands on finite resources. Further it is they which in contrast to established programmes have to prove their worth.

Recognizing that much needs to be done to strengthen these innovative programmes, the World Health Organization considered it desirable to organize a meeting in order to explore the possibility that those responsible for these programmes might provide mutual assistance, in a variety of ways, through the formation of a network of collaborating institutions. This intention is clearly consonant with WHO's overall goal "health for all by the year 2000" on the basis of further developing primary health care. This goal is inseparable from the development and strengthening of innovative community-oriented programmes for the education of health professionals.

Invitations hence were sent by the WHO Regional Office for the Americas to the principals (deans or rectors) of some 20 institutions which were identified by regional offices and headquarters as having some commitment to community orientation and the use of a problem-solving approach.

At the initial meeting, individual programs were presented and discussion was undertaken of common strengths and problems. The collected deans and rectors decided to create a network for information exchange, organization or personal exchanges, and mutual teaching and collaboration. Planning for collaborative efforts began including research, program evaluation, health services research, and mutual solving of common problems and barriers to their form of innovation. To serve these needs, a Secretariat was created based in the offices of the Dean of the University of Limburg at Maastricht, The Netherlands.

Over the next 2 years a series of events marked the important progress of the Network. Many exchanges of faculty and administrative leaders took place. Much material—curricula, planning documents, and articles—was circulated. Task forces began effective work on problem-based learning, evaluation of programs, organizational structures, and how to organize community-based education. Regional liaison officers were named to support the work of the Secretariat and foster local activities. A newsletter was published. Finally, funds were sought and obtained to support these activities from WHO, the government of The Netherlands, the Rockefeller and Kellogg Foundations, and other sources.

In April 1981 a second Network meeting was held at Bellagio, Italy. Most significant at this meeting were the establishment of membership criteria, the deepening of commitment and exchange, and the establishment of an executive committee of the Network to guide it between meetings. Substantive discussions on major topics included coordination of health services and education, obstacles to innovation, and the topics discussed at the initial meeting. Several new schools attended the second network meeting and presented their approaches.

Since then, multiple regional global meetings of the Network have occurred. Forty-four schools have now joined in full (33) or associate (11) status (see Appendix B). Annual workshops have assisted schools interested in exploring or implementing one or the other of these approaches. What began as a tentative meeting of 18 schools has developed into a substantial worldwide activity.

Probably the most important aspect of the Network's work is to facilitate exchange among institutions attempting to accomplish orderly change. The underpinning of such attempts is faculty development, as these changes are made by specific courageous individuals. Some notable efforts at faculty development are presented in Section V of this volume.

## A Look Toward the Future

Many questions occur to thoughtful educators learning about problem-based learning and community-oriented medical education for the first time. Is the initial success an elaborate Hawthorne effect, the positive response seen in any major institutional change?[31] Will such schools produce scientific leaders in addition to health services delivery leadership? What are the economics of these innovations? Do they cost more to deliver? How can students benefit from the inspirational impact of great scientists, scholars, and clinicians if they never hear them talk about their ideas and approaches? Is this fad or fashion, or is it a fundamental shift?

At a deeper level, many are concerned about the inherent reorientation or paradigm shift implicit in these approaches to education. After all, modern medicine for all its inefficiencies and distortions has accomplished wonders. Is it wise to disrupt something so successful and so vulnerable in these times of shrinking resources and attempts to cut back on services?

It seems evident that sufficient momentum has been achieved by these programs that the experiment will have more time to show results. If nothing else, the innovations in evaluation provoke traditional institutions to self-scrutiny, which can only lead to improvements in health for all.

The global divisions between North and South, rich and poor, may come to be expressed in this movement. It is more critical to make such changes in regions of very scarce resources and relatively more difficult to do so in regions where a strong market favors resource allocation in favor of the wealthy. Yet as President Bok of Harvard University explores so elegantly (see Chapter 2), the reasons for these changes ultimately concern the very core of medicine. As such, they may elicit change even in the most conservative or successful settings.

When change occurs, the vision and strength of the men and women who have made these first steps will be remembered. John Evans of McMaster University, Donald Maddison of the University of Newcastle, Fred Katz and Tomas Fülöp of

WHO, Tans Tiddens and Jacobus Greep of the University of Limburg in Maastricht, Kerr White of the Rockefeller Foundation, Moshe Prywes of Ben Gurion University of the Negev, their colleagues, and many others have found a way to begin to restore medicine to its classic role of personal care for the needs of the people.

## References

1. Flexner A: *Medical education in the United States and Canada.* Bulletin No. 4. New York, Carnegie Foundation for the Advancement of Teaching, 1910
2. Lipkin M Jr, Lybrand WA: *Population Based Medicine.* New York, Praeger, 1982.
3. Reiser DE, Rosen DR: *Medicine as a Human Experience.* Baltimore, University Park Press, 1984.
4. Pfifferling JM: The impaired physician: an overview. Chapel Hill, NC, Health Sciences Consortium, 1980.
5. Evans JR: Measurement and management in medicine and health sciences: training needs and opportunities. In Lipkin M Jr, Lybrand WA (eds): *Population Based Medicine.* New York, Praeger, 1982, pp 3–41.
6. Szasz T: *The Myth of Mental Illness.* New York, Delta, 1961.
7. Illich I: *Medical Nemesis: The Expropriation of Health.* New York, Pantheon, 1976.
8. Carlson R: *The End of Medicine.* New York, Wiley Interscience, 1975.
9. Reiser SJ: *Medicine and the Reign of Technology.* Cambridge, Cambridge University Press, 1978.
10. De Vries MW, Berg RL, Lipkin M, Jr: *The Use and Abuse of Medicine.* New York, Praeger, 1982.
11. McKeown T: *The Role of Medicine: Dream, Mirage or Nemesis.* Oxford, Blackwell, 1979.
12. Fuchs VR: *Who Shall Live?* New York, Basic Books, 1974.
13. White KL: "Political arithmetic: integration of cost effectiveness analysis into health systems. In Banta HD (ed): *Resources for Health: Technology Assessment for Policy Making.* New York, Praeger, 1982, pp 156–161.
14. Omitted on proof.
15. White KL, Bullock PJ: *Health of Populations.* New York, Rockefeller University Press, 1980.
16. Banta HD: *Resources for Health: Technology Assessment for Policy Making.* New York, Praeger, 1982.
17. Lipkin M: Disease and illness as processes. In De Vries MW, Berg RL, Lipkin M, Jr (eds): *The Use and Abuse of Medicine.* New York, Praeger, 1982, pp 137–150.
18. Regier DA, Kessler LG, Burns BJ, Goldberg ID: The need for a psychosocial classification system in primary care practice. In Lipkin M, Kupka K (eds): *Psychosocial Factors Affecting Health.* New York, Praeger, 1982, pp 139–150.
19. Kleinman A, Eisenberg L, Good B: Culture, illness and care. *Ann Intern Med* 1978; 88:251–256.
20. White KL, Williams TF, Greenberg BG: Ecology of medical care. *N Engl J Med* 1961; 265:882–892.
21. Katz FM, Fulöp T: *Personnel for Health Care.* Geneva, WHO, 1978.

22. White KL, Henderson MH: *Epidemiology as a Fundamental Science.* New York, Oxford, 1976.
23. Becker H, et al: *Boys in White.* Chicago, University of Chicago Press, 1966.
24. Charap MH, Levin RI, Weinglass J: Physician choices in the treatment of angina pectoris. *Am J Med* 1985;79:461–466.
25. Lipkin M, Quill TE, Napodano RJ: The medical interview. *Ann Intern Med* 1984;100:277–284.
26. Bruner JS: *Toward a Theory of Instruction.* New York, Norton, 1966.
27. Rogers CR: *Freedom to Learn.* Columbus, OH, Merill, 1969.
28. Walsh WJ: The McMaster programme of medical education, Hamilton, Ontario, Canada: developing problem solving abilities. In Katz F, Fulöp T (eds): *Personnel for Health Care.* Geneva, WHO, 1978, pp 69–77.
29. Lodewich L, Gunn ADG: *The Physical Examination.* Lancaster, MTP Press, 1982.
30. Minutes of the First National Meeting, Geneva, WHO, 1979.
31. Schulkey HC, Sheldon A, Baker F: *Program Evaluation in the Health Fields.* New York, Behavioral Publications, 1969.

# 2
# Needed: A New Way to Train Doctors

DEREK BOK

In May 1983, at its final meeting of the year, the Harvard Faculty of Medicine gave its approval to the dean and a group of professors to create an experimental curriculum. Limited at first to 25 students per year, this program has now been incorporated in the core curriculum. The initiative may well be Harvard's most impressive innovation of the 1980s. Instead of merely tinkering with course requirements or shifting hours of instruction from one subject to another, the authors of the program have begun by making a fresh appraisal of the knowledge, skills, and attitudes that physicians today and tomorrow need to possess. On this foundation will be built an entirely new curriculum. Not only does it seek to alter what students learn; it plans sweeping innovations in the methods by which they are taught.

Stirrings of change are evident elsewhere in the United States. In 1982 the Macy Foundation sponsored a major conference that urged far-reaching reforms in the teaching of medical students.[1] The Institute of Medicine has recently come forth with a study on medical education and societal needs.[2] A blue-ribbon committee appointed by the Association of American Medical Colleges has also been studying medical education and has issued a report.

This high-level attention has not come about by chance. Many forces have combined to alter the body of medical knowledge, the way in which doctors practice their craft, and the system of delivering health care services in the United States. It is only natural, then, that educators are starting to wonder how they should respond. As yet, the outcome is difficult to predict. Like ancient China, medical education has experienced many assaults from the outside world without undergoing substantial change. Even so, pressures have now reached a point at which basic reforms are likely to occur. In the pages that follow are considered the forces that have created this opportunity, and the scope and range of improvements needed in medical education.

## Revolution in Medicine

We have grown so used to a world of miracle drugs, open-heart surgery, kidney transplants, and computed tomography (CT) scanning that we can scarcely remember the primitive state of medical science only a few generations ago. Not until this century could patients expect to improve their chances of survival by entering a hospital.[3] Looking back to his boyhood in the 1920s, Lewis Thomas recalls how frustrated his father felt over his constant inability to comprehend, let alone cure, the ailments of his patients. Even during the late 1930s, after entering Harvard Medical School, Thomas recalled that "it gradually dawned on us that we didn't know much that was really useful, that we could do nothing to change the course of the great majority of the diseases we were so busy analyzing, that medicine, for all its facade as a learned profession, was in real life a profoundly ignorant occupation."[4]

Since World War II, the pace of medical discovery has quickened, spurred by billions of research dollars in federal aid each year. The knowledge of physicians has grown enormously; the methods for diagnosing and treating illness have multiplied. With government support, medical school faculties grew fivefold from 1960 to 1980, teaching hospitals transformed into vast temples of research, and laboratories blossomed with equipment of immense sophistication.

As research surged forward, great changes also occurred in the system for delivering and financing health care. In particular, the federal government came to play a major role in making medical services available to all segments of society. With Medicare and Medicaid, the poor and the elderly were ensured access to health care at a total cost to the taxpayer that has come to exceed $80 billion per year. These initiatives expanded the use of medical services by the aged and indigent to such a point that poor people began visiting doctors at rates exceeding those of more affluent individuals. Anticipating this growth in demand, Congress increased the supply of health services by subsidizing hospital construction and medical education. The supply of hospital beds rose by almost 50%, and the number of medical students virtually doubled. As a result of these measures, 90% of the population could count on a reasonable level of medical services by 1980.

Despite these successes, the work of Congress remains unfinished. Still unrealized is a comprehensive system of care comparable to those achieved in other industrialized nations. To our shame, 28 million people are not yet covered by either federal programs or private health insurance. With recent cuts in the eligibility and benefits under federal programs and with financial woes causing retrenchment in many municipal hospitals, patients of modest means are finding it more difficult to get adequate medical services when they need them.

The expansion of health services has also brought new problems in its wake. By the mid-1970s, experts began to warn that the stimulus of government programs had worked too well. Julius Richmond, former Assistant Secretary for Health and Surgeon General, claimed that hospitals now had 150,000 more short-term beds than the nation actually needed.[5] According to the Graduate Medical Education National Advisory Committee, medical schools had expanded to the point that the nation could expect a surplus of 25,000 to 50,000 doctors by 1990.[6] The Institute of Medicine opined that far too many of our doctors were specialists, and far too few were general practitioners.[7]

Worse yet, the methods used by the government and private insurers to pay the cost of care for the aged and indigent carried no incentive to restrain expenditures. As a result, aided by the rapid growth in the number of hospital beds and practicing physicians, medical bills shot up much faster than the cost of living. Whereas the total cost of health care had consumed only 5.3% of the gross national product in 1960, the proportion rose above 10% by 1983, amounting to more than $350 billion per year. No other industrial nation devoted a larger share of its resources to this purpose, and most spent considerably less.

These burgeoning costs in turn have had repercussions throughout the health care system. A host of government rules have sprung up to fix the maximum price the government pays for medical services and restricts the right to construct new hospital facilities. To foster competition, federal officials have encouraged health maintenance organizations, which offer prepaid care at prices below those of Blue Cross and other established insurers. Chains of hospitals operated for profit have also expanded rapidly to take advantage of growing health care markets. More recently, coalitions of corporations, unions, and doctors have formed to search for ways of curbing the rise of health care bills. These developments promise not only to transform the health system but to affect the nature and quality of care itself. For though the initiatives are very different, they do have one thing in common. All of them carry potent new incentives to hold down medical expenditures. The great unknown is whether these incentives can succeed in restraining costs without causing providers to dilute the quality of care.

## Response of Medical Education

With such extraordinary advances in scientific knowledge, not to mention the metamorphosis of the health care system and its attendant policy problems, one would have expected comparable changes in the shape and substance of medical education. In fact, such changes have occurred in the *content* of courses. Instructors have been quick to tuck the latest scientific findings into their classroom lectures and their discussions on hospital wards. The *methods* and the *structure* of medical education, however, have stayed surprisingly constant throughout the postwar period. In order to enter medical school, college students must still take classes in mathematics, physics, biology, and chemistry. Once enrolled, they continue to spend much of the first 2 years listening to lectures on basic science: biochemistry, anatomy, microbiology, pathology, neurobiology, physiology, and pharmacology. During the final 2 years, they still enter the hospital for clinical rotations under the tutelage of professors and house staff, who teach them the arts and skills of obtaining medical histories, finding further information through various tests and procedures, and eventually making diagnoses and prescribing appropriate treatments.*

If the structure and methods of medical education have stayed more or less the same, so also have the criticisms and complaints. Educators have long observed that premedical requirements and prevailing admissions practices push college

*The Second Meeting of the International Network of Community-oriented Educational Institutions for Health Sciences, Bellagio, Italy, 1980.

students into majoring in science and stir anxieties that distort the course selection and even the extracurricular activities of many undergraduates. For years, these comments were largely anecdotal. Research, however, confirms the diagnosis. A survey of undergraduates in leading liberal arts colleges revealed that premedical students experience greater stress than students interested in other occupations and are more likely to alter course selections and extracurricular activities to favor their chances of admission to medical school.* Fifty-three percent of the premedical students in this survey thought that a substantial minority of their fellow students disliked them, and 24% believed that instructors expressed negative feelings toward them. Forty-five percent of all undergraduates who dropped their plans to become a doctor did so because they did not wish to enter a profession with a group of students who seemed so grimly purposeful and ambitious. Still worse are the persistent reports of cutthroat competition, buttressed by a study of 400 medical students among whom 88% admitted having cheated at least once during college.[8] (The results of this are especially ominous as they revealed a positive correlation between cheating in college and dishonesty in the process of patient care.)

It is difficult to overcome such pressures completely so long as there are many more aspiring doctors than places in our medical schools. Even so, except for experiments by a few schools, most of them financed by the Macy Foundation, one is struck by how little medical faculties have done to improve matters by reviewing their admissions practices and premedical requirements.

The problems of the first 2 years of medical school have also changed little over the past few decades. Much of the instruction still consists of lectures in which a procession of teachers relate large quantities of scientific material to a passive student audience. The sheer weight of this material has jumped dramatically with the cascade of discoveries that followed the work of Crick and Watson on the structure of DNA. Thus far, however, faculties have typically reacted by packing their lectures more densely and cutting back on laboratory classes and independent study to make room for still more lectures.

In response to student complaints, faculties have tended to increase the number of electives or provide a bit more contact with "live" patients – palliatives that do not really attack the underlying problems. Increases in faculty size, far from encouraging more tutorial and small group instruction, have led professors to specialize more narrowly and expect lighter teaching loads. Thus course today are commonly divided among many lecturers in a long disjointed "parade of stars" in which the professors, one by one, appear before the students to describe new developments in their specialty. Because more and more of these instructors have received their degrees in basic science rather than medicine, their classes often seem to have little relation to the patient care that attracted most of their

---

*Although the study has not been released, these findings were described by the principal investigator, C. Hess Haagen, of Wesleyan University, and were reported in the *Boston Herald*, March 2, 1983. The study involved 1064 students at Amherst, Bowdoin, Swarthmore, Haverford, Williams, and Middlebury Colleges and Wesleyan University.

students to medical school in the first place. Worst of all, the lecture system encourages a static, passive attitude toward education that emphasizes memorization instead of the active, inquiring cast of mind required to keep up in a rapidly changing field.*

After the first 2 years, medical education turns highly practical. Students begin their clinical rotations in the hospital, learning the rudiments of surgery, medicine, pediatrics, and other fields of practice. At this stage the instruction is much more relevant to the students' professional lives. The tedium and abstraction of the first 2 years give way to the total absorption of working with live patients. However, new complaints come to the fore. Despite the huge increase in the size of the clinical faculty since World War II, students believe that they get too little instruction from professors and too much from hospital residents and interns only slightly older than themselves. They often find the content of rotations unpredictable, the objectives vague, the feedback far from adequate.

More experienced critics expand on these complaints. Commenting on the quality of teaching in the wards, they claim that students are forced to play too passive a role with insufficient opportunity to practice the skills of seeking out information, making tentative diagnoses, testing their hypotheses with further information, and eventually reaching a conclusion. They likewise complain that students have too little exposure to the psychosocial aspects of patient care and too little discussion about preventive measures or the problems of conserving costs when gathering information and prescribing treatment.

A final criticism that applies throughout the curriculum is the lack of attention paid to the nonscientific side of medicine. Only a few medical faculties require their students to take a course in medical ethics, the history of medicine, behavioral science, or the organization and economics of health care. Granted, such subjects have now been introduced as electives in almost all schools, but these offerings rarely have much status in the curriculum or gain reinforcement by being integrated systematically into the clinical rotations. A look at the Harvard Medical School illustrates the problem. At present, Harvard students must take 6 of their 134 required credits from courses listed under Behavioral Sciences, Social Science, or Preventive Medicine, categories that include such offerings as Medical Ethics; Social History of Medicine; Literature and Medicine; Organization of Health Care; Forensic Pathology; Psychiatry and the Law; Culture and Illness; Religion and Medicine; and Science, Sex, and Gender. Such requirements carry a message that all these courses together are of slight importance in the total curriculum, that each is equally relevant to the practice of medicine and that none is important enough to be required of every doctor. With this

---

*A more scathing critique has been delivered by a distinguished scientist, J. Michael Bishop, who teaches basic science at the Medical School at the University of California, San Francisco. "What emerges are physicians without inquiring minds, physicians who bring to the bedside *not* curiosity and a desire to understand, but a set of reflexes that allows them to earn a handsome living." Speech delivered to the annual meeting of the American Association of Medical Colleges, Nov. 8, 1983.

equivocal endorsement, in an environment dominated by science and research, small wonder that only 3 or 4 students in each class of 165 actually choose to take more than the bare minimum of these subjects.

## Obstacles to Change

These criticisms of medical education have been repeated many times; most have been heard for more than 70 years. In fact, a group of Harvard professors in 1847 made all the familiar arguments against the overuse of lectures when they opposed a move by the American Medical Association (AMA) to lengthen the curriculum. Abraham Flexner, the father of modern medical education, restated these points and also called insistently for efforts to balance medical science with greater concern for the psychological and social aspects of health. Professors early in this century even questioned the effects of premedical requirements on undergraduate education when prerequisites were first imposed.

This record provokes an important question. Why has medical education changed so little in the face of such persistent criticism, especially during an era when the field of medicine has changed so much? One important reason is that teaching stands low on the totem pole of medical school incentives. Academic advancement, professional recognition, and public acclaim go to those who succeed in research; and if the rewards of prestige favor science, the material incentives favor patient care. Teaching hospitals need academic physicians who can attract patients and fill beds, and rapidly growing faculty practice plans offer a great deal of money to clinicians who can do just that. Many earn more than $150,000 a year, and incomes of $300,000 to $400,000 are not unknown for part-time clinical professors.

Lured by such attractive incentives, few faculty members develop a strong interest in teaching, and most spend little time at it. Moreover, among the various types of students who pass through medical schools and teaching hospitals, ordinary medical students rank well down the list in terms of the amount of time and attention professors are willing to give. The scientists who make up the preclinical faculty are chiefly concerned with their doctoral students and postdoctoral fellows, who are wholly dedicated to research. To the clinical faculty, residents and fellows often seem more interesting than medical students, as they are more advanced and committed to the very specialties their professors practice.

In this environment it is not surprising that medical education resists change, especially in the most prestigious, research-oriented schools. Basic reforms require work—to change pedagogic styles, to develop new instructional materials, to endure the frustrating trials and errors of developing novel ways of teaching. Because none of the typical incentives and rewards of academic medicine reinforces such activities, few professors devote the time required. In addition, medical schools command less influence among their faculty members than other academic units in the university. Professors owe obligations to their hospital, where they work and receive their salaries; to their departments, which depend far more on patient fees and federal research funds than on the medical school; and even to their professional societies, which confer prestige on their members and often declare their own views on medical education. Amid these competing loyalties, most medical deans have little leverage to engineer major educational reforms.

There is yet another, subtler force at work to inhibit change. In all professions, formal education is shaped to fit the prevailing sense of how practitioners go about resolving the characteristic problems of their calling. The Harvard Business School faculty molds its curriculum and teaching to instill what Fritz Jules Roethlisberger has described as "the administrative point of view."[9] Law professors, especially during the critical first year, teach their classes to help students learn to "think like a lawyer," i.e., to identify legal issues in human situations, to marshal the evidence and arguments on every side of each issue, and then to determine which solution best fits the legal precedents and policy considerations that bear on the problem at hand. So long as the prevailing conception stays unchanged, faculties are unlikely to alter the curriculum very much.

Medicine has its own idea of what it means to "think like a doctor," even though physicians may be less explicit about it than their colleagues in business and law. At the heart of this conception is a view of human disease as a scientific phenomenon consisting in deviations from a biomedical norm. Such deviations are thought to result from a determinate cause or set of causes that are somatic or biochemical in nature. It is the physician's job to ascertain these causes by powers of observation supplemented increasingly by diagnostic tests and other technological aids, and then to cure the ailment or at least alleviate its effects through surgery, medication, or some other course of action. Doctors cannot always diagnose a disease, as their knowledge is limited. Within the realm of what is known, however, they aspire to each a scientifically certain diagnosis by making all relevant observations and tests, while looking to research to narrow their ignorance through the discovery of scientific truths.

Professor Donald Selden aptly summarized the traditional view in his 1981 presidential address to the Association of American Physicians: "Medicine is a very narrow discipline. Its goals may be defined as the relief of pain, the prevention of disability, and the postponement of death by the application of the theoretical knowledge incorporated in medical science to individual patients."[10]

This conception of the doctor's role has had a marked effect on the nature of medical education. In a profession that emphasizes scientifically determined findings, rather than the rough judgments characteristic of lawyers and business executives, professors are inclined to impart knowledge didactically—as truths to be described rather than problems to be discussed. Matters outside the domain of science command little attention. Although everyone knows that psychological and behavioral factors can influence health, doctors have tended to regard these matters as unscientific and have left them largely to others: psychologists, social workers, public health officials, and the like. It is only natural, then, for medical schools to push such subjects to the margins of the curriculum. Similarly, because ethical issues and patient values have little effect on the scientific determination of disease, they have not loomed large in the thinking of physicians or faculty committees, at least until recently, when the law courts and the media began to make such problems too prominent to ignore. Much the same has been true of other subjects relevant to health, such as the prevention of disease, the cost and equitable distribution of medical services, and the development of health policies and regulations. Because these topics are peripheral to the scientific analysis of illness, they have been either relegated to secondary status in the curriculum or left to other faculties such as public administration and public health.

## New Forces in the Medical Environment

Despite its restricted focus, the traditional conception of the doctor's craft rests on firm foundations. Science has vastly expanded our knowledge of the causes and cure of disease. The progress has been so impressive and its results so abundant that no account of modern medicine could fail to place the application of scientific knowledge at the very center of the enterprise. This empirical support is buttressed by compelling psychological forces. Because medical decisions have such vital effects on human lives and the consequences of error can be so severe, both doctors and patients have strong motives for believing in the accuracy and scientific authority of the physician's judgment. With these achievements and attractions, the traditional concept has much to recommend it. Yet new forces have developed that promise not to downgrade science but to expand the physician's role to encompass added problems and complexities.

The growth of scientific knowledge itself is pressing hard against the familiar notion of what it means to think like a doctor. The constant flow of new discoveries makes impossible demands on human memory. In a world with more than 10,000 scientific journals, the traditional library can no longer succeed in giving practitioners quick, efficient access to knowledge. Already, almost 40% of physicians in one survey said that they could no longer keep up with developments in their field.[11] Thus doctors increasingly need to know how to use the computer to aid them in retrieving useful information.

Rising quantities of knowledge not only place heavier demands on human memory but create new difficulties in analyzing problems. Scientific progress constantly expands the range of alternative diagnoses to be considered and the number of tests that can be given to test the clinician's hypotheses. Keeping these possibilities in mind, assessing the risks of harmful side effects from a growing number of tests and drugs, and calculating the meaning to be derived from larger quantities of data are tasks that burden the most sophisticated minds. In the future, the public will undoubtedly make matters even more difficult by insisting that doctors search for diagnostic information and prescribe methods of treatment in ways that are not only effective for the patient but efficient for society by avoiding unnecessary tests and procedures.

When coping with these problems, most physicians are handicapped by their inability to work effectively with complex, quantitative data. Investigations consistently show that they often detect correlations where none exist, cling tenaciously to estimates based on poor information, and exaggerate the informational value derived from small samples.[12] As problems grow more complicated, such weaknesses become more costly; to avoid them, doctors must become proficient in the uses (and the limitations) of statistics, computer analysis, and decision theory. Thus it is not surprising that a poll of Harvard Medical School faculty and students revealed that the four skills most in need of greater emphasis were "assessing cost-benefit and risk-benefit considerations in the use of therapeutic technology," "avoiding the collection of unnecessary information," "seeking lower cost solutions to clinical problems," and "using accepted principles of statistical inference from samples." (These findings were taken from unpublished reports submitted to the Planning Group for the New Pathway.)

Even more revolutionary are efforts to devise computer programs to diagnose illness and thus supplant physicians in the most central of their thought processes. For a few conditions, e.g., rheumatic heart disease, machines can already perform better than physicians. As yet, however, there is little prospect that computers will displace human judgment for a wide range of illness. What *is* likely is that machines will supplement the human mind by storing and manipulating large quantities of relevant data and by supplying an independent source of diagnoses to enable doctors to check their own judgments. Once again, therefore, physicians will continue to need their traditional skills but will have to know how to make effective use of computers as well.

New technology intrudes in yet another way by confronting doctors with a wider and more complicated array of ethical dilemmas. Now that life-sustaining techniques can prolong vital functions long after conscious feeling has disappeared, doctors ask if there is any point, let alone moral duty, to maintain life on such austere terms. Complicated operations may save a child but at a cost so great that one can no longer avoid the problem of deciding what price to place on a human life. Prenatal diagnosis may lead to moral problems if parents request abortions in order to avoid having children of a particular sex. There is no escape once dilemmas of this sort arise. With the rapid growth of malpractice litigation, not to mention investigatory journalism, such issues cannot be ignored any longer, even by the most scientifically inclined physician.

Another significant development is the growing awareness of the importance of psychological and behavioral factors in medical practice. Some statistics help to illustrate the point. Between one-third and one-half of all patients who visit primary care physicians have no physical (or biomedical) ailment at all. Yet studies show that physicians are much more likely to overlook significant emotional and cognitive disorders than physical ailments and symptoms.[13] Shame, guilt, and other psychological factors also affect what patients say to their doctors. In fact, studies of patient interviews indicated that up to one-half of all prior hospitalizations and other significant medical incidents are not communicated.[14] Doctors who fail to detect these psychological and social considerations can easily misperceive the nature of the case before them and resort to unnecessary surgery, overuse of drugs, or needless diagnostic tests—with no relief for their patients. Through lack of empathy and concern, they can drive ill and disabled people to experiment with fads, "miracle" cures, and other treatments of dubious value.

Psychological and social factors may also affect the incidence of disease itself. For example, studies suggest that acute grief can suppress the immune system and thus render a person more susceptible to illness; conversely, conjugal love and support appear to lower the risk of angina.[15,16] Doctors themselves can influence the course of sickness and cure by their behavior toward patients. Thus a series of studies have revealed how efforts to prepare patients to cope with impending surgery can shorten the period of hospitalization and recovery.[17]

Investigations have also shown that more than 30% of all patients fail to take the medicines or follow the treatments their doctors prescribe. Studies have revealed that more than half of such persons do not even understand what they were told to do and that their doctors are usually at fault.[18,19] Presumably, even more people might follow their prescribed treatment if doctors were more adept at persuading them to do so. By virtue of their expertise and their involvement with people at particularly vulnerable times in their lives, doctors are strategically placed to persuade patients to follow treatments and change their habits in life-enhancing ways. As psychologists have revealed, however, physicians can exert such influence effectively only if they take the time and develop the skill to engage their patients actively in an effort to understand the need to alter their behavior.[20,21] In other words, effective practice again requires an understanding of psychology as well as biomedical science.

The final force pressing in on the doctor is the nationwide concern over rising health costs. This problem is bound to grow over the next generation. On the one hand, expenses will continue to be pushed upward by increases in the aged population and in the number of doctors. On the other hand, government, corporate employers, unions, and large insurance carriers have become concerned enough over spiraling medical bills to resist with determination. A major battle is clearly in the making. Government regulations will probably become more intrusive. Health maintenance organizations, government agencies, coalitions of employers, unions, and carriers, even for-profit hospital chains will press increasingly for lower costs. To achieve their ends, these organizations will try to limit the doctor's authority over patient care by imposing checks on decisions to hospitalize patients, to set the length of hospital stay, or to order the use of expensive procedures and tests. In order to avoid unwarranted restrictions, let alone contribute to the national effort to contain rising costs, physicians will have to know more about the issues of health care policy and administration.

Transcending these developments and drawing from them all is a growing change in the perception of how physicians go about making their characteristic decisions of diagnosis and treatment.[22] Fewer doctors are now inclined to think of themselves as simply arriving at logically determined conclusions by applying scientifically tested truths to experimentally derived data. The world today seems much more complicated. Doctors are constantly forced to make educated guesses based on imperfect information. Diseases often have multiple causes, not all of them scientific in nature. The information physicians receive, the symptoms they observe, and the outcome of the treatments they prescribe can be affected by the ways in which they act and interact with patients. The decisions they make are limited not only by gaps in biological knowledge but by bureaucratic rules and economic pressures. In short, the doctor's world cannot be restricted to science or neatly divided between the known and the unknown. Considerations of many kinds are often jumbled together to form a picture full of uncertainties, requiring the most delicate judgments and intuitions.

This conception of the doctor's craft may not be entirely new, but it is surely understood more widely and more vividly than ever before. In its wake come many questions. How does one make wise judgments or probabilistic estimates from various kinds of imperfect data? If doctors do not simply act on scientific truths but often take calculated risks, how much should they tell their patients and how big a role should the latter play in deciding what chances to take with their own health and well-being? Because looking for evidence costs money — more than $20 billion is spent each year on diagnostic tests alone — how much information should clinicians seek and how can they search for data in a more cost-effective manner? Finally, if the doctor's behavior helps determine what patients reveal about their ailments, how quickly they recover from an operation, or whether they follow a prescribed treatment, how can physicians conduct themselves to exert the most constructive influence?

Confronted by such problems, doctors could easily react by clinging resolutely to their traditional role as applied scientists seeking accurate biomedical explanations for a patient's disease. After all, it is difficult enough to cope with the mounting complexity of the biosciences without having to take account of computers, decision trees, health care regulations, ethical constraints, and the vagaries of patient psychology. However, is there a viable alternative?

Conceivably, doctors could try to avoid these complications by delegating responsibility to others. Hire philosophers, as a few hospitals have done, to deal with difficult ethical dilemmas. Leave the psychological problems of patient care to psychiatrists, social workers, and members of the clergy. Find more skillful administrators in the hospitals to cope with government regulations, and trust the AMA to make sure that public officials do not encroach too far on the doctor's prerogatives. Refer the statistical manipulations and data analysis to computer experts who can advise physicians on request.

Tempting though this response may seem, it is bound to fail in the end. The point is not that social workers, administrators, lobbyists, ethicists, and computer analysts are incapable of helping. Indeed, they must help. The critical decisions, however, cannot be cut into separate parts and entrusted permanently to specialists. Eventually, a physician must take the pieces and fit them together to form a coherent plan of action. Only doctors can decide what to do with alternative computer diagnoses after giving due weight to their own observations and impressions. Rarely is a doctor able to delegate the final decision about whether the knowledge to be gained by another test is worth the cost. Physicians normally know more than anyone else about their patient's condition and thus are best able to prepare the patient to make intelligent judgments about alternative treatments. Similarly, physicians often command greater respect than priests or social workers when convincing patients of the steps they need to follow to cure their present disease or avoid future illness.

In sum, there is no substitute for doctors who can understand and integrate a range of subjects quite outside the body of bioscientific knowledge. Those who acquire this proficiency serve their patients, and the public, better. However, it is no longer a question of whether physicians *choose* to respond. The world outside forces them in this direction. Hospital chains and health maintenance organizations are bound to employ an increasing share of the nation's doctors. In a more competitive environment, these organizations will want to hire practitioners trained to gather information economically, to make cost-effective decisions, and to motivate patients to comply more willingly with health-preserving regimens. The rising flood of relevant information will compel doctors to use new technological aids. Law courts and newspapers will push ethical issues to the fore, and those who ignore them will be penalized. In today's environment, then, small wonder that medical schools are beginning to think about basic educational reform. The blunt fact is that most of their students today are receiving an education that is far too narrow to prepare them for the challenges that await them in their working lives.

## The Nature of Reform

Before examining the changes medical schools might consider, let us remind ourselves of the several aims that educational reform should strive to achieve. The most obvious goal is to make improvements in medical education that increase students' ability to serve their patients well after they become doctors. One important way of achieving this aim is to give more attention to neglected areas of knowledge, e.g., ethics, patient psychology, computer applications, methods of prevention. It is also useful to search for better ways to train students to perform traditional tasks. Despite the progress in medical science and technology, many studies have revealed that doctors make a disturbing number of major diagnostic errors. For example, a survey of 100 autopsies at a prominent teaching hospital disclosed such mistakes in 22% of the cases.[23] In almost half of these instances, a correct diagnosis would have indicated a change in the treatment that might have prolonged life. Other studies have shown erratic performance when carrying out routine tasks. Thus a survey of 249 patients in the outpatient clinic of a teaching hospital revealed that internists often neglected simple high-yield procedures, e.g., examining the prostrate or asking for a urinalysis (omitted 20% of the time), ordering blood glucose analysis (omitted 30% of the time), and testing the stool for blood (omitted 40% of the time).[24] According to the authors, "The internists who failed to perform these simple high-yield procedures were at the very least unsystematic and at the worst neglectful."[24] Training students to be more thorough and more skillful in carrying out such tasks may reduce the number of errors and improve patient care.

Beyond helping students become more proficient, faculties should try to avoid making the educational experience more disagreeable than it needs to be to accomplish its purposes. At present, medical schools are not pleasant places for all of their students. This judgment emerges clearly from accounts by students and faculty alike. After all, what is one to make of the long-standing complaints about the pressures felt by undergraduate premedical students and the tedium and frantic memorization associated with the preclinical years? Persistent dissatisfaction on this scale hardly seems inevitable. Nor is it fair to justify the status quo as some sort of test or initiation rite that strengthens the character of students. On the contrary, there is good reason to look for ways to improve on the present situation, for the time given to medical training takes up years of a human life, years that have a value quite apart from whether a better doctor emerges at the end.

Finally, medical schools must do their best to prepare students to address the problems afflicting our health care system. As we have seen, these problems are serious. In particular, 28 million people still lack reasonable access to medical services; yet the total bill for health care in the United States is already enormous and continues to climb much faster than the cost of living. No consensus has yet emerged on how to overcome these deficiencies.

We must be careful not to expect too much of medical training in our search for effective solutions. No country believes more strongly in higher education than the United States, and no country is quicker to attribute national problems to failings in our universities. Business schools are blamed for our declining competitiveness abroad, schools of education for the sagging performance of our youth on standard achievement tests, and law schools for the surfeit of litigation. In reality, however, the causes are almost always more complex. Medical schools cannot ensure proper care for the millions not covered by existing public and private programs. Nor are they well equipped to prescribe how many doctors the nation needs. No single institution can do much to limit the supply of new physicians or persuade them to work in underserved rural areas. Contrary to popular belief, careful studies even suggest that neither medical school teaching nor the nature of the curriculum has much effect on decisions by students whether to enter primary care as opposed to specialty practice or academic medicine.* Although medical faculties can play a modest supplementary role, only government can devise the policies we need to ensure a proper number and distribution of doctors.

Medical schools can make more significant contributions along various lines. To begin with, faculties can offer better instruction in preventive medicine. As

---

*Funkenstein DH: The prediction of the career choices of students at graduation from data collected on them at admission and matriculation to medical school, 1958–1974. Unpublished paper on file at the President's Office, Harvard University. Dr. Funkenstein's study suggested that career decisions were affected primarily by changes in social ideology outside the medical school and by changes in funding patterns affecting the renumeration available for different careers. Because changes in career choice throughout this period tended to occur simultaneously among students at different stages in their training, Funkenstein concluded that the nature of the training itself did not seem to have been a significant factor.

much as half of all illness in the United States could be avoided through changes in behavior brought about by voluntary adjustments in life style or by preventive measures on the part of government and private organizations. The latter are primarily the responsibility of the state, acting through appropriate rules and incentives. Education and persuasion can bring individuals to avoid smoking, excessive drinking, dietary deficiencies, inadequate exercise, unknowing exposure to health hazards, and many other forms of dangerous behavior. In this endeavor, the media and the schools have important roles to play. It is physicians, however, who have a special competence to discover risks that patients unwittingly run in their daily lives. They also have a special status and authority that helps them persuade individuals to alter their habits. Yet prevention currently receives only 1.5% of the total teaching time in the medical curriculum. One should not exaggerate the impact of more instruction; we know too little about the process of changing human behavior. Even so, there is little doubt that doctors could learn to be more effective in detecting avoidable causes of disease, more competent in using epidemiological techniques to identify community measures for prevention, and more adept at persuading patients to minimize needless risks. With a greater number of primary care practitioners and the growth of health maintenance organizations and other community-based institutions for health care, the opportunities for doctors to make such contributions seem destined to increase.

Faculties can also prepare physicians to curb inflated costs by eliminating needless tests and procedures. Individual practitioners typically make decisions involving diagnosis and treatment that call for expenditures of hundreds of thousands of dollars each year. One cannot imagine a company in which executives could purchase goods and services in these amounts without knowing the price of what they bought. Yet investigations show that most doctors do not know (within 25%) what laboratory tests actually cost.[25] Other inquiries have detected enormous variations among similarly situated physicians in the use of laboratory tests and the prescribing of drugs.[26] Fortunately, continued efforts to educate doctors about costs seem to produce impressive economies.[26,27] The potential savings are not trivial. Americans spend more than $25 billion each year on drugs and tests. Moreover, according to one Presidential Commission, unnecessary hospitalization may consume up to 20% of all hospital days; 50% to 65% of all prescribed antibiotics seem unwarranted or incorrectly administered; and billions of dollars are lost each year in useless chest x-ray studies or pointless respiratory care treatment and tests.[28]

If we are to minimize such excesses, the government must fashion appropriate rules and incentives, but these initiatives will not work well unless physicians understand them and agree to cooperate. The success and failure of any regulations depend on how they are implemented in hospitals, health maintenance organizations, and clinics—and those who direct these institutions are typically doctors. Moreover, the struggle to control medical costs in a manner consistent with proper care will ultimately be won or lost by a host of separate decisions that practitioners make in treating individual patients. On this battleground, the doctor inevitably has the upper hand. No government inspector and no hospital trustee can readily overrule the judgment of a trained specialist in matters that involve the health and even the survival of human beings.

Finally, although physicians have great influence in treating individual patients, the public is reluctant to pay the price of allowing everyone access to a health care system in which doctors are free to spend whatever they wish. For this reason, if we are ever to guarantee adequate health care to all, we must somehow find a way of joining the administrator's concern for reasonable cost with the physician's preoccupation with the needs of individual patients. This situation can hardly occur if doctors know nothing of costs and the problems of organizing and administering the health care system. On the contrary, medical schools must do their utmost to prepare physicians who have the understanding as well as the sensitivity and judgment to reconcile the need to serve the patient with the responsibility to avoid unnecessary expense.

## Premedical Education

If reform is to go forward, it should start at the college level, for it is there that students first begin taking courses to advance their medical career. At present, the impact of medical schools on the undergraduate curriculum is, in Lewis Thomas's words, "baleful and malign."[29] Some premedical students are competitive to the point of alienating their fellow undergraduates. Many change their courses and extracurricular activities to suit the supposed demands of medical admissions committees. All face requirements that bias them toward majoring in science and convey the misleading message that medicine, at bottom, is simply a matter of applying scientific knowledge.

In order to address these problems, universities need, first of all, a change in attitude on the part of both medical schools and faculties of arts and sciences. Medical faculties fail to recognize that their admissions requirements are not simply private matters but policies that significantly affect the undergraduate experience. They should acknowledge this fact and accept an obligation to make their influence as benign as possible. Arts and sciences professors, because they dislike having students take their courses to fulfill another faculty's requirements, often turn their backs and teach their classes as though the premedical requirements did not exist. This practice only makes matters worse, as the required courses come to include much material that cannot be considered truly necessary to the preparation of a doctor.

A useful step would be for representatives of both faculties to work in concert, first to agree on the minimum of knowledge needed to enter medical school and then to devise courses that cover the necessary material. Because students are forced to try to satisfy the requirements of all the schools to which they apply, an even better approach would be to launch this effort on a broader basis under the auspices of the Association of American Medical Colleges. Discussions should proceed on the shared assumption that medical school requirements are an undesirable intrusion on the college curriculum and should therefore be kept to a bare minimum. This obligation implies a conscientious attempt to devise pre-medical courses that do not include material irrelevant to becoming a doctor. It also calls for a serious effort by the medical faculty to find space for important subjects in its own curriculum and avoid asking colleges to supply courses that medical schools themselves should offer.

Although it is difficult to know what will come of such an effort, preliminary estimates in our own Faculty of Arts and Sciences suggest that the necessary scientific knowledge might be fitted into two year-long courses. Such compression would cut in half the time presently needed to fulfill the prerequisites for medical school. It would lower the requirements to a level approaching the amount of science that should be taken in any event by all undergraduates, regardless of whether they apply to medical school, as part of a liberal arts education. It would reduce the current pressure to major in science, as students concentrating in other fields could now fulfill their premedical requirements without using up virtually all their undergraduate electives. In these ways, such a modification would significantly lessen the distortions of the premedical requirements on the educational choices of college students.

Another useful step for medical schools would be to cease the practice of expressly basing admissions in part on the applicant's grade average in science courses—the so-called science GPA. Granted, science is fundamental to medicine, and medical schools can scarcely be indifferent if an applicant does significantly worse in science than in other undergraduate courses. Current practice, however, conveys a message that science is all-important and that the more taken the better. No amount of verbal reassurance by admissions officers has served to alter this perception. The result is that many undergraduates take more science courses than they might otherwise have chosen in an effort to impress the admissions committees.

A final possibility would be for college faculties to develop more courses in the humanities and social sciences that involve medicine. Philosophy departments could consider a course in medical ethics. Economics departments might provide an offering in health economics. History of science departments could give instruction in the history of medicine. Corresponding offerings are conceivable for departments of sociology, psychology, and even political science. Such courses are of interest to a wide range of students and can be taught in a manner thoroughly in keeping with a liberal arts education. They offer a broader view of medicine that should help undergraduates make more informed decisions about whether to pursue a medical career. They may also convey the useful message that medicine is more than science and help aspiring doctors adjust to a world in which their profession must cope with a wider set of pressures and concerns.

## Preclinical Education

The principal aim of improving the preclinical curriculum should be to do what other professional schools did many years ago: reduce the amount of factual information conveyed in the classroom and employ teaching methods that emphasize problem solving and the mastery of basic principles rather than memorization of detail. In order to reach this goal, basic scientists and clinical faculty must work together to agree on the basic concepts and material that students need to learn. The number of lectures can be sharply cut back, and professors can teach their material as much as possible through problem-based discussions, tutorials, computer-aided instruction, and other methods that actively challenge their students and teach them how to learn by themselves. Finally, professors can amend their examinations to conform with the new objectives by testing the students' powers of analysis and not simply their ability to recall vast quantities of information.

By taking these steps, a faculty could enhance students' interest, improve their ability to reason creatively and rigorously, and soften the jarring contrast between the intellectual stimulation of the last years of college and the tedium produced by endless lectures and constant memorization during the preclinical years. Faculty members may object that such reforms cut out too much scientific information that is important to physicians and essential for passing the National Boards. These objections are shopworn and unconvincing. Information that is truly important can be communicated in written form. There is no reason to waste the limited resource of classroom time by repeating the material orally. Moreover, one must be skeptical about expansive definitions of "essential" information. With advances in sciences, much of what seems essential today will be outmoded tomorrow. Dean Burwell was only partly facetious in stating to Harvard medical students: "Half of what we have taught you is wrong. Unfortunately, we do not know which half."

Many experiments have likewise shown how little information students actually recall from lectures a week, a month, a year after they are given. According to Duncan Neuhauser, a study at Case Western Reserve has found that second-year students will have forgotten 90% of the factual items they have learned by the time they graduate.[30] Worse yet, cognitive scientists tell us that learning factual details often makes it more difficult to remember the really important concepts.[31] These findings suggest that preclinical teachers do better to concentrate more on helping students master fundamental ideas by actively discussing how to apply them in various contexts.

Furthermore, to echo a host of distinguished critics from Abraham Flexner to Michael Bishop, the most important reason for teaching basic science is not to convey quantities of facts but to instill a set of *attitudes* that carry over into clinical practice—a taste for defining problems, creating hypotheses, and testing them rigorously. What disappoints these critics is that the very effort to cram "all the essential information" into the heads of passive students tends to produce the very opposite of the active, inquiring scientific mind that every physician should possess.

Even if the faculty acknowledges the need for reform, the necessary changes may be long in coming. Professors will find it difficult to agree on which concepts and knowledge are truly fundamental and which can be cut away. It is a daunting task under the best of circumstances. It is made more difficult by the fact that many basic scientists have little idea of what a practicing doctor needs to know, and they regard efforts to reduce the number of lectures they give as a sign of disrespect for their subject. The challenge of mastering new methods of pedagogy is also formidable. Many professors *think* that they can teach by the discussion method. If one observes them, however, they often do little more than ask true/false questions that test students' memory rather than challenge their powers of reasoning. Instructors are also inclined to give the answer when the correct response does not come quickly from the class, thereby depriving students of the valuable experience of struggling through to a conclusion by themselves.

It is no simple matter to prepare faculty members to use new forms of instruction, especially when they have few good models from their own student days. Fortunately, however, much progress has been made in training people to teach. Not only can one find written materials or develop seminars for the purpose; even better ways have been developed through the use of videotape to enable instructors to observe themselves in the act of teaching with the help of an experienced critic. Through these techniques, most people can make surprising progress in perfecting their ability to lead a stimulating discussion. All that remains is to find the motivation and the will — ingredients that must be supplied by leadership backed by adequate rewards.

The preclinical years are also the time to begin an effort to expand the students' knowledge by introducing subjects such as medical ethics, psychology, statistics, computer use, and formal methods of decision-making. We have seen how important these subjects have become in enabling physicians to discharge their responsibilities. Experience also suggests that able teachers can accomplish much to help students acquire competence in these fields. It is certainly possible to train people in the use of statistics, computers, and formal methods of decision-making. As for medical ethics, no one could pretend that a course can turn every aspiring physician into a virtuous human being. Even so, competent instruction using cases and discussion can help students become proficient in perceiving ethical dilemmas when they arise and in thinking about them in a manner that is rigorous and informed. Well conceived courses can also acquaint students with the causes of rising medical costs and the methods for trying to bring them under control, just as training in cost-benefit analysis and better strategies for acquiring information can help students learn how to minimize unnecessary expense when caring for patients.

The teaching of psychology may present greater difficulty, as many complexities of human behavior are still beyond our understanding. Even so, students can certainly be taught to talk more clearly and persuasively to patients about medications and treatments. Instructors have likewise shown that they can train students to interview more effectively and to improve their skill in detecting significant psychological and cognitive disorders. At a deeper level, students can also learn the elements of what is known about the impact of psychological and social factors on human illness and rehabilitation, not to mention the effects of personality factors on the willingness of patients to cooperate fully with physicians.

Most faculties already offer courses on almost all these topics. The problem is to assign them their proper place in the curriculum. In the ethos of the contemporary medical school, with its strong emphasis on biomedical science, subjects such as decision analysis, statistics, patient psychology, ethics, and health care policy must be required and given ample time if we expect more than a few students to study them seriously. Faculty members will complain that there is no room to force these courses into an overloaded curriculum. Students will resist any inroads on their opportunities to take electives. Yet space can and must be found, whether it comes from elective slots or from the time freed by pruning unnecessary detail from the basic science courses. After all, many faculties have experimented with a 3-year curriculum, and doubts are often expressed at other schools about the value of the final year of study. These straws in the wind suggest that there is room to substitute new material for existing courses if such changes are important to serve the needs of medical practice. The subjects just described surely meet this test. No longer peripheral, they have moved toward the center of our emerging vision of how physicians must think in order to function effectively in the modern world.

## Clinical Instruction

The great strength of the clinical years is the vivid reality that comes with learning in the hospital and caring for the sick. Nothing holds students' attention more raptly or motivates them more strongly than the presence of real patients in need of help.

Yet the very strength of the clinical years is also the source of the greatest problems. Because much of the teaching takes place in the hospital, its content is shaped by the exigencies and peculiarities of patient care. What students learn typically depends on the ailments of the patients who happen to be in the ward at that moment—and in a teaching hospital these ailments are likely to be far more complicated and rare than those that ordinary doctors see in community hospitals and ambulatory settings. The quality of instruction on the ward also reflects the overriding responsibility for patient care. Those who teach, especially the house staff, are often weary from their responsibilities and are subject to interruption at any time to serve some compelling patient need.

The principal problems of clinical teaching, then, are rooted in imperatives of care that can easily lead to improvisation and a lack of orderly structure. Adequate structure requires that each rotation have clear objectives fixed in advance to define the basic material and skills that students should master. Adequate structure means that ways are devised and ample time provided to convey the desired material and teach the designated skills within the period of rotation. Finally, adequate structure implies that students know the objectives in advance, receive reasonable feedback to monitor their progress, and obtain sufficient evaluation to see if they achieved the goals prescribed. Too often these qualities are lacking on the wards of our teaching hospitals.

Similar problems are evident in the style of clinical instruction. When walking through hospital corridors, one is struck by the variable, unrehearsed quality of the teaching. Sometimes patients are seen and talked to, sometimes not. Bits and pieces of information are conveyed on the spot as problems develop and new data arrive from the laboratory or the night nurse. Much information is conveyed didactically or demonstrated at the bedside. Instructors do pose questions to students on occasion, but usually to test their knowledge rather than to train their powers of analytical thought. Too rarely does one hear a genuine, sustained dialogue that challenges students to elicit relevant data, venture hypotheses, and move toward a final diagnosis by trial and error. Ethical issues, cost considerations, and psychological problems pop up occasionally but seldom receive thorough discussion. House staff and faculty specialists are rarely well versed in these subjects and often lack time to discuss them in detail amid the pressing responsibilities of patient care.

It is difficult to overcome these problems fully in the context of a teaching hospital with its bustle of busy people and its compelling, unpredictable demands. Yet even in this setting, something can be done to achieve greater structure. Senior faculty can set objectives that are understood by all and offer adequate opportunities for feedback and evaluation (as Harvard departments have tried to do in recent years). Required readings and occasional lectures can help ensure that basic information is conveyed and understood.

Although these measures are useful, the tensions inherent in clinical teaching become more acute as faculties accept the need to broaden their training to place more emphasis on subjects such as ethics, patient psychology, prevention, and cost-effective strategies for making diagnoses and prescribing proper treatments. Many studies have shown that integrating such material into clinical training is essential if these subjects are to make any lasting imprint on the minds and behavior of medical students. However, patients who enter the hospital may not have problems that illustrate the topics in optimal fashion, nor does the house staff always have the ability to teach such subjects well. To some extent, these difficulties can be overcome by more readings and seminars and by extending clinical instruction to ambulatory settings that expose students to a broader range of human afflictions. Still better would be some pedagogic method that could serve the needs of order and structure without giving up the vivid realism of actual patient care.

Simulations of various kinds offer useful ways to help surmount this problem. Whether the simulation takes the form of a written script or uses actors who play the part of doctor and patient, students can learn to ask appropriate questions and to frame hypotheses and test them until a correct diagnosis can be found. The same method can be transferred to a computer with the great advantage of allowing each student to practice as much as desired at any hour of the day. Better yet, one can program the computer to ask questions of its own in order to form a Socratic dialogue that forces students to think more deeply and devise thorough but efficient strategies for obtaining the data to reach a proper diagnosis. Obviously, simulations cannot and should not replace the experience of serving and learning on the hospital ward, with its compelling immediacy and reality. As learning technology develops, however, it is not farfetched to assume that such methods will play an increasing role in helping faculties cover a body of important material that is growing too large and diverse to be fully and effectively captured in the hospital setting.

## References

1. Friedman CP, Purcell EF (eds): *The New Biology and Medical Education: Merging the Biological, Information, and Cognitive Sciences.* New York, Josiah Macy Jr. Foundation, 1983.
2. Institute of Medicine: *Medical Education and Societal Needs: A Planning Report for the Health Professions.* Publication No. IOM-83-02, July 1983.
3. Starr P: *The Social Transformation of American Medicine.* New York, Basic Books, 1982.
4. Thomas L: *The Youngest Science: Notes of a Medicine-Watcher.* New York, Viking Press, 1983, pp 13, 29.
5. Richmond J, Kotelchuk M: The effect of the political process on the delivery of health services. Unpublished paper, 1982, p 18.
6. Wills J, Garrison L, Jacoby I: *Modeling, Research, and Data Technical Panel. Report of the Graduate Medical Education National Advisory Committee to the Secretary, Department of Health and Human Services,* Vol. 2, 1980.
7. Institute of Medicine: *A Manpower Policy for Primary Health Care: Report of a Study.* Publication No. IOM-78-02, 1978.
8. Sierles F, Hendrickx I, Circle S: Cheating in medical school. *J Med Educ* 1980;55:124–125. [The study involved a survey of 400 students at the Stritch School of Medicine, Loyola University in Chicago, and the University of Health Sciences at Chicago Medical School.]
9. Roethlisberger FJ: *The Elusive Phenomena: An Autobiographical Account of My Work in the Field of Organizational Behavior at the Harvard Business School.* Boston, Division of Research, Harvard Graduate School of Business Administration, 1977.
10. Seldon D. Quoted by Filner B, Weisfeld V, Parron D: Infusion of new fields into medical education, *Medical Education and Societal Needs.* Washington, DC, National Academy Press, 1983, p 148.
11. Singer J, et al: Physician attitudes toward applications of computer data base systems. *JAMA* 1983;249:1610.
12. Berwick DM, Fineberg HV, Weinstein MC: When doctors meet numbers. *Am J Med* 1981;71:991.
13. Cohen-Cole SA: On teaching and the new (and old) psychobiology, in: Friedman CP, Purcell EF (eds): *The New Biology and Medical Education: Merging the Biological, Information, and Cognitive Sciences.* New York, Josiah Macy Jr. Foundation, 1983, pp 133–134.
14. DiMatteo MR, Friedman HF: *Social Psychology and Medicine.* Cambridge, MA: Oelgeschlager, Gunn & Hain, 1982, p 106.
15. Medalie JH, Goldbourt U: Angina pectoris among 10,000 men. *Am J. Med* 1976; 60:910.
16. Bartrop RW, et al: Depressed lymphocyte function after bereavement. *Lancet* 1977;1:834.

17. Langer EJ, Janis IL, Wolfer JA: Reduction of psychological stress in surgical patients. *J Exp Social Psychol* 1975;11:155.
18. Hulka BS, et al: Communication, compliance, and concordance between physicians and patients with prescribed medications. *Am J Public Health* 1976;66:847.
19. DiMatteo MR, Friedman HF: *Social Psychology and Medicine.* Cambridge, MA, Oelgeschlager, Gunn & Hain, 1982, pp 40, 48–49, 82.
20. Lewin: Group decision and social change. In Maccoby, Newcomb, Hartley (eds): *Readings in Social Psychology.* 1958.
21. Bass Wilson F: The pediatrician's influence in private practice, measured by a controlled seat belt study. *Pediatrics* 1964;33:700.
22. Bursztajn H, et al: *Medical Choices, Medical Chances: How Patients, Families, and Physicians Can Cope with Uncertainty.* New York, Delacorte Press, 1981.
23. Goldman L, et al: The value of the autopsy in three medical eras. *N Engl J Med* 1983;308:1000.
24. Goetzl EJ, et al: Quality of diagnostic examinations in a university hospital outpatient clinic. *Ann Intern Med* 1983;78:481, 487.
25. Skipper JK, et al: Physicians' knowledge of cost: the case of diagnostic tests. *Inquiry* 1976;13:194.
26. Schroeder SA, et al: Use of laboratory tests and pharmaceuticals—variation among physicians and effect of cost audit on subsequent use. *JAMA* 1973;225:969.
27. Lawrence RS: The role of physician education in cost containment. *J Med Educ* 1979;54:841.
28. President's Commission for the Study of Ethical Problems in Medicine and Biomedical and Behavioral Research: *Securing Access to Health Care: A Report on the Ethical Implications of Differences in the Availability of Health Services,* 1983, pp 1986–1988.
29. Thomas LT: How to fix the premedical curriculum. *N Engl J Med* 1978;290:1180.
30. Neuhauser: Don't teach preventive medicine: a contrary view. *Public Health Rep* 1982;97:220.
31. Larkin JH: Learning and using large amounts of knowledge: the role of basic science. In Friedman CP, Purcell EF (eds): *The New Biology and Medical Education: Merging the Biological, Information, and Cognitive Sciences.* New York, Josiah Macy Jr Foundation, 1983, pp 185, 188.

# 3
# A Medical School for the Future

Davıd Maddison*

The success or failure of the "Newcastle experiment," as it is sometimes called, will undoubtedly have repercussions on medical education throughout Australia, and indeed to some extent throughout the world. Australia's newest faculty of medicine, at the University of Newcastle, admitted its first class of 64 students in March 1978. The methods of establishing the program, selecting students, appointing staff members, and assessing student performance exhibit many novel features, which are already attracting international attention. The basic philosophy of the school and the objectives it sets out to achieve seem to be universally applicable.

## Basic Philosophy for Medical Education

For a dean and his foundation professorial colleagues, there is (or should be) an inherent challenge in the development of a new medical school: It provides an unusual opportunity to influence the shaping of medical education so as to prepare practitioners for effective performance of the tasks that will confront the doctor of the future. The foundation professors at Newcastle agreed that if the school lacked a coherent basic philosophy, it would almost inevitably fall back into the easy groove of "doing its thing" in a traditional way. Very early in the life of the faculty, therefore, the first group of staff accepted the challenge of facing these vitally important issues.

1. Without sacrificing the need to provide quality care for individuals, the school would need to place greatly increased emphasis on the care of total populations: those who sought assistance and those who did not, those who labeled themselves "sick" and those who declined to do so, the hypochondriacs and those who lived in reckless disregard of their own health, the affluent and the disadvantaged, the indigenes and the immigrants.

2. There was a need to respond, in a positive, enlightened, but still essentially scientific way to the increasing clamor for greater evidence of humanity and

---

*Deceased.

"caring" and for more effective communication between patient and doctor in this highly technological age. Our collective previous experiences in medical schools made it apparent that even some senior and highly traditional medical educators were complaining that clinical medical students and young graduates seemed unable to establish effective communication with their patients.

3. Nevertheless, the scientific method had to remain central to the practice of medicine and thus to medical education; but positive action would be needed to close the gap between academic and research medicine, on the one hand, and the problems of the patient in the community, on the other hand. It would also be necessary to ensure that "science" in medical education would embrace more than the traditional biological and laboratory sciences.

4. Due attention would have to be paid to the implications of the frequently repeated statement that patterns of illness were steadily changing, most obviously in the developed world, the natural corollary being that doctors would need to foster a preventive attitude; health education would need to gain importance, for control of the diseases of the future seemed less and less likely to be achieved by manipulation of the environment, the essential element being alteration in the behavior of people. The doctor, then, would need increasingly to think of himself as an educator, and must be appropriately prepared for this role, for better-informed and less deferential patients would demand more appropriate explanations and a much greater degree of involvement in the management of their own illnesses.

5. The new medical school should direct attention to those aspects of the diseased human condition that tend to have been ignored because they have been regarded as distasteful, messy, or unrewarding. The problems of drug dependence and geriatrics are obvious examples.

6. Medical graduates of the future would need to achieve much greater clarification of what is truly a health problem and what is not and arrive at a much more sophisticated appraisal of the place of the doctor in modern society. Students and graduates would need to be concerned with that immense territory of overlap between health problems and social problems. They would need to recognize that the solution of certain major environmental problems might do more to alter patterns of urban morbidity than the efforts of 100 medical graduates. They would need to appreciate that, if a team of young psychologists were to devise a really effective alcohol education program for an adolescent and young adult population, this might do more to affect patterns of illness 20 years later than 100 liver specialists devoting their lives to ameliorating the end results of alcohol excess.

## Faculty of Medicine within the University of Newcastle

The University of Newcastle has been an autonomous institution since 1965, after a period of 13 years during which it was a College of the University of New South Wales. It is a small tertiary institution by Australian standards, with a total student population of approximately 4500 and only seven faculties apart from medicine. Although members of the academic staff had in the past consistently supported the notion that Australia's next medical school should be at Newcastle, some of the same people were now expressing a good deal of concern lest the future financial demands inevitably generated by medical education might become a "drain" on the university's budget and add to the financial problems of other faculties and departments.

This problem has been highlighted by the extraordinarily rapid change that has occurred in the state of the Australian economy (indeed, the state of the world economy, in many respects) between 1973, when the Australian government announced its decision to develop a new medical school in Newcastle, and 1978, when the first class of students was admitted. Moreover, in this short space of 5 years two other developments have taken place that have led to a powerful and critical spotlight being trained on the developing, and still rather fragile, medical school: realization that, first, for a variety of reasons, Australia is likely to have a higher doctor/patient ratio than previously predicted and, second, a rapidly mounting awareness of the extent to which doctors are the prime generators of health care costs, so that any excess of doctors within the system would put an unnecessary burden on the health budget. In strong contrast to the climate of opinion that existed as recently as 1978, there are now some people (including some in quite high places) who are seriously doubting the wisdom of the initial decision to establish the school.

The medical school, however, is by now an established reality; its first major building, to house the medical sciences, has been completed on the Newcastle campus, and construction of the major clinical sciences building on land adjacent to the Royal Newcastle Hospital is complete. Now the medical school is clearly accepted as a going concern and is turning its attention to the ambitious objectives it has set for itself.

## Development of Objectives

Without any doubt the most important task undertaken by the foundation professors was the spelling out, in reasonable detail, of the objectives toward the achievement of which the undergraduate education program would be directed. Virtually all our major educational decisions derive their rationale from a consideration of these objectives. We considered that, without such a foundation, we could all too easily become involved in "change for change's sake"; alternatively, without clear objectives we might uncritically continue certain components of traditional medical education that would be antithetical to our general aims.

After a great deal of painstaking work, we developed a series of 45 program objectives, grouped under six headings, in terms of their relation to: (1) the student's own learning; (2) scientific method and procedure; (3) clinical diagnosis, investigation, and management; (4) attitudes and personal characteristics; (5) community medicine; (6) the doctor/patient relationship.

These objectives have, in effect, nailed our colors to the mast; we have made a public declaration of our belief in the importance of certain commonly neglected aspects of medical education and have declared our commitment to the implementation of an educational program that will ensure that the student, at the time of graduation, will display specific behaviors derived from accumulated knowledge, skills, and attitudes. Some of these objectives crystallize views to which reference is frequently made in discussions of medical education but which are only rarely made so explicit. For example, the graduate (and by this we mean at the time of graduation) will be expected to have demonstrated the following characteristics.

1. Ability and willingness to achieve and maintain responsibility for his or her own learning and for the continuing evaluation of his own performance as a physician; he will have accepted the fact that medical education in its full sense is a lifelong activity and be prepared to invest time in the maintenance and further development of his own knowledge and skills over and above the pursuit of higher professional qualifications.

2. Ability to adopt a problem-solving approach to clinical situations.

3. Ability and willingness to devise and maintain an appropriate management program for patients with chronic, intractable illness, including terminal disease.

4. An approach to all patients that reflects the attitude that the person who is ill is more important than the illness from which he suffers.

5. Awareness that major changes in individual and community health are likely to depend as much or more on change in the behavior of people as on the manipulation of the physical environment.

6. A positive attitude toward the concept of the physician as an educator and an appropriate level of ability and confidence in this role.

7. Openness to genuine yet objective involvement with patients free from undue interference with communication created by psychological defense mechanisms of the type that lead to an aloof, excessively detached approach.

These objectives might be regarded by many as somewhat unusual, at least in the degree of emphasis we are placing on them; a substantial number of the remaining objectives, not mentioned here, would be likely to find much greater acceptance in other, more traditional schools. Note that we have taken the plunge into the area of attitudes. We are unrepentant about this, believing that this dimension of medical education has been neglected for far too long, and moreover that it is the specific area of medical practice, above all others, in which the long-dormant forces of consumerism are currently finding much to criticize.

From the formulation of these objectives evolved all the major developments in our program: the specific structure of the educational experience, the characteristics of the assessments used to monitor student progress, the school's policy on the selection of students, and—very importantly—the academic posts identified as essential for the fulfillment of our aims and the type of person chosen to occupy them.

## Selection of Students

We have adopted an admissions policy that is innovative by Australian standards and that, as far as we know, has certain completely unique features: selecting one-half of the class solely on the basis of their past academic record, and the other half through a carefully defined combination of academic, intellectual, and personal attributes. The task has turned out to be much greater than we anticipated. We estimated that we might receive some 1000 to 1200 applicants, but we were required to process a total of 2250.

Each applicant who meets our academic standards comes to the campus for an extensive series of tests, which select those who will be invited to appear for final interview, a semistructured procedure with clearly defined objectives conducted by a member of the academic staff in conjunction with a medical or nonmedical representative of the local community.

The characteristics we have identified as being essential for our second, non-traditional batch of entrants spring more or less directly from our program objectives. After a great deal of discussion in our Admissions Policy Committee, which included both medical and nonmedical representatives from the local community, we formulated a set of characteristics that we believed were both essential for the effective practice of medicine and reliably measurable. Those aspects of the applicant on which we seek evidence are the following: (1) higher mental abilities considered to be specifically related to the problem-solving approach to medicine; (2) creativity; (3) capacity for empathy; (4) capacity to provide supportive/encouraging behavior; (5) perseverance; (6) flexibility of views and attitudes; and (7) ability to deal with ethically difficult situations in an informed and thoughtful manner. We are not, it should be emphasized, constructing a "personality profile" on each applicant, nor are we using the interview to screen for evidence of personal psychopathology.

One attractive feature of our admissions program is that we collect exactly the same data on every applicant, including those who will ultimately be admitted on previous academic record alone. We should thus be able to compare and contrast student performance throughout the course and, after graduation , of those admitted solely on the basis of their past examination performance and those who, although academically able, have not performed at the same high level in examinations but have displayed important intellectual and personality characteristics. "Performance," it should be noted, will mean much more to us than "success in examinations" during the course.

## Education Program and Its Assessment

If we believe that the graduate should be able to "adopt a problem-solving approach to clinical situations," it follows that the entire educational program should be constructed, from the beginning, around the process of clinical problem solving. From the first term of the first year, therefore, the student is involved with real, live, clinical problems, which he or she is required to understand and manage, obviously at an increasing level of complexity as the course progresses. All learning in the so-called "basic sciences" is derived from study of these problems. The clinical problems themselves have been selected after a close study of detailed Australian epidemiological data, with due regard for prevalence, seriousness, treatability, and preventability.

The consequence of this decision is that the program contains no "courses" in the ordinary sense, the entire approach being an integrated one in both the "horizontal" and "vertical" dimensions. The only exception occurs during the first year, when there are substantial strands of education and supervised practice in the acquisition of basic communication and clinical skills that it has not proved possible to integrate in a completely satisfactory way with the ongoing problem-solving tasks. We are also grappling with the complex issue of introducing the student, from the beginning, to what we identify as the medicine of groups or populations, a vitally important dimension that is not always comfortably integrated into the basic clinical problem-solving sequence.

There are many medical academics who fear that our total commitment to this approach may substantially reduce the student's mastery of the underlying scientific basis of medical practice. They worry lest the student graduate, for example, knowing little fundamental biochemistry, only a few rules of thumb that he has been able to utilize in a slick way to grasp the superficial aspects of the biochemistry of disease. We have been exceptionally fortunate in being able to recruit foundation professors who, drawing on their own experience elsewhere, are more or less completely dischanted with the amount of basic scientific material that the student leans *and retains* during a traditional education program, and who are thus more than willing to commit themselves wholeheartedly to this admittedly somewhat experimental approach.

A great deal depends, of course, on what one means by "science"; there is a respectable argument to be made for the case that the average medical student has had his head filled with what Moran Campbell called "the stories of science," mastering a large number of "facts," many of which turn out in the long run to be of depressingly little value, yet graduating without anything resembling a fundamental appreciation of the scientific approach to disease and to patient management. We have not abandoned the scientific basis of medicine (nor are we in the business of training "glorified social workers," as is sometimes said); on the contrary, we have included in our objectives a highly specific reference to the graduate's need to have demonstrated "an understanding of the scientific method, the reliability and validity of observations, and the testing of hypotheses." We believe, in short, that our graduates will be "strong" in science rather than "weak"; we are equally firm in our belief that the acquisition of the scientific approach has literally nothing to do with the presence or absence of long courses and many hours of practical work in the traditional science subjects. We should also add that we are explicit in including in our concept of "science" those aspects concerned with the behavior of man, and to this end we have appointed a foundation professor and supporting staff in behavioral science.

The advantages of the integrated approach to education via clinical problem-solving are too many to detail in a short chapter. Three specially important aspects must, however, be identified.

1. Bridging the traditional gulf, indeed enmity, between preventive and curative medicine, because when dealing with, for example, coronary artery disease, both dimensions are examined by the student at the same time, so that he sees for himself the essential interrelation between the treatment of sick individuals and the strategies that need to be adopted if morbidity and mortality from coronary disease are to be reduced.

2. Integration of the psychological and social aspects of health and disease with clinical problems as they are encountered throughout the course, which should go a long way toward preventing the disastrous habit, so common among medical students, of isolating these dimensions from the remainder of their understanding of specific disease processes and disease in general.

3. Breakdown of the transparently false antithesis between "basic scientists" and "clinicians." Biological scientists are indeed more, rather than less, visible in this educational program because their involvement is substantial until the very end of the course.

It should also be emphasized that the central task of clinical problem-solving is undertaken throughout the course in small groups, for we are convinced that only in this way can the graduate acquire competence in areas that we rate as being of central importance. Initially the groups comprise medical students only, but their composition is diversified later in the course to include other health professional students.

It is central to our educational philosophy and to the achievement of our program objectives that the student be able to check his or her progress frequently against the standards laid down by the faculty; not only is the student required to reach a certain defined standard at the end of each block (usually a term in duration) but he or she is encouraged to undertake other small, progressive assessments during the block in order to acquire the necessary skill in monitoring his or her own progress. We believe it is self-evident that the results of these assessments, both the end-of-term "summative" assessments and the intraterm optional, or "formative," assessments, should be fed back to the student rapidly and in detail, so that he can immediately identify areas of weakness. Very importantly, assessment is not norm-referenced; that is, results are available on a pass/fail basis; students either reach the requisite standard of performance or they do not. Only in this way, we believe, can we minimize the destructive effects of intrafaculty, dog-eat-dog competition and increase the graduates' ability to work cooperatively as members of a group of collaborating health professionals. We have, however, made the policy decision that during their final year of integrated clinical practice, the students' performance in clinical problem-solving, dealing with a wide range of clinical problems, provides the opportunity for them to be graded as deserving of an honors degree.

## Conclusion

A great deal has changed since 1973, when the Australian Universities Commission in its report "The Expansion of Medical Education" recommended that the University of Newcastle establish a new medical school to assist in the production of more doctors for Australia and thus lower the doctor/patient ratio. We are very much aware that we are setting out to produce more doctors at a time when people are beginning to ask serious questions about the desirability and economic feasibility of such a development; but, frankly, we are not particularly bothered by the accusation that changing circumstances have rendered us redundant. Available manpower figures are, for a start, capable of being interpreted in several ways; and we are less than convinced by the assertion that Australia has, or is likely to have in the near future, "too many doctors." Even if this were true, the answer, in our view, would be for some of the older, larger, and substantially congested medical schools to reduce their student intake, rather than to undermine the viability of our new and different program.

The success or failure of the Newcastle experiment will undoubtedly have repercussions on medical education throughout Australia and indeed to some extent throughout the world. We keep in close touch with schools that have been undertaking somewhat similar developments—notably in Canada (McMaster University), Israel (Ben Gurion University of Negev), and The Netherlands (University of Limburg)—and exchange as much information as we can so that each can learn as much as possible from the successes, problems, and failures of the others. All of us are struggling to a greater or lesser extent with the difficulties of innovation during a period of substantial inflation and consequent cutbacks in government finance and at a time when doctors almost everywhere seem to be regarded with increasing suspicion. Yet "failure," or a substantial retreat from the educational philosophy we have espoused, is not really to be contemplated— for this, we believe, would set back the reforming process in medical education by several decades.

# Part II
# Community-oriented Medical Education Today

MACK LIPKIN, JR.

Pilowski's dictum, communicated to the author after a pithy discussion of problems in his department, states that complaints are proportional to vitality in medical education. The evidence for vitality in medical education is abundant: $6.4 billion spent annually on medical education in the United States[1] and an oversupply of physicians in the educational pipelines in most industrialized countries.[2] So too are complaints abundant. Most criticisms of medicine sooner or later get leveled at the educators, much as the problems of the child are blamed on the parents. Medical education is said to take *wunderkind* and turn them into passive, authority-ridden, rigid, materialistic, dehumanized doctors.[3] They focus narrowly on disease to the exclusion of patient, community, family, ethical values, morality, and epidemiology. On the other hand, they are invasive, causing wasteful and harmful iatrogenic illness. They medicalize the activities of daily life, producing an illness stigma that attaches malignantly to normal phenomena.[4] They do not know normal development and behavior and so are unable to promote health but, rather, proceed on the basis of fear of disease: They fail to prevent illness, perhaps preferring to wait until their disease-oriented services are needed. They drop out, burn out, make poor husbands or wives and poor parents, and they commit suicide often.[5]

It has been noted by many that medical systems themselves fail in major aspects of the mission of medicine. Specifically, it is argued that modern medicine has made a series of systematic errors beginning in the midnineteenth century. At that time the successes of gross and then microscopic pathology produced a spurt of interest in pathology and causes of death. The dominant classification systems of medicine became those of the pathologists, embodied in the international classifications of disease—initially classifications of causes of death. This situation has continued to the present day as physicians are preoccupied with disease and consequently are ineffective in its prevention and in the use of the healthy resources of the people in their own care.[6]

A second series of distortions of the central missions of medicine began with the "scientization of medicine" after the Second World War. As the promise of science perversely became identified with the "triumph" of the production of nuclear fission and the atomic bomb, so governments turned increasingly to view medical progress as resting on increasingly "high," i.e., complex and costly, technology. The reward in medical care systems and in medical educational institutions came increasingly to favor "high-tech" processes and procedures. As this progressed, the costs of medicine increased and consumed increasingly high proportions of gross national products (GNPs). US economists for the past two decades have routinely declared that the proportion of the total economy consumed by the medical sector had become unacceptably high and medicine would soon experience shrinkage and constraint. Yet the projected upper limits have steadily increased as the proportion of GNP consumed by medicine passed 5%, then 8%, and now more than 11%.

With the high cost of medicine has come distortions of resource allocation. At one point, Thailand had a significant proportion of its total annual health expenditures sunk in computed tomography (CT) scanners, whereas the leading causes of death, e.g., malaria, were allocated lesser sums. In the United States, government and other insurance programs pay for coronary bypass surgery—at $10,000 to $25,000 per case—but not for smoking prevention, hypertension screening, or other preventive measures which, demonstrably, could have prevented many of the same cases that ended in this surgery. The status of high-tech programs has led nations to invest heavily in them (e.g., coronary surgery, intensive care units, fetal monitoring) while not treating those problems of their populations, which produce the greatest proportion of the morbidity and mortality.

Similarly, medical education has stressed the frontiers of disease-oriented knowledge since the triumph of the pathologic approach and the Flexner report. This emphasis has resulted in the production of physicians knowledgeable in the uncommon but often ill-equipped to deal with common problems in the least toxic and most cost-effective ways. In the less developed world, the leading physicians and teachers frequently have been trained in industrialized nations in the specialty models prevailing in those settings. As a result, they sometimes have established training programs that directly translate the teaching in their high prestige training programs, with the result that much of the training was irrelevant for the practices entered by their graduates.[7]

Similarly, the decades since World War II have seen an ever-increasing continuation of trends, already evident in the midnineteenth century, toward specialization. Specialization is sometimes justified on the basis of the explosion of knowledge and the inability of anyone to know well more than a narrow area. This view certainly has merit. Presently, to keep up in internal medicine alone, one faces more than 250 new articles each month in the major journals alone. In reality, it is impossible to keep up even in many narrow subspecialities. We now have not only infectious disease specialists but immunology subspecialists. The latter are presently undergoing fission and becoming cellular immunologists and humoral immunologists. (Imagine the problems patients will face when they try to get help for their rhinitis.

Yet the specialists run into practical problems because patients walk into their offices equipped with more than the organs about which the specialist is expert. It has been clearly shown that specialists favor diagnoses in their specialty. They also favor certain diagnostic procedures. A woman with back pain may get lumbosacral spine films from a neurosurgeon, a urine culture from a nephrologist or urologist, a pelvic examination from a gynecologist, a discussion of who is on her back from a psychiatrist. She undergoes a complete physical only from a generalist internist before he sends her to one of the above. Specialists tend to overlook problems in other organ systems and to emphasize pursuit of the obscure while omitting preventive and psychosocial interventions. This approach limits the benefits a patient may expect and raises the cost of care. In resource-limited areas, this is a major problem.

The preceding, exaggerated, rather tongue in cheek description of problems in modern medicine has been familiar to many for several decades. During the 1940s, beginning in several parts of Europe, there was increasing recognition of the growing separation between medical practice and education and the needs of people. In the United Kingdom this awareness was spearheaded by the Royal College of General Practitioners, who demonstrated that much (about 40%) of daily practice could not even be documented using dominant (International Classification of Diseases) classifications. In the United States the pediatricians led the way by recognizing that much of pediatrics is concerned with preventive and well-baby care and that the technically possible elimination of epidemic infectious diseases such as polio, rubella, and diphtheria depended on improving the preventive practices of pediatricians and general practitioners and on improving their penetration of the population.

The growing awareness of the need to bring medicine into balance with the health needs of the population has taken many forms. One is the mushrooming interest of medical schools in clinical epidemiology, the application of sound experimental and quantitative methods to the evaluation of everyday practices of clinical medicine.[8] A second is the application of similar quantitative thinking to issues of resource allocation in health systems.[9] Technology assessment and clinical epidemiology each rest on a rather simple logic. Taken together, they suggest an approach to medical thinking recently termed "population-based medicine." Its tenets are that the mission of medicine is to serve the health needs of the population. In order to do this, it is necessary, first, to assess what the needs of a given population are. The needs of the residents of rain forests in tropical climates are not the same as those of upper-class Brahmins in Boston. Having determined the priority needs of a population, it is necessary to examine the available solutions to meetings or changing those needs. This involves ascertaining what methods are available to deal with a given need and experimentally determining which are the most effective and efficient. Only then can health systems be designed which meet the needs of the population efficiently.[10]

The chapters presented in this section document several aspects of the developments summarized here. *Benor* and colleagues detail the basic principles involved in the concept of community-oriented medical education. They emphasize a health orientation, a community base, concern with a complex view of the natural history of disease and the human life cycle, relevance and integration of materials, and end with a "three-dimensional model" of health problems.

*Zohair Nooman*, former Dean of the Suez Canal University Faculty of Medicine and now Secretary General of the Network, writes about community-oriented education from the perspective of the change agent: Which problems will be faced when implementing a community-oriented curriculum and which solutions are feasible? After this general orientation, *Bollag* and his collaborators give an example of a community problem developed and studied by students. Seven to 14 students, and 2 or 3 faculty members, settled in and studied a village for one month. The detail provided provides a real sense of the power and limits of this method. Bollag and colleagues show both strengths—especially stimulating, broadening of views—and problems—disorganization, complexity and faculty dissension.

Finally, *Ola Alausa*, a Professor of Community Medicine involved in the establishment of a new medical school in Kano, Nigeria, shares in some detail the considerations that provoked the decision to construct a curriculum with its roots in the surrounding community. Of particular interest are the criteria he presents for the selection of work sites for students.

## References

1. Tarlov A. The Shattuck lecture: the increasing supply of physicians, the changing structure of the health-services system and the future practice of medicine. *N Engl J Med* 1983;308:1235–1244.
2. Manard BB, Lewen LS. *Physician Supply and Distribution: Issues and Options for State Policy Makers*. Washington, DC. National Center for Health Services Research, 1983.
3. Becker H, et al. *Boys in White*. Chicago, University of Chicago Press, 1966.
4. De Vries MW, Berg RL, Lipkin M, Jr. *The Use and Abuse of Medicine*. New York, Praeger, 1982.
5. Pfifferling JM. The Impaired Physician: An Overview. Chapel Hill, NC, Health Sciences Consortium, 1980.
6. Lipkin M, Jr. Classification of psychosocial factors affecting health. In Lipkin M, Jr, Kupka K. (eds): *Psychosocial Factors Affecting Health*. New York, Praeger, 1982, pp. xi–xvii.
7. Schroeder SA, Showstack JA, Gerbert B. Residency training in internal medicine: time for a change. *Ann Intern Med* (1986;104:554–561.
8. White KL, Henderson MH. *Epidemiology as a Fundamental Science*. New York, Oxford University Press, 1976.
9. Banta HD. *Resources for Health: Technology Assessment for Policy Making*. New York, Praeger, 1982.
10. Lipkin M Jr, Lybrand WA. *Population Based Medicine*. New York, Praeger, 1982.

# 4
# Important Issues in Community-oriented Medical Education

DAN E. BENOR, STEVAN E. HOBFOLL, and MOSHE PRYWES

The growing interest in community-oriented medicine has aroused a multitude of definitions of this term, sometimes embracing quite different or even conflicting notions. The same could be said about community-oriented medical education. Such an education must be comprehensive, fully combining the teaching of medicine with principles of community structure and behavior. Such education must do more than simply include some components that relate to the community. Operation of out patient clinics, primary care clerkships, and courses in behavioral sciences and epidemiology are all important, yet they are not sufficient to define the program as community-oriented education.

*Community-oriented medicine is first and foremost medicine.* No knowledge of sciences related to community organization and problems can substitute for a thorough, comprehensive knowledge of clinical medicine. Consequently, community-oriented medical education must be based on a curriculum that prepares students to become adequate and up-to-date physicians with the ability to treat the ill, ease suffering, and promote health. Scientific medicine is the basis of community-oriented medical practice and education, as it is the basis for medicine in general (see Chap. 3).

There is a conceptual debate between two major perceptions of community medicine. One views community medicine as a field dealing exclusively with public health issues that are of concern to groups of people but not to individuals, sometimes called "collective care." The other looks on public health problems as but some components, although important, of a more comprehensive approach that includes individual patient care.[1,2] In line with such thinking, Prywes presented a model of integrated community medicine that embraces the care for individuals, their families and the community. He wrote[3]:

This approach aims at finding meeting points between community medicine (collective care) and clinical medicine, in order to bring both closer together in those areas of practice in which a mutual interest is shared[2] . . . relating to the quality of life as well as its prolongation. [3]

In the following pages we are presenting a concept, not describing medical or educational reality. Community-oriented education means more than restructuring the curriculum. No existing school of medicine can be content with what has been achieved so far. As is so often the case, achievement means struggle; in this case it is a struggle for concomitant social change, redirection of resources, and remodeling of the health care delivery system, as well as struggle for a new educational approach.

## Health Orientation

The most fundamental feature of community-oriented medical education is its being health-directed rather than disease-directed. the care for the "quality of life as well as its prolongation" cited earlier[3] means exactly that. Illustrating this point, Antonovsky[4] wrote:

... to ask about health-ease, that is to seek to explain what facilitates our movement toward the most salutary end of the breakdown continuum; is to search for weapons that may be more potent in decreasing human suffering than is any specific disease-preventing or disease-curing factor.

A somewhat similar idea was expressed by Ordonez[5]:

A new conceptual framework has to be developed that considers health and illness on a continuum coordinated by the interaction between the individual as a social being and the environment in which he lives.

Health thus envisioned is in itself an entity; which means something that may or may not exist independently of the fact that disease is absent. It is positively defined by its characteristics rather than negatively defined by the absence of disease. A full discussion of meaning of health is beyond the scope of this chapter. One may wish to adopt the World Health Organization (WHO) definition that health is a state of complete physical, mental, and social well-being. Others may prefer different descriptions. However, health-directed principles must be a central component of community-oriented education. This concept of health can then be extended from individuals to groups and to the entire community.

The concept of health suggests an existence of "community health"[6,7] (see Chap. 3). This concept comprises the sum of health status of the community members as well as the resources which enable the community to cope with disease situations of some of its members. Effective coping, rather than absolute health, may differentiate between healthy and unhealthy communities. This idea implies that community medicine deals directly with allocation of resources, both physical and emotional-cultural; their proper utilization and reorganization of health care systems; evaluation and reevaluation of health needs; and last but not least, relating to, influencing, and remodeling attitudes toward health.

One may easily identify the areas of knowledge required for competence in the above-mentioned areas. The main difficulty, however, is to motivate the physician to feel responsible for much wider and very different areas of concern than those that have been traditionally accepted by the profession. This point was stressed in almost every presentation at the Second Meeting of the Network of Community Oriented Educational Institutions for Health Sciences in Bellagio in 1980.[3,5-9]

The individual physician is not expected to handle the enormous responsibility of health alone. Moreover, community involvement is required if the community is to maintain or improve its health. Three issues stem from this concept. First is the health team notion.[7,8] Second is the need to acquire knowledge in the fields of sociology, social anthropology, psychology, medical economics and management, and epidemiology. Third is the need for the skill of identifying and triggering community resources, including formal and informal institutions, and the ability to work with them on the basis of mutual respect, consideration, and understanding. Judgment-free and cultural-free attitudes on the part of the physician are required, even if these goals are more difficult to achieve than acquiring the necessary scientific knowledge.

## Community Basis

Community-oriented medicine and education must certainly be community-based. Community basis includes both physical and conceptual components, as exemplified in the curricula of some community-oriented medical education programs in various places in the world.[2,6,7-11] The physical one is quite obvious: The cornerstone of community-oriented medical education is the network of facilities providing health care that are located in the neighborhoods, villages, and work places, which are the individual's "life space." The teaching–learning locations may include clinics as well as, for example, homes for the aged, rehabilitation institutions, adult education organizations, and others. Hospitals too should be clearly defined and perceived as one of the major community health institutions, fully interwoven into the health network.

Equally important and more difficult to teach is the conceptual basis of "community," which is characterized by active outreach behavior of the medical professionals. It is the initiative of the health worker to break away from the four walls of the health institution, not waiting for the patient to come for help, but rather to look out for the ones in need, at risk, the underprivileged, as well as for the sick, disturbed, or recovering individuals who need reintegration into their families, work places, and community life.

Without sacrificing the need to provide quality care for individuals, the [medical] school would need to place greatly increased emphasis on the care of total populations: those who sought assistance and those who did not; those who labelled themselves as sick and those who declined to do so, the hypochondriacs and those who lived in reckless disregard of their own health, the affluent and the disadvantaged, the indigent and the immigrants.[6]

The community-oriented physician both provokes and catalyzes social processes concerned with health. These objectives obviously require relevant knowledge from the appropriate fields in the behavioral and social sciences.

However, the community-oriented physician is by no means a social worker, nor is he or she a behavioral scientist. These sciences are *tools* for the specific health care tasks as they are related to medicine—no more (but not less either) than pathology or pharmacology. Learning community structure is the "community's anatomy"; family dynamics are the "community's cellular biology"; "community physiology" is provided by sociology and social anthropology; and "community pathology" is learned through both epidemiology and sociology. Moreover, the student must acquire "community clinical skills" of intervention, utilizing the "community pharmacology" provided by organizational dynamics, public health organizations, epidemiology, and psychology.

The community basis, both conceptual and physical, requires a team approach. One may perceive the team as purely medical, including the physician, nurses, and allied medical professionals. The team may, however, be a health team and thus include, in addition to the medical staff, welfare workers, clinical and educational psychologists, school counselors, and community officials. Various professionals, including hospital consultants, would join or leave the team as required. The physician's position on the team may be that of a leader, a member, a consultant, or even a consumer, depending on the problem at hand, not on the assumed supremacy as a physician.

## Natural History of Disease

The "natural history of disease" model, although not a new concept, serves well in the operational definition of the scope of community medicine and as a focus for organization of the curriculum.[11] The model suggests premorbid and morbid phases and further divides the morbid phase into maintenance, breakdown, and rehabilitation phases. These sequences suggest preventive, curative, and rehabilitative phases of care.

The prevention concept is central to the model and is congruent with the health orientation. It may be noted that the model does not apply necessarily to primary care alone. It also includes a community-oriented cardiologist interested in preventing coronary heart diseases, a surgeon/oncologist who is concerned with early detection of breast cancer, or a pulmonologist who is carrying out an antismoking campaign. However, the areas of preventing work and road accidents, encouraging proper nutrition, and improving the social competence of an individual are less emphasized or even ignored by traditional education and practice. Effective prevention requires broad knowledge of the pathophysiological and immunological processes, knowledge of individual and group psychology and anthropology, the art of redirecting attitudes, and an awareness of available resources. It requires, above all, liberation of the physician's self-perception as a curer of diseases only. Detecting excessive stressors that risk the individual's breaking down and an attempt to decrease them is the "vaccination" of modern ailments, not yet perceived as "immunology" or "immunization" by the medical tradition.

The key word in prevention and therefore a key concept in community medicine is *early*. This idea designates not only timing but also monitoring, observing, and following up. Such continuity of care is carried over to the acute care phase and rehabilitation in the natural history of the disease model. The community-oriented physician, whether primary care doctor or specialist, perceives the hospitalization phase as a short though crucial segment of the continuum of the natural history. While caring for the sick the physician must bear in mind whatever preceded and what will follow the disease – physically, emotionally, and socially.

The rehabilitation phase is often the most neglected stage of patient care in today's medicine. However, when consistent with the health orientation, the rehabilitation phase is a wider concept and not simply postacute management. It includes geriatric treatment of healthy elderly individuals, combating their loneliness and the public ignorance of their problems as well as their diabetes or hypertension. It also may include group care of social ailments such as drug abuse, alcoholism, and family violence.

The emphasis on the natural history of disease assigns a special role to the primary care practitioner in community-oriented medicine.[1,2] Indeed, primary care and community orientation are by no means identical terms.[2,6,7-11] However, although specialty medicine can and should be community oriented, only the primary care physician is capable of moving across disciplines and of providing the required continuity of care.

## Life Cycle

In the previous sections we discussed the developmental processes of health and disease as they relate to community-oriented practice and education. In order to be both health and community oriented, a knowledge of developmental processes of an individual is also needed. This concept encompasses physical, emotional, mental, and social dimensions of the life cycle.

The life cycle is basically a biological process of aging. On this continuum one can point out the periods of infancy, childhood, adolescence, young adulthood, middle age, old age, and death. On this biological continuum concomitant life events of biosocial nature are taking place. These may be, for example, schooling, army service, identity crisis, courtship and marriage, child birth and weaning, menopause, retirement, and mourning. Pediatrics have long ago established the point that a child is not a small adult, and the discipline is not just internal medicine for little human beings. We wish to take this point further: The management of a female patient must be illustrated to the student to be different when the patient is a middle-aged mother of young children than it is when she is a mature single woman of the same age or a middle-aged mother of grown-up children who have left home. These female patients have a different role and a different status in the community, reflected in the amount and kind of social support they harvest both formally and informally. Social context is a culturally dependent variable.

Aging on one hand and sexual behavior on the other are striking examples, yet by far not exclusive. It is the interplay of health–age–society rather than each aspect alone that turns out to be the factor of central importance when making medical decisions, including the decision not to intervene. A community-oriented physician should be aware of this interaction to the same extent any physician is aware of the patient's age. The student must understand that crisis situations may and should at times be "treated" by allowing the developmental process itself to proceed normally, even if sometimes painfully, as in the case of normal mourning. Some other crises could best be "treated" by affecting changes in the environment rather than focusing on the patient.[5] Still other situations may be dealt with by providing emotional support or by education. In some of these situations the intervening agent is the family; in others it is the community through its official institutions.

Consistent with the life cycle model is the evolution of the development of the community itself. Here, in contract to the individual's development, the changes are not biologically linked; yet they still are on a continuum. It is especially true in developing countries, although the ever-growing population mobility in industrial countries makes this dynamism relevant to them as well.[5,7,8]

The developmental dimension again strongly implies health team work and again hints at the changing status of the physician in the team as directed by the problem at hand. Furthermore, the necessary community basis is implied, as is the possible community orientation of the hospital-based consultant.

## Characteristics of Community-oriented Education

There is no one right or wrong educational approach to community-oriented education. Different settings may require different solutions; distinct prevalence of health problems dictates specific priorities; political and financial constraints may alter the strategies; and the availability of sufficiently strong physician role models has a direct bearing on the curriculum. This variability of approaches was recognized by all the speakers at the Bellagio meeting. Moreover, sometimes the curriculum must protect the community orientation of the institution against falling back to traditional practices and emphases. In some other instances the community orientation is rooted deeply enough to allow the curriculum more flexibility in order to achieve additional goals.

Two major general points should be stressed from the outset. The first is the level of institutional commitment to the concept. There is a fundamental difference in the educational approach between a medical school that is primarily committed to community-oriented education and the one in which community-directed learning is but one of several alternative tracks. Such a difference may affect all facets of the program, from the student selection policy to evaluation procedures. From this difference stems the need for clearly stated institutional objectives, which describe the desired behavior of their graduates and define the institutional level of commitment to community-oriented education.[7,11]

The second point, which is of utmost importance, is the level of institutional involvement in the actual delivery of health care to a given community. The service institution necessarily has a different curriculum from one that primarily has teaching responsibilities. The differences may be reflected in many aspects of the education. Yet it may be noted that both the service and the nonservice institutions may have equal commitment to community-oriented education, as illustrated by their institutional objectives.

The educational implications of community orientation are many-fold and far-reaching. Of primary importance is the acquisition, acceptance, and internalization of the proper attitudes toward health and thus a shift in the learner's attention away from disease. This objective is relatively easy to achieve if the general atmosphere in the institution is so directed and the role models act in this manner. Unfortunately, this situation is not the case in most medical schools. Education may compensate for this disadvantage by adopting several principles, as follows.

First is the *early and repeated* exposure to the various aspects of community medicine. Second, there must be concomitant provision of both *an intellectual and a humane challenge* within community medicine. Third, is the emphasis on acquiring the *necessary tools* for proper community practice, which includes both the knowledge base and the opportunities to *apply* this knowledge to real life situations.

Let us consider these points more carefully. The novice student is generally humanistically oriented and perceives himself or herself as "curer."[12,13] The student is also eager to learn, and to absorb information in order to create a meaningful conceptual world. This procedure is part of professional socialization and is accelerated during the first, formative years in the school of medicine. To this state of affairs conventional education contributes two major components. One is praising the objective, scientific truth, reflected by the basic sciences, which are presented and perceived as an end in themselves. The other is the glamor of the hospital care with its scientific aspirations and sophisticated equipment. These two aspects carry the same message: "Real medicine" is in the hospital and the research laboratories—and there alone.

Community-oriented education should try therefore to influence the students' *conceptual formations* in the stage in which they are created. The sciences should be perceived as an important basis of knowledge applied to clinical medicine. Likewise, the hospital must be looked on as a community establishment, integrated into the health care network. The hospitalization periods, which are usually short, may be emphasized vis-à-vis the natural history of disease. Needless to say, the student must perceive that the health needs originate in the homes, work places, and neighborhoods, not in the hospital wards and laboratories. This concept by no means denigrates the importance of the hospital; it simply exposes the student to the hospital in an appropriate context and in proper proportion.

Community-oriented medicine is an especially appropriate framework for meeting the *humanistic challenge* of young students. Teaching and learning interpersonal relationships can be of greater depth and breadth than in a hospital-based setting because such settings lack the environmental dimension and because they are disease oriented rather than person oriented. This idea applies equally to the development of empathetic attitudes and communication skills. Only in community-based medicine can the student fully appreciate the concept and consequences of patient compliance; only there may the student meet the familial aspects of health and disease; only there do the skills needed for health education and for changing one's attitudes toward health hazards have a meaning. Furthermore, in community medicine activities the learner is immediately and directly rewarded by the patient, who thus reinforces empathetic behavior. The humanistic drives of young students may be developed into emotional involvement by bringing the student into homes, the delicate familial matrix, workplaces, schools, homes for the aged, and community clubs. However, this involvement develops if, and only if, the student perceives those activities as medically relevant and needed, if he is provided the knowledge from the appropriate behavioral sciences that allows him to feel professionally competent, and if he feels intellectually challenged in these activities.

The place of social and behavioral sciences in the community oriented curriculum deserves special consideration. First, it is the medically related parts of these disciplines rather than a thorough and systematic coverage that are needed. An overemphasis of these disciplines creates almost instantly a "boomerang effect," in contrast to the case when only the relevant and helpful portions required for solving medical problems are learned. These needed portions are presented in Figure 4.1, which points out their relevance at each level of the community. It should be noted that although the importance of the various disciplines rotate according to the level of the problem, the need for a knowledge of clinical medicine remains relatively stable, making the physician a key player across problems and levels of community.

The general educational principle of *relevance* applies also to knowledge in other fields than behavioral sciences. However, it raises the question of who shall decide what is relevant for community medicine and on which criteria this decision is based. There are several ways to address this question, but the ultimate test of relevance is the applicability of the learned material to clinical reality.[2,8,9]

*Integration across disciplines* of learned subject matter is a major educational concept. It is typical of, though not unique to, community-oriented education. The concept suggests simultaneous learning of the segments of all the areas of knowledge that bear on the problem at hand.[11,14,15] Integration further suggests that considering problem-related rather than discipline-related material may promote learning; it provides the feeling of relevance and thus raises motivation; it calls on synthesis of information central to effective problem-solving; and it emphasizes the applicative nature of the learned information. Interdisciplinary integration has a special importance in community medicine because of the multiplicity of the disciplines involved, because the basic working unit, the health team, is interdisciplinary by definition, and because the patient-problems presented in community medicine encompass so many facets of life. The integrative approach suggests a repeated exposure to patient and community problems

| Physical/Conceptual Level of Community | Health Care Responsibilities | Disciplines of Knowledge* |
|---|---|---|
| Individual | Health screening | Med., Epidemiol. |
| | Patient management | Med., Psychol. |
| | Health education and reorientation | Sociol., Anthropol., Psychol, Med. |
| Family | Family planning | Med., Anthropol., Sociol., Psychol. |
| | Genetic screening and counseling | Med., Anthropol, Sociol., Psychol, Epidemiol. |
| | Health counseling | Med., Anthropol., Sociol., Psychol. |
| | Educational counseling | Psychol., Sociol., Anthropol. |
| | Sexology | Psychol., Med., Anthropol., Sociol. |
| | Child growth and development | Med., Psychol., Sociol. |
| Neighborhood/workplace | Primary prevention | Med., Epidemiol., PH, Anthropol., Sociol. |
| | Delivery of health management | Med., Anthropol., Sociol. |
| | Health education | Sociol., Anthropol., Psychol., Med., O.D., Epidemiol. |
| City/town† country (rural) | Design health services | Med., PH, Econom., Epidemiol., O.D., Anthropol., Sociol. |
| | Health screening | Med., Epidemiol., PH, Anthropol, Sociol. |
| | Public health management | Epidemiol., Sociol., Med., PH, O.D., Sociol., Econom. |
| | Primary prevention | Epidemiol., PH, Anthropol., Sociol., O.D., Med. |
| | Secondary prevention | Med., Epidemiol., PH, Anthropol., Sociol, O.D. |
| Region | Public policy (pertaining to health) | PH, O.D., Econom., Epidemiol., Med. |
| | Design health services | Med., PH, Econom., Epidemiol., O.D., Anthropol., Sociol. |
| | Health screening | Med., Epidemiol., PH, Anthropol., Sociol. |
| | Health education | Sociol., Anthropol., O.D., Epidemiol. Psychol., Med. |

*Anthropol. = social anthropology; Econom. = medical economics; Epidemiol. = epidemiology; Med. = clinical medicine; O.D. = organizational and group dynamics; PH = public health organization; Psychol. = psychology; Sociol. = sociology.

† Including formal and informal institutions.

FIGURE 4.1.

and to general medical themes on an ever rising level of sophistication, in conjunction with the growing ability and will to take actual clinical responsibilities, as exemplified, among others, by the Cuban experience.[5] What emerges is a *spiral model*, in which all disciplines are simultaneously presented from the beginning to the end of the curriculum. Each turn of the spiral exposes the student to a higher level of both knowledge and responsibility, and brings him closer to professional performance.[11]

*Problem-solving* is another concept in medicine in general and is not specific to community medicine. Yet the problems presented to and perceived by the students as clinically relevant are very different in a community-oriented educational framework. To avoid stressing the obvious, we just mention that health rather than disease and a person within a family and an environment rather than the individual alone need to be considered. The earlier the students embark on solving health problems utilizing multifaceted knowledge and skills, the stronger is the acquisition of problem-solving capability. Moreover, real life problems have a greater attitudinal impact than simulated ones and may thus be incorporated into the curriculum. Finally, evaluation of problem-solving capability is essential. One may consider measuring specifically the cognitive abilities involved, e.g., synthesis, analysis, hypothesis generation and evaluation, and others.

Likewise, *self-learning* is a generally accepted educational procedure that is both a method and an end in itself. Facing the "information explosion" and the rapid developments in medicine, the acquisition of self-learning skills and habits is a crucial factor for maintaining competence. In the community-oriented educational institution, self-learning becomes even more essential because it is likely that the community physician—whether family practitioner, primary care taker, generalist, or public health worker—will be working at times alone. Even if he does not, the amount of peer review and supervision is likely to be less than in a hospital setting. In addition, the rapidly developing new medicosocial disciplines offer a specific learning challenge to a community physician. However, there is no one proper way to acquire self-learning capability. Community-oriented education may take into consideration personal learning styles, variability of pacing, and individual preferences when planning its curriculum and thus endorse a variety of alternative learning opportunities.

## Selection of Students

We have already mentioned that the entering students perceive themselves as "curers." Nevertheless, this idea does not exclude possible differences in students' interests in and their inclinations toward the community. Without downgrading the effect of education, we may acknowledge the existence of "preeducational" community-oriented individuals. It is thus suggested that these individuals may be identified by the selection procedure in order to enhance the educational effect.

Furthermore, there are certain personal characteristics that, although indelibly fixed in the applicant's personality, would be very difficult to change. Of these personal traits, some are desirable and may be selected for, whereas others are undesirable and may be selected against. Empathy, sense of responsibility, and intellectual flexibility are among the desirable traits. One may look on community mindedness, social tolerance, and the capability to work in groups as equally important.[16] For these reasons a number of community-oriented programs, e.g., McMaster and Beer-Sheva, have questioned the traditionally accepted selection criteria of scholastic achievements and cognitive abilities that have been shown in many studies to be of no predictive value to later clinical performance.[17–19] Moreover, selection based on traditional scholastic achievements may thus negatively select those individuals who are most desired in a community-oriented medical school.[20,21]

Various empathy and social mindedness scales have been suggested for selection.[16,22] However, personal interviews are still the most common procedure. Personal histories of applicants reflecting involvement with, interest in, and acceptance of responsibilities toward community may be considered as additional admission criteria. Success in clinical studies in a community-oriented medical school may indeed be related to such "prior" behavior and values.

## Summary of the Features of Community-oriented Curriculum

The following list summarizes the characteristics of community-oriented educational approaches and curricula. It should again be stressed that this proposed is by no means a prescription; it is not of an "all or none" nature, and it does not yet exist fully in any of the few community-oriented schools.

1. Exposure of students to a community health networks and workers should start early; actually on commencement of the medical studies. This exposure should be of a repeated nature, continuing along the entire course of studies while students' responsibilities for patient care are gradually developing.

2. The community settings for teaching may include primary care clinics, home visits, schools, workplaces, clubs, homes for the aged, and other settings not generally entitled "medical." However, activities in these settings should be in conjunction with a particular medical problem and for the purpose of solving this problem.

3. The curriculum must stress the concept of the natural history of disease, incorporating preventive, curative, and rehabilitative aspects. The students ought to apply their acquired knowledge in these fields to actual service circumstances.

4. The curriculum should stress the concept of life cycle, including growth and development, psychological and cultural aspects of behavior, aging, death, and dying. Life cycle parameters should be constantly included in clinical discussions.

5. The curriculum should include learning of both knowledge and experience regarding structure, organization, and management of health care systems. This learning may be done in the appropriate sequence, timing and doses as needed for solving actual or simulated health problems. The perception of health care delivery in the eyes of patients may be both experienced and discussed.

6. The curriculum should include epidemiology in both classroom activities and field projects. The projects may be either student initiated or planned or

both. However, epidemiological parameters need to be included in all the clinical considerations.

7. The curriculum has to include a knowledge base in the fields of psychology, sociology, and social anthropology. These areas may be introduced in the appropriate timing and doses as required for solving individual or communal health problems.

8. Basic bio-medical, behavioral, and social sciences may be learned in segments, consistent with the students' level of knowledge and responsibility. These segments may further be interwoven in relation to either an actual patient problem or a more general health problem. Thus a meaningful matrix is created integrating across disciplines both horizontally and vertically.

9. The disciplinary knowledge segment should be repeated over and over again along the course of studies on ever growing levels of sophistication and applicability. A proper "coverage" of the subject matter may be eventually achieved by carefully planing the students' learning experiences.

10. Problem-solving activities should be planned on the basis of either real-life or simulated situations. In these, attention may be paid to the ability to synthesize concepts and knowledge over disciplines and cases.

11. The learning need be active. This implies a definition of students' clinical responsibilities in each phase. It also includes learning of clinical decision-making and its critical evaluation. The expected level of patient responsibility should be made explicit and known to both students and teachers.

12. Self-learning should be encouraged all along the course of studies. It may include directed learning of literature reviews, critical reading, and critical decision-making processes.

13. Student activity may be carried over to research. The research may be interdisciplinary by requirement and may call for involvement of various community agents as well as scientists. Epidemiological research may be used for this purpose.

14. Thorough training in human interpersonal relationships must be introduced early and reinforced along the studies continuously. Communication skills on the level of the health team should be included in the learning of interpersonal skills. Likewise, ways of communication with formal and informal community institutions is another aspect of communication that also includes understanding of organizational dynamics.

15. Health team workers, both medical professional and others, should serve as recognized teachers and instructors, including both classroom and field work. Appropriate appointment and promotion policy may enhance such recognition.

16. The various components of a community-oriented curriculum should be included in all the appropriate student-evaluation procedures, whether intermediate or final, formative or summative.

17. Students may be selected based on their personal characteristics that indicate interest in, involvement with, and care for the community as reflected in their personal history, as well as their empathy, tolerance, and sense of responsibility.

18. Faculty, including allied professionals need be recruited for their inclinations toward both community medicine and the described educational approach.

19. Finally, yet most important, is this concept: The community-oriented medical school defines its institutional objectives clearly, describing the expected behavior of a competent graduate. These objectives should be made known to both students and faculty from their first step into the institution. These objectives should be perceived by students and faculty as directive guidelines rather than intentions.

This list is quite extensive, yet it does not exhaust the possibilities. One may wish to add some points and to challenge others. It may be noted that taking actual medical care responsibilities for a defined community was not included among the educational principles. Nevertheless, it affects dramatically both the educational setup and the general atmosphere in the institution. Finally, the organizational structure of the institution has not been discussed, yet existence of strong departments, and thus departmental interests, may hinder many good intentions and courageous educational policies.

## Three-dimensional Model

We summarize the discussion on community-oriented medicine and education by suggesting a three-dimensional model that demonstrates how community medicine is different from the traditional disease-oriented approach, and what the outcome of a community-oriented educational process should be able to do (Fig. 4.2).

The large cube represents any disease entity. The first dimension of this model is that of the natural history of the disease continuum. The second is the life cycle. The third dimension includes the resources for coping, progressing from individual strengths to familial support to community aid, both formal (institutionalized) and informal. It is argued that any disease entity pronounces itself differently, progresses differently, and leads to different outcomes in each of the small cubicles in the model. As a consequence, the management of any particular disease should take into consideration a proper combination of all three dimensions.

It is further argued that medical tradition pays most of its attention to the disease entity, represented in the model by the entire large cube, and persistently ignores the differences stemming from the interaction between environment, age, life events, and personal and public resources on the one hand and the stage of the disease on the other. Such interaction is presented in our model by the small cubicles. Like the frustrating "Hungarian cube" puzzle, the physician and the community-oriented student must spin the individual elements to achieve a comprehensive composite.

Let us assume, for illustrative purposes, that the large cube represents diabetes mellitus. Is it not the case that an entirely different approach should be taken with

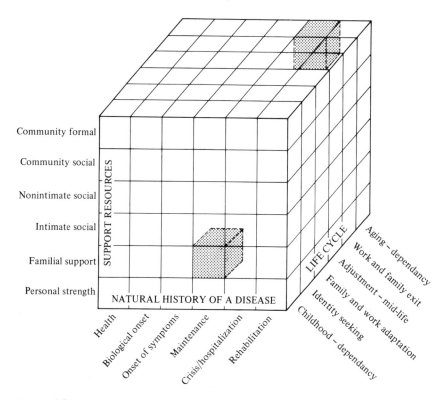

FIGURE 4.2.

an elderly, lonely person who has a full-blown clinical picture than with a second elderly patient who has the same symptomatology but who enjoys the care and the support of a loving family? Still another example might be taken with a lonely, elderly person who lives in a community that provides home care and/or physical shelter versus one in another environment where no welfare facilities are available. Would the physician prescribe the same regimen of diet, insulin injections, and physical restraints in all these somewhat similar cases? The examples given above may be quite simplistic and well perceived by any internist. But will this be as simple in the case of a leukemic child, a young alcoholic, or a nephritic pregnant woman? We suggest that even selecting the drug of choice, not to mention a nonmedical treatment, may be different in each of the multiple possible combinations shown by the model.

Community-oriented medicine, and consequently community-oriented education, is that kind of practice which simultaneously takes into consideration all three dimensions of the health problem. Moreover, a competent community health professional is one who takes measures to influence, adjust, and modify whatever is adjustable on all three parameters for preserving and improving health.

# References

1. Prywes M: Merging medical education and medical care. *Hosp Med Staff* 1973;2.
2. Prywes M: Community medicine – the "first-born" of a marriage between medical education and medical care. *Health Policy Educ* 1980;1:291–300.
3. Prywes M: Medical care and medical education, in: *Bellagio Conference Proceedings*, 1980.
4. Antonovsky A: *Health, Stress and Coping*. San Francisco, Jossey-Bass, 1979.
5. Ordonez C: Toward better coordination between health services and education, in: *Ballagio Conference Proceedings*, 1980.
6. Maddison D: A medical school for the future: the Newcastle experiment. *World Health Forum* 1980;1:133–138.
7. Hamad B: Medical education at the Faculty of Medicine, University of Gezira, Sudan: a new approach, in: *Bellagio Conference Proceedings*, 1980.
8. Mercado A: Some experiences on community-oriented teaching – learning process, in: *Bellagio Conference Proceedings*, 1980.
9. Greep JM: Curriculum design in a new medical school, in: *Bellagio Conference Proceedings*, 1980.
10. Villarreal R: Universidad Autonoma Metropolitana, Xochimilco, Mexico: an interdisciplinary innovation in medical education, in: Katz FM, Fulöp T. (eds): *Personnel for Health Care: Case Studies of Educational Programmes*. Public Health Paper 71, Vol. 2. Geneva, WHO, 1980.
11. Segall A, Prywes M, Benor DE, Susskind O: University Center for Health Sciences, Ben Gurion University of the Negev, Beer Sheva, Israel: an interim perspective, in: Katz FM, Fulöp T. (eds): *Personnel for Health Care: Case studies of Educational Programmes*. Public Health Paper 70. Geneva, WHO, 1978.
12. Becker HS, Geer B, Hughes EC, Strauss AL: *Boys in White: Student Culture in Medical School*. Chicago, Chicago University Press, 1961.
13. Shuval JT: Socialization of health professionals in Israel: early sources of congruence and differentiation. *J Med Educ* 1975;50:443–457.
14. Bouhuijs PAJ, Schmidt HG, Snow RE, Wijnen WHFW: The Rijksuniversiteit Limburg, Maastricht, Netherlands: development of medical education, in: Katz FM, Fulöp T (eds): *Personnel for Health Care: Case Studies of Educational Programmes*. Public Health Paper 70. Geneva, WHO, 1978.
15. Neufeld VR, Barrows HS: The "McMaster Philosophy": an approach to medical education. *J Med Educ*, 1974;49:1040–1050.
16. Hobfoll SE, Anson O, Antonovsky A: Personality factors as predictors of medical student performance. *Med Educ*, 1982;16:251–258.
17. Wingard JR, Williamson JW: Grades as predictors of physicians' career performance: an evaluative literature review. *J Med Educ*, 1973;48:311–321.
18. Murden R, Galloway GM, Reid JC, Colwill JM: Academic and personal predictors of clinical success in medical school. *J Med Educ*, 1978;53:711–719.
19. Hobfoll SE, Benor DE: Prediction of students' clinical performance. *Med Educ*, 1981;15:231–236.
20. Gough HG: Nonintellectual factors in the selection and evaluation of medical students. *J Med Educ* 1967;42:642–650.
21. Benor DE, Hobfoll SE: Prediction of clinical performance: the role of prior experience. *J Med Educ*, 1981;56:653–658.
22. Werner DW, Kagan N, Schneider J: The measurement of affective sensitivity: the development of an instrument. *Ann Conf Res Med Educ*, 1977;16:187–193.

# 5
# Implementation of a Community-oriented Curriculum: The Task and the Problems

ZOHAIR M. NOOMAN

## The Task

For decades, in my country and most other countries, the task of implementing a medical curriculum used to be an easy job that had only a few problems worth mentioning. That is why, a few days after I had settled in my new job as a Founding Dean of the Faculty of Medicine at Suez Canal University, in October 1977, the Secretary General of the University asked me to be ready with the bylaws of the "new" school, which included the curriculum, for the following University Council meeting to be held a few weeks later. His request was completely justified. A few days were more than enough to photocopy the curriculum of any of the 10 existing medical schools, for all were the same and followed the conventional curriculum of the 150-year-old prestigious Kasr El-Aini Medical School of Cairo University, last revised 50 years earlier. But this was not my mandate, and it was almost 4 years later that the Secretary General had the curriculum in his hands. The mandate was to introduce and implement great changes in medical education, which mounted to a complete reorientation to bridge the wide gap between the education of medical graduates at that time and their successful functioning as health care providers who would meet the health needs of the people and serve them efficiently, effectively, and humanely.

The need for this change was acutely felt in Egypt as a compelling national need,[1] a feeling that was certainly augmented by the powerful global movement towards Health for all[2] and the necessity to reorient national health care delivery systems towards primary care to serve that goal. The role of health professions educational institutions in this process has been defined by the almost simultaneously emerging concept of integrated Health Services and Health Manpower Development (HSMD), which indicated that the quality and quantity of health manpower has to be planned in response to the specific needs of the national health system and, through this, to the health needs and demands of the population.[3]

Challenged by the demands of their newly defined role, health educational institutions, including medical schools, had to revise their curricula with the objective of educating graduates who are competent to serve effectively in the

Five institutional goals are recognized at present:

1. To qualify physicians whose primary objectives will be to provide health care in a combined hospital–community system with major emphasis on primary care.
2. To relate medical education to the needs of the society so that the physicians would be able to diagnose and manage the community health problems.
3. To develop and implement with the Ministry of Public Health and other health care delivery bodies an integrated system for comprehensive health care delivery and health manpower development in the Suez Canal Area and the Sinai. Such systems consider the limits of the national per-capita health expenditure at present and in the foreseeable future. The regional health service facilities will be used as the locus for education and training.
4. To develop and provide for health personnel programs of postgraduate training and continuing training.
5. To develop research programs that address primarily the actual health needs of the community.

FIGURE 5.1. Institutional goals of the Suez Canal University Faculty of Medicine.

proper time and proper place demanded by the system (Fig. 5.1). Quoting Füllöp[4]: "graduates of medical programs should certainly be able to: (1) respond to health needs and expressed demands of the community, and work with the community, so as to (2) stimulate healthy life-style and self-care, (3) educate the community as well as their co-workers, (4) solve, and stimulate the resolution of both individual and community health problems, (5) orient their own as well as community efforts to health promotion and to prevention of disease, unnecessary sufferings, disability and death work in, and with, health teams, and if necessary, (6) provide leadership to such teams, and (7) (8) continue learning life-long so as to keep competence up-to-date and even improve it as much as possible."

To create and implement the curriculum that would adequately educate such graduates has become the major task of health sciences education institutions. Far from being a simple task, it is a major undertaking that almost teems with challenging problems. It is our job to identify those problems, work at their solution, overcome them, and avoid giving way under their heavy pressures to the warm comfort of the "conventional."

## The Problems

Medical educational programs that train the above-described graduate are characterized by curricula that "focus on population groups and individual persons, which take into account the health needs of the community concerned."[5] Thus defined, this is *community-oriented education* (COE). The educational activities that constitute the curriculum in a community-oriented educational program, or institution, should obviously be based largely in the community and in close relationship to it in a diversity of health service settings the same as, or closely similar to, those in which the graduates will function as future health care providers. This is the definition of *community-based education (CBE)*,[6] which, in itself, is a tool to achieve the overall goal of community orientation of the whole institution, students, and faculty alike.

## Problem 1: How to Do It?

The answer to this question is that *there is no existing ready-made recipe for community-based education*. Most probably such a *universal* recipe will never exist, or should never exist. Let us explain this further.

• So far, community-based education is being adopted by only a few medical schools, including the members of the Network of Community-Oriented Educational Institutions for Health Sciences. The institutions are all rather young. Although those pioneers have many features in common and do try to share their experiences and learn from each other, there is an obvious and pressing need for comparative studies of the diverse solutions that have so far been developed for problems of planning and implementation, and a more extensive exchange in experience.

• Even when the design of community-based education programs and the mechanisms of integrating them purposefully with the objectives, policies, and structures of the educational system gain more definition and wider agreement, still, by its nature, the implementation of community-based education programs is so intricately tied to the local socioeconomic, geographic, and political environment to an extent that would make universal recipes unworkable and even harmful. The principle will always remain to *adapt* and not to *adopt*.

### BASIC PRINCIPLES AND INGREDIENTS OF A COMMUNITY-BASED EDUCATION PROGRAM[6]

It is true that there is no ready-made recipe, but the ingredients of community-based education, the underlying principles, are well known.

A community-based curriculum should:

1. Reflect—as a whole—the priority health problems and needs of the community.
2. Promote a community orientation from the outset of, and throughout, the curriculum.
3. Foster a holistic approach to health care that considers the needs of the whole person.
4. Foster a high level of health education to the public designed to promote health promotion and prevention of disease.
5. Foster students' problem-solving abilities as well as "learning how to learn," leading to educational self-reliance.
6. Ensure valid assessment of the competencies that students should acquire from community-based education.
7. Promote the health team approach.

Community-based learning activities should be:

1. Geared to planned goals and objectives that derive from explicitly stated expected professional competence.
2. Introduced very early, and must continue throughout the educational program.
3. Viewed not as peripheral or casual experiences but as a standard, integral, and continuing part of the educational process.
4. Involving students in real work and participation in service geared to their training needs.

A COMMUNITY-BASED ACTIVITY VERSUS A COMMUNITY-BASED CURRICULUM

It is important to differentiate between a community-based *activity* and a community-based *curriculum*. A community-based learning activity is an activity that takes place within a community. Field trips and training in the offices of family physicians for weekly half-days or full days for a certain period, or even field projects when performed in an isolated manner unrelated to an other-wise conventional curriculum, are all examples of community-based learning activities. These activities are useful, but they do not constitute a community-based curriculum. A curriculum can be called "community based" if, throughout its entire duration, it includes an appropriate proportion of learning activities in a balanced variety of educational settings in the community and in a diversity of health care services at all levels. The appropriate distribution of the community-based learning activities and their integration and incorporation within the overall educational program are essential characteristics of a community-based curriculum.

## Problem 2: The Challenges in Established Medical Schools

Conventional curricula are not based on the foregoing principles, which imply a new and different orientation of medical education, a genuine change toward relevance to the health needs of the people. The dimensions of reorientation and change are so great that to introduce them in a conventional curriculum, where various disciplines compete for curricular hours, would be a formidable task, a real battle where every professor is willing to fight until the end for the integrity of his or her disciplinary territory. No wonder, because conventional curricula are discipline, rather than community, oriented. The battle usually ends by the defeat of the innovators (however, see Martenson[7]). New schools may need to be established. A real breakthrough may be to create a community-based track that runs in parallel and coexists with the old conventional curriculum.*

---

*Examples of such "parallel innovative tracks" exist in several schools (eg the University of New Mexico Medical School and the problem-based track at Harvard Medical School (USA).

## Problem 3: The Right Leadership—The Right People

At present, the movement of community-oriented education is certainly growing and gathering strength all over the world. Still, however, in a given country or institution, it is a pioneering endeavor to try and materialize a community-based curriculum that is worth its name. All the problems of planning and implementation are surmountable if you have the right leadership and the right critical mass of people who are willing, and able to *do it*. In the absence of these factors, any single problem is enough to force you back to the "conventional." The issues here are commitment, creativity, an imaginative yet pragmatic approach, social awareness and sensitivity, political abilities, perseverance, courage, proficiency in medical education, credibility (both personal and professional), good role modeling, and last—but not least— managerial abilities. Ultimately, it will be the graduates of the community-based education programs who will best carry the implementation of such programs. From now until they grow to lead and man educational institutions, we have to manage through the rough roads of the pioneering phase.

## Problem 4: Collaboration with the Health Sector

Community-based education requires a functioning, stable coordination between the educational institution and the health services. This is crucial for many reasons.

- Priority health problems need to be heavily represented in the curriculum.
- Student's learning-training takes place largely in the various health settings of the community.
- There needs to be a continuum between what happens within the walls of the institution and outside in the community.

The two processes should not be segregated in the student's mind. Likewise, there should be no segregation in the organizational structure, and, most importantly, in the minds of the administrators and the personnel on either side of the fence. There should be no fence. Instead, there should be coordination and integration.[3] Experience, however, shows that the accomplishment of this task is often not only an organizational challenge but also a behavioral one that masks vested interests and professional rivalry. University teachers and health personnel alike need to descend from their respective ivory towers and work together in a coordinated effort to teach and serve. The exact manner in which such a coordination-integration is brought about is dependent on the local administrative, socioeconomic, political, and even cultural and behavioral practices and policies. It may require the establishment of joint committees, contractual relationship, joint appointments, and issuance of new laws or political decisions at the highest level.[5] In every case, however, successful coordination will be brought about if the right people are there, who conceive the rationale and the benefits of coordination and integration and commit themselves to its success.

Collaboration should start early in the planning phase of the educational program and must continue and grow throughout implementations, ie for good. Gradually, and ultimately, a new shape, a new way of life, is imparted to both the educational and service components of health care fostering the meaningfulness of the former and the quality of the latter. This is the essence of the Health Service Manpower Development Concept.

## Problem 5: The Use of the Community–Community Involvement

Community-based educational curricula need to, and do, *use* the community extensively for educating students. Communities do not like to be used. They need to — and should be — served. People will not readily accept the argument that they should be used now for the benefit they get tomorrow from the graduates of community-based education programs. To accept the students they expect to be served now by the students and their teachers. Also, they need to be *involved*, really and meaningfully, and not by lip service, in the planning and implementation of the community-based educational activities. The challenge to curriculum planners is to plan and implement the community-based students' activities in a way that brings about both service to the community and relevance to students' learning-training at the same time. This is possible, for example, by conducting the activities in underserved areas or carrying out a research project to solve a health problem that is deeply sensed by the community. The community may feel that they are overused by the program and also that the program's services are directed only to privileged strata. This would destroy the program which virtually forfeits its objectives.

## Problem 6: Issues in Curriculum Design

1. community orientation should be spelled out explicitly in the institutional goals. Those goals should govern, dictate, and guide the whole life of the institution, from curriculum planning to implementation; the selection of teaching staff, their activities, and criteria for reward and promotion; students' selection — where applicable; learning-activities, and the evaluation system. Figure 5.1 shows the institutional goals of the Faculty of Medicine at Suez Canal University. The goals are prominently displayed at the school's entrance in the hope that they would be imprinted in the hearts and minds of every faculty member, student, and administrator.

2. Community-based activities should not appear as isolated spots in the curriculum. They should permeate the whole curriculum and be planned and geared to provide the major stimulus and medium for good quality learning of the "required" basic, biomedical, community health, and behavioral sciences. The requirements are the competencies that need to be acquired by the graduate to fulfill his or her professional role and should be derived from a task analysis of the expected professional profile. In this sense, it is a competency-based curriculum. This approach has far-reaching implications.

3. Field work is no longer the sole prerogative of community medicine or public health departments. Faculty members from many disciplines should share to define the educational objectives and design the educational activities in their implementation and evaluation. This multidisciplinary effort should also involve the health personnel sharing in students' learning-training. This sharing is crucial to community-based educational curricula and foreign to conventional discipline-based ones. Many barriers, departmental and psychological, need to be broken to achieve successful implementation. This means a different and compatible organizational structure of the medical school itself.

4. Valid performance assessment of community-based student activities and its integration in the overall institutional assessment system are essential. This would be done by designing the valid evaluation instruments, carrying out the evaluation at the actual place of performance and involving the personnel who shared in student supervision and training, and maintaining reliability and consistency of evaluation when activities are being carried out in different places — some of them remote — with different people in different circumstances. These are all considerations that pose problems to be solved by administrators of community-based curricula whose duty is to maintain the institutional responsibility of graduating safe, efficient, and effective physicians who are also community oriented.

In the Faculty of Medicine at Suez Canal University, students, in every phase are not allowed to sit for the end-of-phase written examination unless their field work assessment has been satisfactory.

## Problem 7: How Should Students Learn? Community-based Education and Problem-based Learning

Among institutions that adopted community-based curricula, a few are adopting problem-based learning as an educational strategy as well. The prototype is the Faculty of Medicine at Suez Canal University, where learning throughout the six-year community-based curriculum is solely problem based. Problem-based learning (PBL) is the learning that results from the process of working towards the understanding or resolution of a problem. It is learning by discovery. It is not simply the presentation of problems to students as a focus for learning or an example for application of already "given" knowledge. It is a rigorous, structured approach to learning that is tailormade for medical education.[8] Our experience at Suez Canal University is a living demonstration of the mutual relevance of the beneficial interaction between the two strategies to the education of the student to acquire the right competencies required for the "Doctor of Tomorrow."

Thus, students' learning is triggered by and results from either written problems that they work up together in small groups (group learning) in the classroom, as well as from actual individual and community health problems they encounter in their work as a team during their community-based field activities. Both written and real problems would stimulate their enquiry and drive them to pursue knowledge and skills in the library, the laboratory, and from subject-matter experts both within and outside the school. Students follow the same steps of problem definition, analysis, hypothesis generation, formulation of learning objectives, collecting information, synthesis and testing "solutions" followed by self, peer, and tutor evaluation, whether handling a classroom or a field problem. They acquire problem solving as a way of thinking, an attitude, a way of life. At times classroom problems are derived from actual problems appearing in the students' reports on their field work. The sense of reality, continuing novelty, and stimulating variation in the learning experiences brought about by this approach cannot be missed. Besides, the competencies of problem solving, self-directed learning, critical thinking, critical appraisal of evidence, self-evaluation, working in a team, and learning from each other are deeply entrenched in the students' mind and behavior.

Problems to be presented to the students are selected and formulated according to certain criteria. These criteria deal with common individual or community health problems that are manageable, they could also be biomedical problems. Besides being stimulating, the expected educational objectives that would be derived by students should fall within the planned objectives and competencies of the educational phase.

## AN EXAMPLE OF A COMMUNITY-BASED, PROBLEM-BASED EDUCATIONAL EXPERIENCE

The problem: Schistosomiasis is the most prevalent endemic disease in Egypt. It is prevalent all over the Nile Valley, infection being acquired by contact with the snail–intermediate host-infested canals found throughout the valley. Schistosomiasis has never been reported in the indigenous Bedouin population of Sinai that has so far been deprived of Nile water. The need for development of the peninsula has prompted major irrigation schemes to be planned based on extending water canals eastward underneath the Suez Canal. Already, an area east of the Bitter Lakes is being cultivated on Nile water through a canal that has been dug several years ago. More extensive irrigation schemes are underway. The questions asked then were:

• How far did the expected, although so far never reported, transmission of schistosomiasis afflict the inhabitants?
• Have preventive measures been taken? If not: what measures could be taken to protect the people in this situation and to be recommended for the larger schemes to follow?
• Could infected persons if identified be treated?

This was the problem selected by a group of fourth-year medical students at the Faculty of Medicine at Suez Canal University as a subject of their 6-week elective study period. The students identified the problem, planned their study, defined and covered the areas of knowledge and skills to learn to be able to conduct the study, prepared a budget and itinerary, prepared the community for their study,

mapped the area and, together with Ministry of Health technicians, searched for
the snails in their expected habitat and diagnosed the infected ones. Next, the students examined urine and stool samples from all the available inhabitants, interviewed the infected ones and examined them under supervision of their tutors,
referred seriously sick people to the hospital. The students analyzed and interpreted their data, discussed them with each other, and filed a written report that
they discussed with their faculty and supervisors. The students reported that the
canals were infested with infected snails and that Bedouin inhabitants who have
never crossed to the Nile Valley were already infected and never treated. The students prepared a program of health education that they conducted while distribut-
ing the specific antischistosomal drug to the patients. The students studied and
discussed with the health authorities the recommended preventive measures to
prevent transmission of infected snails in the current and prospective irrigation
schemes.

## Problem 8: Where Should Students Learn?

Basically, community-based education can be conducted wherever people live
and work. In the Faculty of Medicine at Suez Canal University, around 25 sites
are being used for regular field training. These are mostly rural and urban health
centers but also include general hospitals, infectious disease hospitals, and health
insurance clinics. But community-based education activities also include projects
such as community surveys, community diagnosis, and action plans that would be
conducted in households, factories, a whole village or urban sector, or on
representative samples of the population.

The factors to consider in the definition and selection of the sites or setting of
community-based education activities are many and include:

• Relevance of the learning experiences to be gained in this site to the educational
  objectives of the particular phase of the curriculum.
• The feasibility of organizing the community-based education activity. The
  factors to be considered here include collaboration of the local health service
  personnel and of the community itself, available facilities, accessibility, logistics, cost of transportation, accommodation, etc.
• The need of the local community for service. The proportionate exposure to the
  various level of care—primary, secondary, and tertiary—is a function of the
  competencies that need to be acquired and would be certainly heavier on the
  primary care side but not excluding tertiary care. The "Natural History of
  Health Problems" approach (9) could be helpful in that respect. Students would
  be given supervised responsibility of groups of patients and families from a
  given community. Under close supervision of their teachers, students would
  proportionately base their learning activity first at the level of the whole
  assigned population, then at the level of those who come into contact with
  health care in an ambulatory service, then those who are admitted at least once
  to a hospital (10%) and finally those 1% who are admitted to a university

tertiary care hospital. In this way the types of health problems confronting a given community would determine the types of training settings.

## Problem 9: A New Role for Teachers

Teachers of community-based educational programs, particularly those adopting problem-based learning as well, have different tasks to perform, unaccustomed as they are by their colleagues working in conventional discipline-oriented, teacher-centered programs.

- *Teaching*: Instead of being a teacher actively teaching, it is the students who are actively learning. The teacher's role is to plan the educational activities, make the learning resources available to students, supervise and facilitate the learning process as a class or field tutor, and evaluate the students. Other educational activities include training of health personnel on educational methods and upgrading their professional skills. Teachers need to be trained for these new functions.
- *Service*: Instead of confining their practice in sophisticated tertiary care hospitals, with which they are mostly comfortable, here teachers have to extend their services to primary care sites and share the same practice environment with regular health service personnel.
- *Research*: Educational and administrative activities often compete with research to occupy the time of faculty members leaving little time for the latter. Faculty members may be frustrated because they need to do research for their academic satisfaction and career development.
- *Administration*: Many new jobs appear on the organizational chart of community-based institutions. They are needed to run the extensive outdoors community-based field activities, such jobs can usually be performed only by faculty members.

Hence, recruitment and retention of faculty in community-based education programs could be a major problem that threatens the quality or even survival of the program. This is accentuated by the faculty-intensive nature of community-based education curricula. Imaginative solutions to this problem that would create an appropriate reward system that would foster the faculty qualities and activities are needed.

Every effort should be made to involve nonfaculty suitable health personnel to take part in students' training and supervision. Their "teaching" abilities could be enhanced by joining the "tutor training workshops" offered to the regular faculty. Many of them are stimulated by the presence of students to resume reading or join postgraduate courses to refresh and upgrade their professional skills. The medical school should encourage, facilitate, and open such opportunities to health personnel. This not only facilitates students' learning but also serves to upgrade health delivery through community-based education.

Our experience has shown that it takes a few years of teething problems and growing pains before a steady state is reached when the faculty find themselves comfortable with their mastery and control of the educational process. Their comfort is strongly augmented by their satisfaction with the fine product growing in their hands – their students. At that time, the faculty discover that they do have time and opportunity for more fascinating research in which they join in multi-disciplinary teams, often including their students to address fundamental community health problems.

### Problem 10: Management and Organization

The administrative system and organizational structure of an institution adopting community-based education needs to be adapted to the peculiar needs of the program.

- Mention has already been made of the need to establish a functioning stable relationship with the health service sector. This has its administrative and financial implications.
- A matrix structure is needed to coordinate and integrate educational, service, and research activities of the institution and direct their movement towards the institutional goals, in which the departments would follow the vertical axis and the committees the horizontal one. It is particularly crucial to avoid a conflicting authority of departments and committees. The friction could be damaging and the whole process and output would suffer.
- Students and faculty community-based activities need an appropriate management system that guarantees adequate control and flow of information and the provision of support services at the proper time in the proper place.
- The logistics of providing transport, accommodation, sometimes small libraries and various materials required for the educational process in several places scattered over wide and sometimes remote areas, and the required funds pose management problems to be solved.

Each institution should find out how best to manage the operation of its program within the available resources. At present, there are no universal recommendations that can be adopted everywhere. Whatever the system, however, a valid and affordable program evaluation mechanism should be built in the system from the very beginning.

## Conclusion: Working Together to Solve the Problems

This chapter highlighted the magnitude and seriousness of the efforts needed from all of us to add value to our profession as physicians and educators and to bring relevance, for our selves and for what we do, to serve the needs, demands, and expectations of our people.

# References

1. The 1st Fayoum Conference on Medical Education, Fayoum, Egypt, April 1978. A national meeting arranged by the Action of Medical Education, of the Supreme Council of Universities, The Physicians' Syndicate and Ministry of Health.
2. Primary Health Care, Report of the International Conference on Primary Health Care, Alma-Ata, USSR, 6-12 September 1978, WHO "Health For All" Series No. 1, 1978.
3. An integrated approach to health services and manpower development, Report of a Ministerial Consultation. Teheran, 26 February–2 March 1978, WHO/EMRO. Technical Publication No. 1.
4. Fülöp T: Problem-based learning in the mirror of the great social target – Health for all. In Schmidt HG, De Volder ML (eds): *Tutorials in Problem-based Learning*. Assen/Maastricht, Van Gorcum, 1984, pp 9–15.
5. World Health Organization: A network of community-oriented educational institutions for health services. Report of a meeting held in Jamaica (HMD/79,4) Geneva, 1979.
6. Community-Based Education of Health Personnel: Report of a WHO Study Group, World Health Organization, Geneva, 1986.
7. Martenson D: *Educational Development in an Established Medical School*. London, Chartwell-Bratt, 1985.
8. Barrows SH, Tamblyn RM: *Problem-Based Learning*. New York, Springer Publishing Company, Inc., 1890, p 1.
9. White KL: Final report of Institutional Workshop on Community-Oriented Education in the Health Sciences, Oaxtepec, Morelos-Mexico, Jan. 25–29, 1982, p 38. Network of Community-Oriented Institution for Health Sciences and Universidad Autonoma Metropolitana-Xochimilco, Mexico.

# 6
# Medical Education in Action: Community-based Experience and Service in Nigeria*

U. BOLLAG, H. SCHMIDT, T. FRYERS, and J. LAWANI

Most medical schools in the developing world have been modeled on their counterparts in industrialized countries of the Northern Hemisphere. Their educational programs are not really focusing on the health problems (communicable diseases, malnutrition, and population growth) of poor, warm climate countries.

In Nigeria, for instance, this approach results in a health care situation in which graduated certified doctors find themselves unaccustomed to assess and evaluate the health needs and priorities of their own country and its people. They are incapable of providing effective health education or implementing preventive programs. They are ill-prepared to work in the slums of the cities or to manage a rural health care team.

Problem-based, student-centered, and community-oriented learning were basic to the construction of the medical curriculum of the Faculty of Health Sciences, University of Ilorin, Nigeria.[1] The recommendations of the Academic Planning group and the Working Party on Education of the National University Commission that new medical schools be oriented to the environment and produce students with a sense of service and a strong inclination toward broad community care and preventive medicine were used as additional guidelines. The COBES (community-based experience and service) educational program, directed at renewal of both the methods and content of medical education reflected these recommendations and is described herein.

## Design and Objectives of COBES

Twice a year and throughout the second to fifth years of their medical studies, small groups of students, each accompanied by two or three staff members (called supervisors/tutors) settled in a village or other community for 1 month. Five sites were chosen, two in the outer parts of Ilorin town (urban setting) and the other three spread over Kwara State (rural setting).

*This chapter is based on an article with the same title, published in *Medical Education* 1982;16,282–289, reprinted with permission.

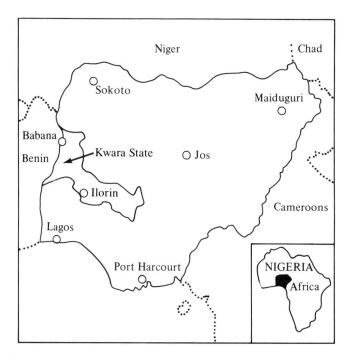

FIGURE 6.1.

Forty-two students entered the program initially (October 1978). Some of the more unusual objectives of COBES were to (1) sensitize the students to community health needs from the beginning of their student career, (2) assist community health efforts and prepare the students to work in any community, and (3) develop team spirit toward promotion of community health and create individual habits of study.

Each of the five groups adopted its own work style, so long as the limited objectives for the first posting (COBES placement) were fulfilled. Each group estimated population size and produced a simple representative map of its areas of work. Each group was to consider aspects of two major health problems, malnutrition and infectious disease. Groups were free to study contributory factors to those problems, e.g., sewage disposal, sources of water, major occupations, housing, and diet. Each group collected and analyzed data and made deductions in the form of a written report at the end of each COBES placement. The general goal was to have the students scratch the surface of the problems during their first COBES placement and have them investigate each problem in more detail during subsequent postings.

One group of seven students was living in Babana, a small village in the northwestern district of the Borgu Local Government area, some 400 km away from Ilorin (Fig. 6.1). Depending on the season, the roads were more or less motorable, so that communication was unreliable, transport slow, and referral for health care from peripheral dispensaries insecure. Public services were poor, and in many places the illiteracy rate was well above the Nigerian average and diseases due to nutritional deficiencies were widespread. Ethnic, cultural, social, and religious variations were prominent.

In the following paragraphs we let the Babana group speak through fragments of their basically unedited reports and thus illustrate learning situations originating from COBES.

## What Was the Community?

We thought that we had to visit the community leaders first in order to learn about the community. We presented ourselves to the local chief (Sariki) and explained to him the aims and objectives of our medical school. It was essential to get his consent for the use of available facilities such as school rooms and health clinics. He even granted us permission to visit houses, talk to families, and study family cases. We further met with the local health workers in an attempt to receive first-hand impressions and information about the prevailing health problems; we learned that diarrhea, cough, and high fever accounted for most of the diseases. It became obvious that the two trained health workers of this remote rural place were carrying out a hugh amount of work and had to make do with very little in terms of equipment and facilities. We then met with the headmaster and teachers of the local school. We and our tutors offered our possible services to the school, e.g., in the form of an assessment of the pupils' health status. The headmaster anticipated that we might experience language problems in communicating with the local people and therefore put a well educated woman at our disposal as an interpreter.

We were eager to know more about the local patterns of health and disease but found ourselves stuck again with questions that had to be answered first: What kind of people made up the community? What kind of work did they do? What did they earn? What were their beliefs and customs?

Babana, the district capital, was mainly inhabited by the Bokos, the principal tribe in the area. Other tribal groups such as the Yoruba, the Hausa, and some Ibo could be looked on almost as immigrants, and they made up for roughly half of Babana's population. Marami, a village some 11 km away from Babana, was much smaller than the latter. Its population consisted almost exclusively of Bokos. The Fulani, on the other hand, were seminomads; they were scattered over the savannah, and their habitat was geared to the availability of water and food for rearing their cattle.

The total population of Bokos in Babana, Marami, and among the Fulani in neighboring camps of the district stood at 408, 281, and 252, respectively. When we analyzed the groups by age and sex, several points were noteworthy. The ratio between 0 to 1 and 2 to 4 years age groups was 1:4. From this ratio we inferred that most deaths among the less than 5 years age group had occurred during the first year, and that there had been no fatal epidemics for the past 4 years. For the 5 to 9 years age group we counted nearly twice as many boys as girls in Babana and Marami. Trying to explain this phemonenon, it struck us that we were concerned here with the school-age group, and these uneven distributions applied only to the two places that had schools. The situation reflected the idea of these rural people that there was no use in future housewives being educated. None of the youngsters in the Fulani camps we visited were reported to go to school. We know that the Fulani rear cattle mainly, which, along with the pattern of lifelong wandering from pasture to pasture, accounts for the absence of Fulani at school.

The fact that there were always more female than male individuals in the group over 10 years age was explained by the trend of young men moving out to seek their fortune, whereas young women awaited motherhood and marriage, and by the fact that men have more than one wife.

When we visited the same community again in April 1979, at the end of the dry season, we were astonished by the changes in the population composition. The number of the Fulani, for example, had decreased by about 30% as a result of the scarcity of food and water. The number of children in the 2 to 4 years age group had also decreased, whereas the children of 5 to 9 years had increased. We attributed this difference to the fact that the exact age of the children was unknown to the parents and that errors might therefore have been incorporated because we tried to separate those less than 5 from those more than 5 years of age. In other words, environmental and cultural factors seemingly influenced the accuracy of our statistical numbers.

To conduct a census of the people was difficult for other reasons. Not knowing the local language was one of them. Apart from the fact that not all the English words had equivalents in the local language, an additional difficulty was that the answers not only depended on the addressee's understanding of the questions but also on the interpreter's understanding. We found out that we had to ask people questions about themselves and that we confused the people when we asked big, general questions; for example, "Do you raise small animals?" was a poor question, whereas "How many chickens does your family have this year? How many cows? How many sheep? could be easily answered.

Another difficulty was that mothers exhibited emotional stress when having to answer questions about their dead children. Therefore we avoided this subject as much as possible. Finally, parents found it easier to hand us data about children present at the moment than about those who happened to be absent.

## Nutritional Status of Children

Malnutrition was seen as a possible health problem affecting one community more than another — and thus arose the idea to conduct a survey and compare the status of nutrition between the children living among the Bokos in Babana and Marami, and the Fulani children.

Prior to the survey we were briefed by our tutors on simple ways to measure the nutritional status of children. The results of this survey have been described elsewhere.[2] There were no learning resources other than some basic readings and a few articles pertinent to the topic.[3,4] We had no weighing scale because of financial constraints and thus were unable to weigh the children. However, by means of colored arm bands, we measured the mid-upper arm circumference of the children, and by means of a simple tape we measured their height.

Although we were able to ask the families about the availability of food (food production, opportunities to buy and sell food) and feeding patterns and although we were able to record our measurements, we experienced considerable trouble in the interpretation of our figures. However, we learned more about medical statistics and more specifically about the use of standardization to give reliable age/sex specific rates[5] between the first COBES rotation in October 1978 and the second in April 1979.

We repeated the nutritional survey during our second COBES rotation in April 1979; not only could we demonstrate that there had been fewer malnourished children in the 5 years age group (assessed by the mid-upper arm circumference) at Babana than in the other two communities in October 1978, but also that the dry season had caused the gap to become wider. Fulani children suffered most from the effects of the dry season. The question to be answered was why Babana had maintained monopoly of the first position on the nutrition chart.

Babana had the singular advantage of being in possession of the only major market, so that regardless of the season there had never been a shortage of food in Babana. The place enjoyed further advantages: Even when water was scarce in the surroundings, Babana had a stream that did not completely dry up during the dry season. Finally, Babana had the only dispensary in the district and was benefiting from the direct influence of the government in that a few state governmental facilities had been established there (court, police post, power house, and a maternity health center).

## Guinea Worm Infestation in Dekala

We had seen cases of guinea worm infestation in October 1978, and during our second COBES rotation in April 1979 the community of Dekala, a hamlet situated some 35 km west of Babana, called for our help. It was a ideal learning situation for us; guinea worm infestation, a problem suffered by the people on one hand could be coupled with the stated objective to look into the problem of infectious diseases during COBES on the other. The transmission cycle of guinea worm infestation (source, vector, host) was known to us from the reading that had been assigned by the tutors prior to leaving for Dekala.[6]

All of the 109 cases reported were located at Dekala; 52 male subjects and 57 female subjects were found to be infected. Thus the disease did not seem to distinguish between the sexes. Among those infected, the ages ranged from 2 to 60 years, but only three children less than 5 years of age were included. We attributed this finding to the fact that the very young were not yet sent to fetch water and therefore did not get in close touch with the source of the infection. The site of infection usually was on the lower extremities and sometimes on the breasts in female patients and the scrotum in males patients.

Interviews held with some members of the community disclosed that the guinea worm infection was believed to have been introduced from a neighboring hamlet through intermarriage. By further inquiries we learned that there were two families, one of them the family of the Sariki, who had not had any guinea worm infections. These families boiled their drinking water. As a matter of fact, the Sariki had a transistor radio and had listened from time to time to broadcast lessons. That is how he had learned never to drink any unboiled or untreated water. We wondered whether the power of the Sariki as leader of the community could not be used to change the hazardous habits of his people. We argued further that the presence of medical professionals from a university would certainly have a favorable effect on the credibility of his educational talk. Fortunately, he agreed with our idea and so gathered all the villagers under a huge tree and delivered a speech to them emphasizing the necessity of boiling any water for drinking purposes.

The only water source at Dekala was a dirty pond. Microscopic examinations of a specimen of the water showed the causative agent of the disease, *Cyclops*. We mounted our microscope on the bonnet [hood] of our vehicle and encouraged the people to look at the organism responsible for all their suffering. Now they were even better able to grasp the Sariki's warning never to wade into the pond with the contaminated water.

Many patients presented with superinfected wounds where the worm had found its way out. We cleansed the lesions and in some cases administered antibiotic drugs to control secondary infection.

At the end of the day one of the tutors demonstrated how a tiny fraction of Dettol sufficed to kill the *Cyclops*. If this measure was to be applied in regular 2- to 3-month intervals, and if all infected people were treated successfully or the worm was absorbed or extruded, dissemination of the disease could be stopped. We instructed the teacher in the village to repeat the disinfection of water with Dettol, a bottle of which we left with him.

## Discussion

The activities as described by the Babana group of students make it possible to draw three conclusions. The first is that the learning process can be greatly facilitated by direct, concrete confrontation with health problems. The guinea worm episode shows particularly how both parasitological and epidemiological knowledge can be acquired and integrated in the context of joint preventive and curative actions; the acquisition of knowledge is intimately related to the use of such knowledge. It has been shown that generally speaking a learning situation of this kind leads to the acquired knowledge being better memorized and being used with greater flexibility.[7]

TABLE 6.1. Documentation of learning as reflected in the students' statements

1. We have been able to interact with the community, and we have been able to gain some knowledge about the people's way of life, which will help us in the future COBES postings, e.g., methods of approach to the community.
2. We have been able to identify some of the people's health problems and needs, which will enable us to plan ways of helping them in future.
3. COBES enabled us to have a broad view of the scope of problems a doctor would encounter in a rural community. This view has obvious advantages if one is posted to a rural community later in life.
4. We have had the benefits of seeing health problems in real life and their relation to the community such that when we read about them in our course, we will have a better grasp and understanding.
5. We have had the opportunity to do creative work, tackling problems as they arise, formulating possible hypotheses from observations.
6. The problems and challenges we saw open to a medical doctor stimulated our interest more toward the study of medicine.
7. We have been able to work harmoniously as a team, making constructive suggestions and criticism where applicable.

The second conclusion is that COBES gives students the opportunity to observe health and disease in relation to the environment and the people's habits, both intricately intertwined. The students came to appreciate the influence that the local food situation had on the state of nutrition of the children; they themselves perceived the hazard infected people created for the community when they waded into the pool from which water was drawn for drinking. Such insight makes it more logical and desirable to interfere effectively at an early stage for the benefit of people's health. Medical education of the traditional kind usually implies that students are shown only the final stage of the process of a disease — the sick person who is admitted to a hospital. This approach may result in the students seeing their task as future doctors to be concerned with the curing of individual patients only. The guinea worm experience clearly shows how incorrect and pointless such an attitude would be.

The third conclusion is that education that prompts students to engage actively in their studies appears to be highly motivating. This idea was evidenced by the enthusiasm with which the students prepared themselves and the satisfaction they found in performing their tasks. The students were given the opportunity to comment on COBES and were asked to state specifically what had been gained by the study project. Table 6.1 contains a selected list of students' quotations.*

The statements of the students brought out what they thought they had gained by their studies in COBES. Whereas they served the faculty by providing valuable feedback, provision had also been made for more objective evaluation. The proximity of students and tutors during the postings made it easy to exchange ideas, pass on knowledge, and correct mistakes in an ongoing and informal way. Moreover, each student's performance was evaluated by a Likert-type five-point

---

*Appendices 1 and 2 to this chapter contain short reports of a third- and a sixth-year student reflecting upon COBES and its central importance to their learning.

Student's name _____
Group leader _____
                              (staff)
Date of posting _____
Place of posting _____

| 1<br>unsatisfactory | 2 | 3<br>satisfactory | 4 | 5<br>distinction |
|---|---|---|---|---|

Please mark X in the appropirate box below

|  | Mid-posting | End of posting |
|---|---|---|
| 1. Appearance and general behavior | ☐☐☐☐☐ | ☐☐☐☐☐ |
| 2. Punctuality | ☐☐☐☐☐ | ☐☐☐☐☐ |
| 3. Attitude toward the COBES program | ☐☐☐☐☐ | ☐☐☐☐☐ |
| 4. Relationship to other students | ☐☐☐☐☐ | ☐☐☐☐☐ |
| 5. Relationship to people in the community | ☐☐☐☐☐ | ☐☐☐☐☐ |
| 6. Collection of data | ☐☐☐☐☐ | ☐☐☐☐☐ |
| 7. Presentation of data | ☐☐☐☐☐ | ☐☐☐☐☐ |
| 8. Interpretation of data | ☐☐☐☐☐ | ☐☐☐☐☐ |
| 9. Ability to relate findings to solving community health problems | ☐☐☐☐☐ | ☐☐☐☐☐ |
| 10. Student's critique of his own approach to the problems | ☐☐☐☐☐ | ☐☐☐☐☐ |
| 11. Ability to suggest new approaches to the solution of problems | ☐☐☐☐☐ | ☐☐☐☐☐ |
| 12. Contribution to group discussion | ☐☐☐☐☐ | ☐☐☐☐☐ |
| 13. Performance in crisis situation | ☐☐☐☐☐ | ☐☐☐☐☐ |
| 14. Assessment of the student's written report | ☐☐☐☐☐ | ☐☐☐☐☐ |
|  | TOTAL SCORE | ☐ |

Remarks by the group leader _____

Student's comments on his own performance. (The group
leader is to discuss the performance with the student
concerned, at mid-posting and end of posting and enter
here relevant points which might come out of the discussion.)

Date _____     Signature of the group leader _____

FIGURE 6.2.

scale.[8] An abbreviated form for the evaluation of students' performance is shown in Figure 6.2. The written reports served as another device for assessment of the work done by the students during COBES. These records went into a permanent file. Finally, a plenary was organized in Ilorin after each COBES rotation, with all students and tutors being present and the groups presenting their findings to each other. Apart from serving as teaching/learning sessions, these meetings constituted an opportunity for the students to voice their complaints on any aspect of COBES and make proposals for improvement.

However, it was thought by staff and students alike that the extent and complexity of the COBES program made evaluation a difficult enterprise. Clearly, more precise learning objectives were needed for COBES before succinct evaluation criteria could be developed.

The COBES program constituted an experimental situation in the first year of a new faculty. Elements of confusion, ill-definition, disagreement, and error were inevitable. A fundamental problem arose from the incomplete negotiation of role sets for tutors. The personal insecurity inherent in a situation such as COBES can be particularly threatening to professional people accustomed to being thoroughly competent (and accepted as such) within their own specialist field. For example, in Babana students regularly needed the assistance of staff members not present at the station. The distance to, and the poor accessibility of, Babana made it unattractive for many of the staff to teach on the spot. Nor was there great enthusiasm to share the students' primitive living conditions for any period of time.

A second major problem was the rather serious doubt and uncertainties on the part of some staff members with regard to the value of the COBES program. At the time of the second COBES placement the program was already faced with the question with which any educational innovation is confronted: Does this innovation lead to the desired goals? The faculty did not take the time to present this question explicitly for reflection and thereby lost the active participation of a number of its Nigerian staff members. As a consequence, the program had to rely on expatriates to a greater degree than was acceptable to ensure its continuity.

The need to form a COBES planning team became obvious after the first two placements. Such a team might work out academic proposals for the whole 5-year program in terms of learning objectives and principal themes that would be common to all groups. Every specialty represented on the teaching staff could submit detailed proposals for their own potential contributions, which would facilitate the integrated program that COBES reflected.

The lack of resources (finances and manpower) greatly hampered the educational input of COBES. It was thought that each COBES area should develop a resource bank of its own, including: (1) standard equipment for clinical investigation, simple laboratory tests, and storage of specimens; (2) a small library of reference books relevant to the student's work in the area; (3) collections of papers and reviews to be used as resources for specific projects; and (4) copies of reports and data from all previous student work.

Nonexpert area tutors would require specialist assistance from many disciplines represented in the teaching staff; topics for instruction and in-service training would include area management and liaison, student guidance, problem and task definition, resources management, project monitoring, and continuous evaluation.

# Conclusion

A sound and modern philosophy about education as such does not suffice to bring about the desired changes in students who in the future are to organize and run the health care system in rural and urban areas. A society that is willing to alter its health care system should not rely exclusively on the idealism of a few who are prepared to work among the poorest and most deprived populations. Working in the bush should also be attractive to nonidealists. One of the authors of this report (H.S.), by that time an external consultant of the Faculty of Health Sciences, interviewed students about COBES and discovered that although the students in question support wholeheartedly the teaching staff's educational philosophy they doubted that they would later appreciate spending long years working under primitive conditions. This problem remains a key issue in medical training and manpower planning for developing countries.

*Acknowledgments.* We would like to praise the spirit of motivation and sacrifice of all the students who were involved in COBES. We would also like to thank our Nigerian colleagues of the Faculty of Health Sciences, Unilorin, from whom we have learned a great deal about health and disease in Nigeria. We are grateful for the contributions to this chapter made by the following students of the Faculty of Health Sciences, Unilorin: C.A.D. Adigun, N.I. Agwu, J.O. Awobusuyi, K.A. Awolola, M.O. Chukwumweike, I.A. Nwosu, and H.A. Ukpeh.

# References

1. Neufeld VR, Barrows HS: The McMaster philosophy: an approach to medical education. *J Med Educ* 1974;49:1040.
2. Bollag U, Bennike T, Adigun CAO, et al: Problem based medical education in the community: a student nutritional survey in Nigeria. *Int J Epidemol* 1980;9:375.
3. Shakir A, Morley D: Measuring malnutrition. *Lancet* 1974;1:758.
4. Arnold R: The "Quac stick"; A field measure used by the Quaker service team in Nigeria. *J Trop Pediatr* 1969;15:243.
5. Barker DIP: *Practical Epidemiology.* Edinburgh, Churchill Livingstone, 1976.
6. Parry EHO: *Principles of Medicine in Africa.* Oxford, Oxford University Press, 1976.
7. Mayer RE, Greeno JG: Structural differences between learning outcomes produced by different instructional methods. *J Educ Psychol* 1972;63:165.
8. Best JW: *Research in Education.* Englewood Cliffs, NJ, Prentice-Hall, 1977.

# Appendix I
# A Student's Reflections on COBES

OMNI D. MARCUS—THIRD-YEAR STUDENT

## Introduction

"What is COBES?" This is the major question that recurs thoughtfully in the mind of any medical student entering the Faculty of Health Sciences of the University of Ilorin for the first time. Within the first month of enrollment, they soon learn, either at their posting site or in the introductory class, that COBES is an abbreviatory word for Community Based Experience and Service. This is a faculty program whose overall philosophy is to produce doctors with a great sense of service and a strong inclination to broad community care and preventive medicine.

During this program, groups of students are sent to different communities in Kwara State (some as far as 400 km away) where they reside for a total period of 14 weeks in three separate postings. While at these posting sites, each group, supervised by members of the academic staff, is engaged in studying different aspects of the community in relation to the occurrence, transmission and periodicity of diseases. Such aspects include culture, religion, socioeconomy, environmental sanitation, etc. Usually, an introductory course covering epidemiology, biostatistics, parasitology, microbiology, map reading, and the basic sciences often precedes the first posting.

The highlights of some of the observations recorded between 1978 and now are presented as follows:

## Shao Group

The major problem identified by the group at Shao (the posting site of this group) was onchocerciasis (riverblindness). The Shao community, being situated in a valley with fast-flowing streams, is physically conducive for the breeding of Simullium Damnosum, vector of Onchocerca Volvulus. Coincidentally, the most extensive farming activities occur in these valleys. Thus, farmers are being exposed regularly to the bites of black flies. This disease is readily recognizable among persons 30 years and above as leopard skin on their legs. The prevalence of this dermal depigmentation was found to be highest among the male adults who constituted about 80% of the farming population. Consequently, the prevalence of blindness and visual impairment were correspondingly highest in this economically active group.

The community has no knowledge of the association between black flies and leopard skin. Their general perception was that dermal depigmentation was due, directly, to aging.

## Babana Group

The high prevalence of dracunculiasis (Guinea-worm infection) in this community was the most striking observation made by this group. The rampantness of this infection was related with the problems of water scarcity, poor water management, and ignorance. Infection was reported to be highest during the peak of the dry season and at the onset of rainfall. The intermediate hosts (*Cyclops*) with guinea-worm larvae in them were identified in the pond water drunk by the people. Over 80% of the infections were located on the legs. Multiple infections were common and the rate of incapacitation was very high. Thus, farmers could neither prepare their lands and plant their crops at the onset of the rains nor harvest their crops, if any, during the dry season. Therefore, in the Babana district, guinea-worm infection constitutes a major socioeconomic problem. Also, it was noted that secondary infection resulting from ignorance and unsanitary methods of local management of the infection was responsible for the severity of the disease in this community.

## Mopa Group

At Mopa, endemic goiter was observed to be highly prevalent, especially among the women. Whereas the group associated this problem with insufficient amount of minerals (iodine) in the community water sources, the natives attributed it to witchcraft.

## Pakata Group

The rampantness of gastrointestinal infection in this community, although with pipe-borne water, was reported to be largely due to poor environmental sanitation. Sewage disposal system is poor or totally lacking. This affords promiscuous contamination of food with flies and other vectors. This is borne out of the fact that the highest incidence was recorded during the period when certain fruits (eg mango, gmelina) ripen and are visited by flies.

# Conclusion

The selected reports given here are a few of the numerous efforts and observations made by students during their interaction with the community. Other investigations carried out include nutritional survey, anthropometric measurements, health and socioeconomic problems of smoking, and use and misuse of drugs and alcohol. On the basis of the general experience, and the achievements, of the early exposure to the community through COBES, the students have been able to identify the major community health problems, to assess the influence of human factors in the transmission and dissemination of certain diseases and to appreciate the relevance of relating health program efforts with the percep-tion of the community with respect to endemic diseases. Therefore, these understandings provide sufficient background to recommend health educational programs and preventive measures for the communities concerned.

Concisely, this early exposure stimulates the awareness of the student to the community health needs, gives him or her the background to establish a relationship between the patient and the patient's background; motivates the student to contribute to and assist community health efforts, and enhances the student's appreciation of the relevance of demographic studies (including culture and socioeconomy) in planning a community health program.

# Appendix II
# My Impression of COBES

ODIGIE I. PIUS – SIXTH-YEAR STUDENT

There is a great evidence that COBES is a learning process that aims at sensitizing the "young doctor" to community health needs whose end embraces a prompt, effective, ready acceptance, and understanding of treatment offered to patients in terms of available resources. When the COBES posting first began in October 1978, the very first day of our training in the medical school, little did we know that this program was going to triumph over the tempted prejudice and likely disadvantages that inevitably arose and that was to make ours different from the methods of approach adopted by the old medical schools. Perhaps it suffices to say that although in its primary phase, COBES has provided an opportunity of taking a "bird's eye" view of the community in terms of health services, social influence, and gaps in the health needs of the communities we studied. There are limited and terminal objectives of this program that should aid in the day-to-day assessment of students in terms of the extent they have achieved the goals of this program.

It is quite clear that the limited objectives of COBES are designed to help us assess our own evaluation of the program. These objectives are not isolated as they are fundamental tools for achieving the terminal objectives. The limited objectives of the first posting have as a primary focus the use of a survey map in collecting vital statistical data that are invaluable in determining the health needs of the community. This employs a reasonable estimate of the population as a fundamental tool for assessing the health needs and of designing a plan of establishing the priorities of health problems of the community. The environmental influence on the health of the people is of foremost importance to us.

The terminal objectives of COBES call for prior recognition of the health needs of a community and its total integration with a delicate and dynamic sensitivity of the "new doctor" to the health needs of the community and subsequent improvement of the community health standards. The ultimate goal, therefore, is to create an atmosphere of balanced relationships that will not only ensure an adequate knowledge of the background of a patient when determining the course of his or her illnesses, but that will also combine the glory of team spirit in determining the influence of culture and socioeconomic factors on the health needs of the community in question.

By taking part in these extensive programs, the new doctor soon finds that he or she develops a paradoxically surprising individual attitude of voluntary habit of study and of providing solutions to health problems that have an immediate bearing in improving the community health standards. This will, in turn, sensitize him or her as a socioeconomic and cultural determinant on the consequences of health and disease. However, this will require the student's seeking help from other professionals in real-life situations.

Undoubtedly, COBES aims to eliminate the difficult task that has always been to strike at a balance between giving service as near as possible to where the patient lives and at the same time concentrating on giving the best hospital services in terms of available resources. Looking at these objectives vividly, it is not unlikely that it will make a substantial change in the final analysis on the responsibility of the new doctor, ie shifting his or her responsibilities from the old concept of white-coat, office-chair assignment to active participation in community health planning and services. The doctor will then be equipped with enough experience to work in any community anywhere in the world.

Quite often, there is a temptation to think that these COBES groups lack problems. However, there are salient features and remarkable evidences to show that this is not quite true. There is no doubt that from the very onset, students posted to these COBES Sites have experienced lots of difficulties, but our success has been due largely to our capacity of solving problems arising in the community. In such critical conditions, we have relied on the community effort and the selfless services of our faculty supervisor for appropriate solutions.

Some of the stark realities in these COBES sites were actually very shocking. Contrary to expectations, it was not all that rosy, but we had endeavored to cope adequately well. It is hoped that students will continue to endeavor to solve problems arising where possible as we have always done, but we also hope the Faculty will continue to intervene by providing basic necessities and fundamental tools at these COBES sites. The relationship between students, faculty staff, and the community must be a balanced one. The fact that students and lecturers have learned to live as part of the community in good team spirit is strictly speaking the mystery that keep the COBES groups going.

The first posting was very exciting. One of its advantages has been the provision of an environment that provided opportunity of learning by observation and participation. Another important social advantage has been the good reception and cooperation of the people without which our efforts would have failed. Perhaps one more thing is in providing a field of integration of thoughts.

The second posting was even more dramatic. Recognition of common community problems like sanitary facilities, the idea of animal sharing human accommodations, while the activities of the butcher takes place in the open air, all create primary arousal of interest in community study.

Besides all these, the health team assess from time to time the effective improvement of health planning that is, in fact, very difficult. The importance of health education cannot be overemphasized—by convincing people to modify their habits (which are harmful to their health and well-being), we can teach them to live fuller and more enjoyable lives. All these realities enumerated above are only a small part of the whole story.

Finally, I am optimistic that COBES will emphasize the prevention of disease and maintenance of health and at the same time bring into this country a sound health care system. Perhaps I should add that the generality of COBES, if properly managed, would offer the population the best possible service. It is worthwhile noting that such a dynamic program like COBES could be a potential means of providing the best preventive measure of community diseases, establishing a drastic change, and a total eradication of major infections in these communities and its environment at large—especially in a developing country like Nigeria.

# 7
# Community-based Medical Education in Nigeria: The Case of Bayero University

OLA K. ALAUSA

Medical schools in developing African countries have been modeled on after their counterparts in Western industrialized countries such as Britain and the United States. Consequently, medical education programs set up in Africa have not focused on the health problems that occur in less-developed health care settings.

In Nigeria, for instance, the first three decades (1948–1977) of medical education were dominated by the teaching hospital model because it was generally assumed that the most effective use of medical technology and highly skilled manpower (such as doctors, pharmacists, and nurses) was through clinical diagnosis and treatment in a few centralized medical centers. The dominant model of medical education in Nigeria has resulted in less than 40% coverage of the population, the majority of whom live in the rural areas. In addition, it has produced a health care situation in which newly graduated and certified doctors undergoing their one-year National Youth Service (NYSC) find themselves unaccustomed to assess and evaluate the health needs and priorities of their own country and its people. The majority of these medical graduates are incapable of providing effective health education or implementing the primary health care policy program of the government to the greater Nigerian population who live in conditions of rural and urban poverty. This population is exposed to health problems, quite different from those of the West (Table 7.1).

Overemphasis of the hospital-based model of medical education and medical care overconcentrates scarce resources in a few centers, distorts the perception of the priority health needs, and creates a system inaccessible to, and alienated from, most of the population. This often leads to dissatisfaction among highly trained physicians who cannot get appropriate tools to work with (and therefore seek employment in rich countries) and discourages self-reliance in peripheral health workers. With the increasing demands by the various communities in developing African countries for improvement and extension of good quality health services, particularly with the adoption of the primary health care concept as the vehicle for achieving the social goal of health for all by the year 2000, reorientation of medical education has gained greater significance. For instance, medical schools in Nigeria are now required to be involved in the training of

TABLE 7.1. The major disease entities in Nigeria.

1. Disease of poverty and underdevelopment
   a. The diarrhea–pneumonia–malnutrition complex
   b. Water-related diseases—Guineaworm, schistosomiasis, onchocerciasis, etc.
   c. Meningococcal meningitis
   d. Leprosy
2. Tropical diseases
   a. Vector-borne parasitic disease—malaria
   b. Vector-borne viral disease—yellow fever
   c. Trachoma
3. Childhood preventable communicable diseases
   a. Measles
   b. Poliomyelitis
   c. Whooping cough
   d. Tetanus
   e. Tuberculosis
4. Diseases associated with inadequate obstetric care
   a. Birth injuries
   b. Prematurity
   c. Neonatal infections
   d. Anemia in pregnancy
   e. Toxaemia of pregnancy
   f. Vesicovaginal fistulae
   g. Postpartum haemorrhage
   h. Puerperal sepsis
5. Other major causes of morbidity/mortality
   a. Road traffic accidents
   b. Snake bites
   c. Sickle disease
   d. Mental illness
   e. Liver diseases
   f. Diseases of the aged (including neoplasms)
   g. Hypertension
   h. Diabetes mellitus

doctors and other health professionals who are aware of their role in the health care delivery system of the country. In addition, health institutions are expected to search for new models of health care delivery that are less expensive and more easily accessible by the general population. It is now becoming clear, for instance, that for proper medical training, it is essential for the medical schools to cooperate more closely with government officials responsible for the health care delivery system, in order to define appropriate and relevant objectives for medical education relevant to the country's needs.

## Institutional Objectives of Bayero University Medical School

Bayero University, Kano, is situated in the northern part of Nigeria. It has adopted a community-oriented and community-based educational philosophy, as will be elucidated by its objectives, stated as follows:

On successful completion of the MB–BS program, the graduate of the Faculty of Medicine, Bayero University, Kano, would have developed attitudes and acquired knowledge and skills to be able to:
* *Practice as a general practitioner in an urban or rural community:* By use of clinical skills, including personal interview and physical examination, and by

means of appropriate but simple laboratory, radiological and other investigative procedures, diagnose and take an initial decision on every patient who presents to him or her.

Perform minor surgical procedures and lifesaving emergency procedures in General Practice, whether in an urban or rural setting.

- *Perform professional services within the concept of Primary Health Care System* Detect, define and diagnose community health problems and proceed to plan and implement projects including health education aimed at preventing or remedying such problems.

Whether in the practice of preventive or curative medicine, take into account the role of interpersonal relationships in families and communities and the social, cultural, and traditional factors that might have a bearing on health and disease.

Function as an active member in a primary health care team and organize immunization programs, control programs for epidemic and locally endemic diseases, and run maternal and child-health and other comprehensive/community health-care clinics.

Function as an agent of change in a community, inspiring the participation of individuals, families, and communities in programs designed to bring about socioeconomic development.

- *Develop personal characteristics required of a professional doctor:* Maintain a high level of personal integrity, sense of responsibility, compassion to the sick, and devotion to duty.

Uphold the ethics of the profession in his/her relationship to patients and colleagues.

Possess adequate management capabilities to be able to play leadership roles in the health care team.

- *Undertake postgraduate or continuing medical education:* Take part in postgraduate programs to acquire higher or specialized degrees to become hospital specialists, teachers in medical schools, or health management experts (health administrators).

Engage in self-educational programs by means of reading books and journals and by the use of audiovisual materials and thus keep in touch with advances in medical science and practice.

To achieve the principles outlined in the philosophy of the medical at Bayero University, Kano, the curriculum has the following characteristics:

1. *Learning is integrated and student-centered.* As medical science is a rapidly progressing and ever-changing body of knowledge, it is important for medical graduates to be able to pursue a continuing education by the process of self-learning. When students arrive at the medical school, they are hardly able to learn by themselves. In the secondary schools and colleges, they are used to being taught, or in other words "spoon-fed." As a result, the students' expression of their knowledge is mainly in the form of recall of facts. At the level of the medical school, didactic lectures will be reduced to the minimum, and students will be exposed to a learning process through problem-solving, analysis and interpreta-

tion of data, and actual performance of various skills in the course of their training. This training in self-education would equip medical graduates of Bayero University, Kano, with the necessary attitude and ability to undertake continuing education throughout his or her career as a medical practitioner.

2. *Learning to be community oriented and community based.* Training programs are to be geared towards the community. Community participation in the development and implementation of the community-based health programs of the faculty are essential. Therefore, the faculty will cooperate with identified social and cultural groups in the various communities where its medical educational programs are located. This will easily be achieved through the formation of Community-Health Committees in the areas. A Community Health Committee has the following functions:

(a) To organize a cross-section of the community (eg, traditional leaders, influential groups, teachers, traditional health practitioners, and other people in the community interested in health and social development) into a cohesive group for the purpose of determining the health problems and types of disease in the community, the problems associated with health-care delivery, the priority health needs of the community, and possible solutions to these problems through community action.
(b) To promote the health of the community by: stimulating interest in community health and health-related programs motivated by educating the community in health-related matters and other aspects of socioeconomic development.
(c) To encourage intersectoral cooperation.

TABLE 7.2. Educational objectives for CBMES Program, Bayero University, Kano.

At the end of the course, the student should be capable of:
 1. Planning and executing a simple estimate of the demographic characteristics of a defined community.
 2. Identifying, and consulting with, the important people in the community in order to plan, promote, implement and evaluate health programs through maximum community participation.
 3. Identifying the major factors associated with health problems in a defined community and appreciating the influence of cultural and other socioeconomic factors in the determination of health problems in different community settings.
 4. Investigating identified community health problems and prescribing rational and realistic solutions to them, based on the prevailing socioeconomic status of the community.
 5. Establishing a cordial relationship between patients and the communities from which they come and educating the communities in their pursuit of good health.
 6. Understanding the organizational structure and functions of the various health institutions in the community, also noting the relationship to the overall health services in the state and the country.
 7. Identifying and correcting inadequacies in the various health-delivery services in a defined community.
 8. Working harmoniously with other health personnel for the overall socioeconomic development of the community.
 9. Planning a comprehensive health care program for a defined community.
10. Documenting the health activities in the community of operation.

TABLE 7.3. Criteria for selection of areas for community-based education and service (CBMES) program in Nigeria.

  I. Be a well-defined community, with similar sociocultural background
     1. Well-defined but nonhomogeneous in both language and religion
     2. Well-defined but nonhomogenous in *either* language *or* religion
     3. Well-defined and homogeneous in both language and religion
 II. Be of manageable size in population and land area
     1. Less than 5000 people/more than 25,000 people and less than 200 houses/more than 1200 houses
     2. 5001 to 10,000 people and 201 to 700 houses
     3. 10,001 to 25,000 people and 701 to 1200 houses
III. Availability of health facilities
     1. Available (community owned/government owned)
     2. Available and functioning efficiently (community owned/government owned)
     3. Available, functioning well, and owned by the medical school.
 IV. Accessibility of community
     1. Footpath/unmotorable road
     2. Untarred but motorable road
     3. Tarred good road
  V. Distance to the medical school
     1. Over 60 kilometers away
     2. 16–59 kilometers away
     3. 0–15 kilometers away
 VI. Availability of suitable accommodation
     1. Not available
     2. Available for hire (100%) to medical school
     3. Available at partial rent to medical school community
     4. Available and free to the medical school (donated by community)
VII. Water supply
     1. Not available
     2. Occasional supply but inadequate for daily use
     3. Continuous supply but requires treatment before drinking
     4. Continuous supply and wholesome
VIII. Electricity supply
     1. Not available
     2. Occasional supply (some hours of the day)
     3. Continuous supply
 IX. Receptiveness of the community
     1. Nonhospitable people
     2. Indifferent people
     3. Hospitable/warm people
  X. Establishment of community health committee
     1. Not available
     2. Available but not active
     3. Available and active
     4. Available, active, with regular financial and material contribution toward health projects

Maximum score for any community chosen is 30 points (i.e., 3 × 10).

TABLE 7.4. First community-based medical posting.

1. Projects to be executed by students: Community health diagnosis of a defined community
   (a) Situation analysis
   (b) Baseline data collection
2. Specific learning objectives
   a. Identify and interview the important people in the community
   b. Produce a simple map of the area
   c. Produce a simple census and construct the demographic characteristics of the community
   d. Survey the existing social facilities available in the community
      (1) Health facilities, including data on disease patterns
      (2) Educational institutions
      (3) Religious institutions
      (4) Water supplies, environmental sanitation facilities, electricity supplies
      (5) Road network
      (6) Recreational facilities, social organizations
   e. Observe the life pattern of the people and their major occupations
   f. Survey the health needs of the people
   g. Describe the various relationships between man and his environment in the community
   h. Conduct health-related studies, under the guidance of the faculty supervisors (optional)
   i. Write a report of the community-based experience
   j. Present the report to a joint student/staff/community meeting

# The Community-based Medical Education and Service (CBMES) Program

The CBMES program is spread over a 5-year undergraduate curriculum. A total of 32 weeks is spent by students outside the medical school/teaching hospital setting. These 32 weeks are divided over six clerkships in various communities. The educational objectives for the CBMES program are listed on Table 7.2. The two clerkships during the preclinical years are carried out in defined communities (CBMES posting sites) that have been selected based on the criteria outlined in Table 7.3. (Each number represents a score. The numbers are added. The higher the final score, the better suited the community for use as a posting site.) Subsequent placements are carried out during the clinical years in the same CBMES sites by the same group of students. However, students are exposed to a range of health facilities (health centers, district hospitals, etc) in order to implement certain specific educational objectives in the CBMES program.

The first CBMES posting, which specific learning objectives are outlined in Table 7.4, gives the students an opportunity to explore cultural, social, environmental, and demographic aspects of health and disease before these students become socialized as doctors. In subsequent postings, defined and identified health topics are studied, often linked to major health problems in the community (such as malnutrition, infections, parasitic infestations, epidemic diseases, etc), or nationally recognized health problems (such as smoking, road traffic accidents, hypertension, family planning, immunization, etc). This approach ensures that the program is also problem based and student centered.

During the latter stages of CBMES postings, the students become involved in the planning and provision of primary health care to the community, under the supervision of registered medical practitioners. Evaluation of students is based on observations during field activities (focusing on skills and attitudes) by the supervising staff, oral presentation and written reports by students, and written examinations at the end of each posting. These assessments will constitute the in-course, continuous evaluation with an eye toward the professional examinations.

In conclusion, it appears to be possible to design and implement medical curricula adapted to the health needs of the population and using the scarce resources available in Nigeria in an optimal manner. The task, however, requires an imaginative, creative group of people who believes in its mission. Given the present financial constraints, it is not always easy to find appropriate medical staff, because a faculty appointment often interferes with the maintenance of private practice.

# Part III
# Problem-based Learning: Rationale and Examples

HENK G. SCHMIDT

Problem-based learning is an instructional procedure that, in contrast to conventional education, transfers control over the learning process from the teacher to the students. In this approach to learning and instruction, students are encouraged to formulate and pursue their own learning objectives and to select the learning resources most adapted to their current information needs. A major accent in this system is that teachers contribute to this learning process only by providing suggestions for further study, not by requiring prespecified learning activities. Thus, problem-based learning can be described as a *student-centered* approach to learning, as opposed to the traditional teacher-centered approach.

In this section, practical and theoretical issues concerning problem-based learning as an approach to health professions education are discussed. We start by describing the method in order to provide the reader with a perspective insight in the learning process of students under the problem-based learning regime. Subsequently, some historical comments are made emphasizing the different roots back to which problem-based learning can be traced. An overview of Part III concludes this introduction.

## Short Description of the Approach

Problem-based learning is characterized as follows: A small group of students, usually no more than eight, to meet together twice a week, is confronted with *problems*. A problem commonly consists of a description of a set of phenomena or events that require an *explanation*.[6] This explanation can take the form of a description of the processes, principles, or mechanisms that underlie the phenomena. In medical education, the problems used are often clinical ones in which the phenomena to be explained are a patient's symptoms or complaints. For example: "A 55-year-old woman is lying on the floor writhing in pain. The pain occurs in waves and extends from the right lumbar region to the right groin and the front side of the right leg." Such a presentation is, however, not always used. Nonclinical problems can also be explored in problem-based learning, such as in the following example: "If, for an extended period, you sit on a chair in the same position with your legs crossed, your legs may fall 'asleep.'" That is, when you stand you will experience discomfort or numbness and trouble with walking and standing. After a short while, usually a few seconds, these phenomena disappear."

The task for the small group is to come up with explanations for the presented problem of phenomena. For the first example, this explanation could be found and described in terms of gastrointestinal or urogenital system function. The second example would most probably include the description of the nervous system as well as aspects of locomotion. Students accomplish this task by *analyzing* the problem. First, they discuss it thoroughly and at length, attempting to understand it using prior knowledge and common-sense reasoning. In this stage of analysis, it is expected that questions will emerge about aspects of the problem that are poorly understood or unsatisfactorily explained. Thus, a list of questions, differences of opinion, and other issues emerge. These questions become the *learning goals* that are pursued in the students' subsequent, individual, self-directed studies. Answers to the questions are sought using appropriate texts, handbooks, resource persons, and general faculty who are experts in a particular area, as well as searches of current literature and the use of audiovisual aids. In a follow-up session the newly acquired information is exchanged and *synthesized*. Students check whether they are now able to provide better, less superficial explanations for the problem or to raise more sophisticated questions. If a clinical problem is under investigation, the group may attempt to formulate questions for the patient, or suggest physical examinations and laboratory tests that are indicated in order to arrive at a differential diagnosis. The tutor, a teacher who attends the small-group tutorials and facilitates the learning process whenever necessary, may play the role of the patient and be interviewed. Other means can also be used to give students the opportunity to apply the knowledge acquired. Chapter 8 by Schmidt provides a detailed description of this process.

## A Historical Perspective on Problem-based Learning

The problem-based approach was developed in the early 1970s by medical teachers at McMaster's University in Hamilton, Canada, including Howard Barrows, John Evans, and Victor Neufeld.[5] Barrows who has been the most prominent proponent of the method since, writes that in the 1960s he became disappointed with the effectiveness of traditional medical education. Students often appeared to have acquired substantial amounts of knowledge but did not seem to be capable of applying this knowledge when required. He became convinced that medical students should build up and anchor their knowledge around clinical problems. Clinical problems would be formulated as brief descriptions of the complaints and symptoms actually presented by patients to their physicians. It would be the students' task to analyze problems of this kind and to establish what information they would need to solve them. Barrows expected that information from various disciplines would thus be integrated by the learners and that the knowledge structures produced would be "problem centered." He further asserted that this procedure would familiarize students with the physician's reasoning process. Finally, because acquisition of knowledge throughout their study would be self-directed and independent, the problem-based approach would help the students to learn how to detect and fill gaps in their own knowledge. If the process continues after graduation, a positive attitude toward lifelong learning is fostered and coupled to mastery of self-education.

Problem-based learning has borrowed, both in its procedure and in its underlying assumptions, from two somewhat older approaches to education: the *case study* method, practiced at the Harvard Law School,[4] and the *discovery-learning* approach.[3] Barrows' preference for concrete descriptions of patients as a stimulus for learning and his emphasis on the physician's problem-solving competencies as the ultimate goal of medical education appears to be clearly influenced by the case-study method. The emphasis on problem analysis prior to information gathering and the emphasis on self-directed learning activities was strongly influenced by Bruner's views on learning. The *combination* of both approaches makes problem-based learning a unique attempt to solve some of the pressing, persistent problems that plague higher education. Chapter 10 addresses this issue.

At present, problem-based learning in medical education is found in North America at the University of New Mexico, Albuquerque, New Mexico; Mercer University, Macon, Georgia; McMaster University, Hamilton, Ontario; and Harvard University, Boston, Massachusetts. Other schools committed to problem-based learning include Suez Canal University, Egypt; the University of Newcastle, Australia; and the University of Limburg, The Netherlands. The University of Limburg, in addition, has a school of law and faculty of economics that apply problem-based learning in their curricula.

## Overview of Part III

This section opens with a chapter by Henk G. Schmidt, an educational psychologist from the University of Limburg in The Netherlands. Schmidt discusses principles of learning that may apply to problem-based learning. According to Schmidt, problem-based learning is a useful instructional tool because it stimulates students to activate prior knowledge and elaborate on that knowledge, processes considered basic to all forms of cognitive information processing. In addition, he believes that using problems derived from professional practice may encourage an important cognitive process, called "encoding specificity." By means of a tutorial group, working on a problem, he shows to what extent these principles of learning apply to problem-based learning.

The chapter by Roderick Neame, a physiologist at the University of Newcastle, commences with the description of what he sees as some of the major shortcomings of traditional medical education. He argues that traditional education excessively emphasizes tertiary care, neglects the development of attitudes and other personal characteristics among students of medicine, fails in preparing them for continuing education, and lacks a coherent educational philosophy. He then discusses the learning processes of students in a problem-based curriculum and the way in which knowledge from different disciplines is integrated around what he calls "priority" problems. A priority problem is a clinical situation that a newly qualified doctor in contemporary practice should recognize and be able to manage. A problem should be serious, appropriate medical care should be able to play a significant role; it should be common in the community and should have implications for prevention. These "priority" problems should, in Neame's views, present the core of a medical curriculum.

Finally, the late Jack Sibley outlines the curriculum of McMaster Faculty of Health Sciences, the first medical school that implemented the problem-based approach on a large scale. He describes the different "phases" a McMaster's student has to work through and formulates the educational objectives of problem-based learning as an instructional tool. In Sibley's conception, the main objectives are that students learn to identify and define health problems at both an individual and a community level, to examine the underlying physical, biological, and behavioral mechanisms of health problems, to develop the clinical skills and knowledge required to manage health problems of individuals and communities, and to become self-directed learners. Subsequently, he discusses some of the common questions raised by the problem-based approach. Do students really learn science in this way or do they only confront themselves with applied clinical knowledge? Why is integration of knowledge important? Can a problem-solving approach be used in large classes or are small-group tutorials always necessary?

## References

1. Barrows HS: A specific, problem-based, self-directed learning method designed to teach medical problem-solving skills, self-learning skills and enhance knowledge retention and recall, in Schmidt HG, De Volder ML (eds): *Tutorials in Problem-based Learning.* The Netherlands, Assen, Van Gorcum, 1984, pp 16–32.
2. Barrows HS, Tamblyn RM: *Problem-based Learning.* New York, Springer-Verlag, 1980.
3. Bruner JS: Learning and thinking. *Harvard Educ* 1959;29:184–192.
4. Fraser CE: *The Case Method of Instruction.* New York, McGraw-Hill, 1931.
5. Neufeld VR, Barrows HS: The McMaster Philosophy: An approach to medical education. *J Med Educ* 1974;49:1040–1050.
6. Schmidt HG: Problem-based learning: Rationale and description. *Med Educ* 1983; 17:11–16.

# 8
# The Rationale Behind Problem-based Learning*

HENK G. SCHMIDT

The goal of this chapter is to describe the process of problem-based learning in the light of current theories of human information processing. First, three principles of learning are discussed. Second, a detailed account is given of how students transform a problem into a series of learning activities using a systematic working procedure. Finally, the extent to which these activities, undertaken within the problem-based format, fit the principles of learning will be assessed.

## Three Conditions That Facilitate Learning

In order to be able to evaluate the characteristics of problem-based learning a frame of reference is needed. It can be provided by the information processing approach to learning.[1] According to this theory, three principles play a major part in acquiring new information: activation of prior knowledge, encoding specificity and elaboration of knowledge.

1. Learning, by its nature, has a restructuring character. It presupposes earlier knowledge that is used in understanding new information. For instance, by studying an article about defense mechanisms against infections, a student applies knowledge he already possesses in order to understand the new information. A first-year medical student, while reading and interpreting the article, will probably make use of his secondary-school knowledge of biology, perhaps supplemented with common sense knowledge on bacteria, viruses, influenza and vaccinations. A fourth-year student, in studying that article, will use his immunological and microbiological knowledge, acquired earlier. This prior knowledge and the kind of structure in which it is available in long-term memory, will determine what is understood from the article and this, in turn, will define what is learned from it.[1,2] This relationship between prior knowledge and learning could be demonstrated with first- and fourth-year medical students, who read the same article and have the same amount of reading time elaborated prior knowledge

*Parts of this chapter have been published as "Problem-based Learning: Rationale and Description. *J Med Educ* 1983;17:11–16 and are reprinted with permission.

will enable them to process the new information more easily. Instructional methods, however, differ in their capacity to induce activation of relevant prior knowledge.[7] Only in as far as they help students in activating relevant knowledge they will facilitate the processing of new information.[6]

2. The second condition that facilitates learning has been derived from the work of Tulving and Thomson.[14] They state that successful retrieval of information on some point in the future is promoted when the retrieval cues that are to reactivate the information are encoded together with that information. In other words, the closer the resemblance between the situation in which something is learned and the situation in which it is applied, the better the performance. This phenomenon is called *encoding specificity*. It is practiced during clinical lectures or clerkships, where students acquire knowledge related to patient problems that have characteristics in common with what students will encounter in later professional life.

3. The third condition has to do with elaboration of knowledge. Only recently did psychologists discover that information is better understood, processed and retrieved if students have an opportunity to *elaborate* on that information.[3] In education there are many ways in which this condition is fulfilled. Students can elaborate on information by answering questions about a text; by taking notes,[9] by discussing subject matter to be learned with other students,[11] by teaching peers what they have first learned themselves,[4] by writing summaries,[15] and by formulating and criticizing hypotheses about a given problem.[13] According to Reder,[10] elaborations provide redundancy in the memory structure. Redundancy can be viewed as a safe-guard against forgetting and an aid to rapid retrieval.

In conclusion, in order to optimize learning, education should help students in activating relevant prior knowledge, provide a context that resembles the future professional context as closely as possible, and stimulate students to elaborate on their knowledge. If one or more of these conditions are not met, the quality of instruction will suffer.

## Problem-based Learning: Description of the Process

To assess the extent that problem-based learning meets the requirements stated above, it is necessary to take a closer look at it.

The process of problem-based learning starts with a problem such as the following:

A plumber sees his doctor with the following complaint: "During a hard cough this morning I suddenly tasted blood in my mouth. As this has occurred more often these past few weeks, I'm become a bit anxious."

The task of a group of students is to explain these phenomena in terms of underlying processes. Explanations take the form of physical, biological or psycho-social mechanisms that may be underlying the phenomena concerned.

While working on the problem, the study group uses a systematic procedure to analyze the problem, to formulate learning objectives and to collect additional information. This procedure consists of seven steps (Table 8.1).

TABLE 8.1. Steps involved in problem-based learning.

Step 1: Clarify terms and concepts not readily comprehensible.
Step 2: Define the problem.
Step 3: Analyze the problem.
Step 4: Draw a systematic inventory of the explanations inferred from step 3.
Step 5: Formulate learning goals.
Step 6: Collect additional information outside the group.
Step 7: Synthesize and test the newly acquired information.

1. The first activity in relation to any problem should be clarification of terms and concepts not understood on first sight. Use may be made of group members' relevant knowledge. In some instances also a dictionary is of help, whereas in others the first step consists in reaching agreed opinion about the meaning to be attached to the various terms. In the latter case, therefore, the aim is consensus about the interpretation rather than clarification of terms. If a group of students dealing with the "oral blood loss" problem should be unfamiliar with a plumber's duties, the dictionary will inform them that he engages in the "installation and maintenance of water-conduits and sewerage systems in and about the building."

2. The second step aims to produce an exact definition of the problem. The group as a whole has now to reach agreement about which interrelated phenomena should be explained. More often than not problems do not present difficulties in this respect. Occasionally, however, a problem is intentionally structured to tax students about the recognition of symptoms. Some problems consist of a series of secondary, independent problems; these must be identified as such before further completion is possible, i.e. the question to be answered in order to define the problem is: Which phenomena have to be explained?

3. Analysis of the problem calls for careful perusal of the text to gain a clear impression of the situation described, which results in ideas and suppositions about the structure of the problem. These are either based on students' prior knowledge or are the result of rational thought. Hence, analysis of the problem substantially consists in recapitulation of group members' opinions, actual knowledge, and ideas about the underlying processes and mechanisms. The group does not confine itself to activation of prior knowledge ("I've read somewhere that . . ."), but also tries to formulate relevant hypotheses by reasoning ("Could it be that. . .?").

Most of the time a kind of free association-round is held, in which each individual is allowed to verbalize ideas freely before the ideas, knowledge and suppositions are scrutinized, accepted, complemented or modified. This procedure is often referred to as the "brainstorming" technique. Application of analytical efforts of this kind to the oral blood loss problem may yield the following line of thought, illustrated by a verbatim transcript of an actual problem-analysis by a group of Dutch first-year medical students.

Could we have a case of lung cancer here? The site of origin of the oral blood need not be the lungs at all. Injury in the throat or in the mouth itself may have occurred. But how?

(Coughing subjects blood vessels to a pressure increase: people who cough vigorously often turn red in the face. Does that not point to a ruptured vessel? For that matter, why does one cough? The reason may be the presence of an irritant in the air passages, an inspired peanut, or phlegm. Coughing is a reflex mechanism for clearing the respiratory tract and expelling foreign bodies.

People suffering from tuberculosis sometimes cough up blood. The plumber has now had this for 2 weeks, the oral blood loss, I mean. I wonder if he has actually been coughing much longer. Perhaps he is a smoker. But why this blood? I can imagine that the sudden explosive expulsion of a stream of air results in such a high air pressure that something gets damaged. A tumor? It might well be the obstruction creating the coughing stimulus. Being a plumber, he frequently works in draughty rooms and spaces. He may also have caught a severe cold then, an inflammation of the mucous membrane in the respiratory system caused by a virus or something similar. In my opinion, certain glands in the mucous membrane secrete an abnormal amount of mucus to protect the body against the virus. But what about the blood?

By the way, cancer of the lung is a growth of malignant cells, malignant lung tissue. It expands in the lungs, so that they can no longer function properly. Well, I am not sure about the exact process. Tuberculosis? That is a disease brought about by the tubercle bacillus. A type of inflammation of the lungs.

4. In the fourth step a summary is produced of the various explanations of the problem. In the above analysis, several general descriptions of biological phenomena were advanced. The first one relates to the students' ideas about the origin of the coughing ("a reflex mechanism activated to clear the respiratory tract and expel obstructions"). The second covers the possible connection between coughing and a bleeding ("I can imagine that the sudden explosive expulsion of a stream of air results in such a high air pressure that something gets damaged"). The other descriptions refer to the many obstructions that may affect the air passages ("inflammation of the mucous membrane," "cancer of the lungs," "tuberculosis"). The systematic inventory might yield the scheme shown in Figure 8.1.

A representation such as this acts as a summary and structures the product of the problem-analysis.

The point is now reached when the assumed processes and mechanisms referred to in the analysis are to be studied more extensively. To what degree can the expressed knowledge and ideas be considered correct and complete? Study priorities have to be established because, as a rule, there is not enough time to pay adequate attention to all aspects involved.

5. The fifth step, therefore, requires formulation of learning objectives. These are the answers to the questions evoked by the problem analysis phase, to gain a more profound knowledge of the processes forming the crux of the problem. In the example cited the following questions might arise:

What physiological mechanisms are involved in the coughing reflex?
In what way does draught affect the air passages?
How does bleeding result from coughing?
What causes mucous membranes to become inflamed and what does the membrane look like in this state?

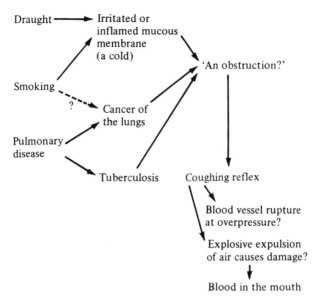

FIGURE 8.1. Schematic presentation of the oral blood loss problem.

What is the effect of smoking on the respiratory tract?
What is lung cancer?
What is tuberculosis?

 The group selects the objectives on which it will concentrate its activities and, if necessary, agrees on a distribution of tasks. Finally, it tries to find out which learning resources might supply the required answers.

 6. The sixth step consists of individual study. The group members individually collect information with respect to the learning objectives. The source explored may be literature, but other tools may also serve. For instance, audiovisual aids might be employed. Experts can be consulted about aspects of the problem not yet clarified.

 7. The process of problem-based learning is completed by synthesizing and testing the newly acquired information. The students inform one another about their individual findings, supplement this knowledge, and correct it where necessary. It is then established whether the group is now capable of giving more detailed descriptions of the fundamental processes causing the problem. Often new questions are proposed in the course of this exchange of information. In that case the group may decide to take up again the process of problem-based learning—now at a deeper level of understanding—starting with the fourth step. However, it may prove equally effective in that phase to exploit the newly acquired knowledge by tackling a different, though related, problem in order to find out whether the group can now perform the analytical and explanatory task in a faster and better way.

## Discussion

In the first section of this chapter, it was stated that instructional methods should stimulate students by activating relevant prior knowledge, providing a learning setting as similar as possible to the setting in which the acquired knowledge is to be used (encoding specificity), and by giving students opportunities to elaborate on their knowledge. Does problem-based learning meet these conditions?

To meet the requirement that problem-based learning should lead to the activation of relevant prior knowledge, attention must be paid to the characteristics of the problems being used. Written problems will activate relevant prior knowledge only if they have the following features:

1. They should consist of a neutral description of an event or a set of phenomena that are in need of explanation in terms of underlying processes, principles or mechanisms.
2. They actually do have to lead to problem-solving activity. If students are asked to study "the heat-regulating mechanism of the human body," this task will not lead to activities such as described in the preceding section. But the following problem will do so: "You have been playing a game of tennis. You've a red face and are wet all over your body. How can these phenomena be explained?"
3. Problems have to be formulated as concretely as possible.
4. Problems should have a degree of complexity adapted to students' prior knowledge. If a problem is not complex enough, it will not be recognized as a problem. If it is too complex, students will think that it is no use trying to solve it.

The second condition that facilitates learning (encoding specificity) is met by the problem-based learning approach insofar as problems are used that have a close resemblance to problems that students will come across in later professional life. Barrows and Tamblyn[5] and Neame[8] further specify this condition by proposing that problems should be chosen:

5. That have the greatest frequency in the usual practical setting.
6. That represent life-threatening or urgent situations.
7. That have a potentially serious outcome, in terms of morbidity or mortality, in which intervention—preventive or therapeutic—can make a significant difference in prognosis.
8. That are most often poorly handled by doctors in the community.

The third facilitating condition, giving students opportunities to elaborate on their knowledge, is augmented during group discussion, when students provide each other with opportunities for amplification and change of existing knowledge structures. When students try to explain the blood loss problem by hypothesizing possible processes responsible for the phenomena observed, they are not merely reproducing knowledge acquired at some point in the past. They are using this knowledge as "stuff for thinking." In doing so, previously unrelated concepts become connected in memory, newly produced insights change the structure of their cognition, and information supplied by peers is added. The same applies to the last step of the problem-based learning procedure where newly acquired information is exchanged, critically discussed and eventually applied. These are the activities that can be viewed as elaboration processes.

In conclusion, problem-based medical education at least carries the promise of providing students with a learning environment more adapted to their needs and more in line with principles of learning, than conventional education usually has to offer.

## References

1. Anderson RC: The notion of schemata and the educational enterprise: general discussion of the conference, in Anderson RC, Spiro RJ, Montague WE (eds): *Schooling and the Acquisition of Knowledge.* Hillsdale, NJ: Erlbaum, 1977.
2. Anderson RC, Biddle WB: On asking people questions about what they are reading, in Bower GH (ed): *The Psychology of Learning and Motivation*, Vol 9. New York, Academic Press, 1975.
3. Anderson JR, Reder LM: An elaborative processing explanation of depth of processing, in Cermak LS, Craik FM (eds): *Levels of Processing in Human Memory.* Hillsdale, NJ: Erlbaum, 1979.
4. Bargh JA, Schul Y: On the cognitive benefits of teaching. *J Educ Psych* 1980;72: 593–604.
5. Barrows HS, Tamblyn RM: *Problem-based Learning*. New York, Springer Publishing, 1980.
6. Mayer RE: Instructional variables in text processing, in Flammer A, Kintsch W (eds): *Discourse Processing.* Amsterdam, North-Holland Publishing Company, 1982.
7. Mayer RE, Greeno JG: Structural differences between learning outcomes produced by different instructional methods. *J Educ Psych* 1972;63:165–173.
8. Neame RLB: How to: construct a problem-based course. *Medical Teacher* 1981; 3:94–99.
9. Peper RJ, Mayer RE: Note taking as a generative activity. *J Educ Psych* 1978;70:514–522.
10. Reder LM: The role of elaboration in the comprehension and retention of prose: a critical review. *Rev Educ Res* 1980;5:5–53.
11. Rudduck J: Learning through small group discussion. *Society for Research into Higher Education*, Guildford, England, 1978.
12. Rumelhart DE, Ortony E: The representation of knowledge in memory, in Anderson RC, Spiro RJ, Montague WE (eds): *Schooling and the acquisition of knowledge.* Hillsdale, NJ: Erlbaum, 1977.
13. Schmidt HG: Activation and restructuring of prior knowledge and their effects on text processing, in Flammer A, Kintsch W (eds): *Discourse Processing.* Amsterdam, North-Holland Publishing Company, 1982.
14. Tulving E, Thomson DM: Encoding specificity and retrieval processes in episodic memory. *Psych Rev* 1973;80:352–373.
15. Wittrock MC: Learning as a generative process. *Educ Psych* 1974;11:87–95.

# 9
# Problem-based Medical Education: The Newcastle Approach

RODERICK L.B. NEAME

There have been radical changes in the patterns of disease in the community, in life style, and in the structure of society in recent years. Indeed the principal causes of morbidity and mortality today are quite different from those of 50 years ago. Over a similar period there have been major advances in the science and technology of education. There has also been a massive expansion of knowledge relating to medicine, components of which have been included in curricula, often by simple addition without deletion of less relevant material. The predominant causes of illness today in industrialized nations are related to life style, behavior, the environment, substance abuse, and socioeconomic status,[1] yet these areas are grossly underrepresented in conventional curricula.

There is a pressing need today for doctors to become involved in primary care and rural practice, and to show active interest in cost containment and disease prevention. Their training, however, prepares them far better for careers in tertiary care, urban practice, and curative medicine, and there is little evidence of significant emphasis on cost containment. Frequent reviews of medical education, starting from that of Flexner,[2] have pointed out defects in the conventional system. Many authors[3-5] have highlighted the fact that there is little if any correlation between success in medical school examinations and in the subsequent clinical environment. Such findings, however, have been ineffective in bringing about significant change in the process of medical education.

To the scientist there is but one logical conclusion. Conventional medical education is not specifically related to community health needs, future clinical practice, or prevailing disease patterns.

This chapter identifies some of the principal problems and deficiencies of conventional approaches to medical education and outlines an integrated curriculum based entirely on clinical problems designed to overcome these problems, from both philosophical and practical points of view.

## Problems of Conventional Medical Education

There have been numerous reviews of medical education that have identified shortcomings of the existing system and have outlined directions for the future.[6-10] A recent in-depth study[11] of the conventional structure of preclinical studies concludes: "there is little evidence that the existing preclinical courses are essential to high quality medical practice; mastery of them seems to confer little benefit." Some of the issues that have been of particular significance in the development of the philosophy of the medical school at Newcastle, New South Wales, are summarized in the following paragraphs.

1. *Philosophy.* There is all too often no coherent philosophy behind an offered course.* There is therefore no basis on which to decide what material to present, in what way, or when. Without a philosophy there can be no coherent basis for planning, and the curriculum inevitably becomes a goalless sequence of disjointed experiences strung together through ad hoc decisions based on educationally irrelevant or counterproductive considerations.

2. *Objectives.* Many courses have no stated objectives. Frequently neither staff nor students are able to determine how the segments relate to clinical practice. In addition, when students do not know what is expected of them, objectiveless courses give rise to extreme anxiety when assessment looms near. There is often no need to do much more than present students with objectives for them to learn: stating objectives detracts nothing from their importance. Rather, it reveals them for discussion and improvement.

3. *Aims.* The stated or implicit goals of most conventional schools are oriented almost exclusively toward content, factual knowledge, or technical skill. Little systematic attempt is made to develop understanding, help students learn how to use knowledge, and develop the areas of knowledge relating to clinical reasoning, problem-solving, and other process skills essential to the effective practice of medicine.

4. *Assessment.* Assessment is usually based on factual recall, thus reinforcing the students' tendency to concentrate on rote learning of lists, rather than development of understanding and the ability to use information appropriately.

5. *Noncognitive attributes.* Little emphasis is placed on defining or developing desirable noncognitive characteristics in the students. Such areas as professionalization, management skills, attitudes, and personal characteristics are all but ignored.

6. *Relevance.* Some of the material included in the medical curriculum is of doubtful relevance to achieving the goals of undergraduate medical education because it is too detailed or specialized, of questionable validity, or outside the appropriate boundaries of a medical curriculum.

7. *Timing.* Much of the remaining material is presented to the students with inappropriate timing. That is, material is presented at a time when the students can appreciate neither its significance to clinical practice nor its importance or relevance. The best time to learn about fluid movements and edema, for example, is when confronted by a patient with pitting ankle edema or ascites.

8. *Subject and time allocation by discipline.* The traditional and long-established disciplines (e.g., anatomy, biochemistry, surgery) retain the lion's

---

*The term "course" is used here to signify curriculum rather than a single course (meaning a related sequence on one subject).

share of the curriculum. The newer disciplines (e.g., immunology, community medicine, general practice, behavioral science, and clinical epidemiology), whose importance to contemporary practice is undisputed, received relatively small allocations of curricular time.

9. *Fragmentation*. The autonomous discipline approach to medicine dictates that the student receive fragmentary and unintegrated training. Student knowledge is conceptualized along disciplinary lines without a clinical frame of reference. One cannot reasonably expect a student to integrate in his or her head the extensive knowledge acquired piecemeal. Particularly when the teachers do not do this, do not indicate that integration of knowledge is important, and make no attempt to assess other than in a disciplinary fashion. Integration requires collaboration and coordination. Frequently academics are unable to collaborate with their own peers.

10. *Interdisciplinary areas*. One special consequence of the disciplinary approach to education is that interdisciplinary areas (e.g., life style-related illness, substance abuse, environmental illness), which are of enormous importance in society, are largely ignored.

11. *Tertiary bias*. Tertiary care is normally given strong emphasis by basing activities in or around a tertiary care institution; by exposing students exclusively, primarily, or preferentially to tertiary care role models; and by having few if any primary care staff members. When aspiring to model their own professional activities on those of such teachers, several things happen. They become dependent on the logistic support of a major hospital. They are indoctrinated with the testing style of practice. Thus primary care loses credibility as a career choice except among the most humanistic or contrary students. Such attitudes are subsequently difficult to erase.

12. *Process skills*. The didactic instructional style fosters the unthinking and noncritical acceptance of material presented. Little attempt is made to promote active learning, which has significant advantages as an educational strategy over passive learning, or to inculcate an attitude of responsibility for the students' own learning.

13. *Clinical reasoning*. The skill of clinical reasoning similarly receives little systematic attention. Many clinicians believe that it is an art or a skill that is innate and cannot be learned. This view has little to recommend it and certainly is not supported by studies of reasoning. Educationally, the main problem seems to be the lack of an appropriate model of clinical reasoning to use as a basis for development of educational experiences, for assessment of students, and for feedback on their performance.

14. *Continuing education*. One of the challenges of professional education today is to prepare the graduate for a lifetime of continuing education. Much knowledge acquired as an undergraduate is soon proved inaccurate and out of date. New information is rapidly generated. Graduates must be able to keep up with the changes. They need to know how and be willing to continue to learn.

15. *Evaluation*. Perhaps the most distressing failure of conventional schools is their lack of interest in systematic evaluation. Without information on what is actually taking place in the school (education, research, and service), there is no

rational basis from which to plan change. Without information on health care, manpower, disease, and the external environment, there is no basis from which to select the changes that are desirable. Without objectives, there is no yardstick by which to measure achievement of aims.

The above briefly outlines some of the cogent reasons for seeking a new approach to medical education. Conventional approaches are wanting. Their deficiency becomes greater, not less, with the passage of time because their management and organizational patterns are all too often inappropriate to their needs, are inflexible, and have consistently failed to adapt to changing patterns of society, disease, and student need.[12-13]

## Systematic Development of a Curriculum

Implicit in the preceding analysis of the deficiencies of conventional medical education are the desirable features that a curriculum should exhibit. Many groups in society have legitimate concerns about the characteristics of doctors: government departments (health, economy, education), the medical profession, allied health professions, community health care consumers, medical academics, universities, and so on. When planning the curriculum at the University of Newcastle, Australia, information from all of these groups was obtained by a Delphi questionnaire technique. This information was then synthesized into aims for the faculty. Thereafter the input of community groups has been maintained through their involvement in all major decision-making bodies of the Faculty.

In a series of working papers[14] the goals, aims, philosophy, and policies of the Faculty were initially elaborated between 1975 and 1979 initially by Founding Dean David Maddison and subsequently by those of the foundation staff present on campus. These working papers emphasized a logical and systematic approach to development and implementation of all Faculty activities. Far from being a fossil record, they are looked on as statements of intent, and are amended and extended as operational circumstances require. The development of a coherent educational philosophy and of objectives, research and professional service programs that link the school explicitly with the community, appropriate staff recruitment and student selection policies, and many other highly relevant issues are discussed and stressed in these documents.

The systematic approach to undergraduate educational activities is outlined in Figure 9.1. The sequential phases of planning, implementation, and evaluation are represented as descending the figure: The review phase completes the iterative cycle. The aim is demonstration by the students that they have achieved the objectives; learning and assessment are therefore products of the same educational objectives. Student competence is certified in the context of these objectives. The effort that goes into specifying the objectives is therefore thrice justified. The program objectives are the basis of student learning, certification of competence, and program evaluation and review.

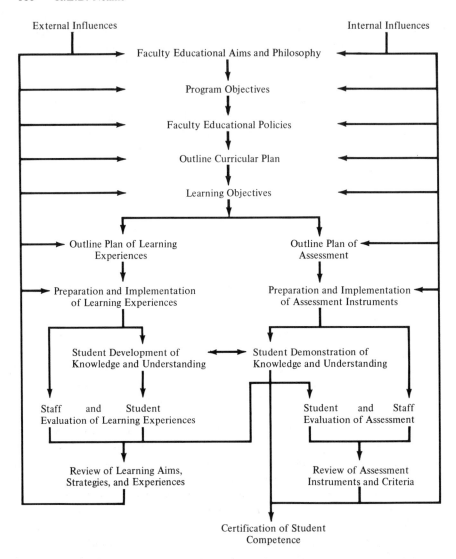

External Influences                                                          Internal Influences

Faculty Educational Aims and Philosophy

Program Objectives

Faculty Educational Policies

Outline Curricular Plan

Learning Objectives

Outline Plan of Learning                         Outline Plan of
Experiences                                      Assessment

Preparation and Implementation                   Preparation and Implementation
of Learning Experiences                          of Assessment Instruments

Student Development of          Student Demonstration of
Knowledge and Understanding     Knowledge and Understanding

Staff      and      Student                      Student    and    Staff
Evaluation of Learning Experiences               Evaluation of Assessment

Review of Learning Aims,                         Review of Assessment
Strategies, and Experiences                      Instruments and Criteria

Certification of Student
Competence

FIGURE 9.1.

Initially, the 45 objectives for the Undergraduate Medical Program, specified in Working Paper VI, were divided into six domains. These had to do with the students' own learning (Nos. 1–6), scientific method and procedure (Nos. 7–9), clinical diagnosis, investigation and management (Nos. 10–23), attitudes and personal characteristics (Nos. 24–26), community medicine (Nos. 27–40), and the doctor–patient relationship (Nos. 41–45).

As a result of detailed review, in 1985 a revised set of Programme Objectives was drafted (Working Paper XVII), reaffirming the commitment of the Faculty to the original goals, but making minor amendments to them in the light of experience. The objectives were reassorted and the original 6 domains were altered to 5 of more equal size. These related to professional skills, relationships, and communications (Nos. 1–14), critical reasoning in medical care (Nos. 15–20), identification, prevention, and management of illness (Nos. 21–32), population medicine (Nos. 33–41), and self-directed learning (Nos. 41–45).

These domains of objectives provide a clear statement from the Faculty identifying those areas that are considered professionally essential. This emphasis is reflected in the assessment policies of the Faculty, which require that every student demonstrates competence in every domain in order to graduate. Excellence in one domain cannot compensate for deficiency in another. Within each area the objectives are interdisciplinary, laying considerable emphasis on the development of algorithmic knowledge, i.e., the knowledge that constitutes the "driver" program or organizer whereby factual information can be applied and used. Thus the emphasis is on clinical competence rather than on the underpinning basic knowledge itself.

Further documents outline the educational framework and strategies (No. IX), assessment practices (Nos. I and X), and use of problem solving (No. XI). Great emphasis is placed on integration between disciplines and between years. The use of small groups is also elaborated, as is the emphasis on development of skills in relation to teacher-independent learning and clinical reasoning. The vital role of program evaluation is stressed through establishment of a group responsible for this function (together with a resource function for medical education) and the specification of how the data obtained are to be used.

## Problem-based Learning: An Educational Strategy

The concept of a problem-based approach to learning in medicine has previously been outlined: the general conceptual basis is well covered by Barrows and Tamblyn,[15] and this is supplemented by a further volume on operational issues.[16] The Faculty of Medicine adopted this educational strategy because the aims and goals elaborated by the Faculty, which were based partly on a recognition of the deficiencies of conventional schools, would not be as easy to achieve by any other approach.

Among the many potential advantages that were anticipated from the successful development of a course based on problems, which was integrated and community-oriented, were the following:

1. The relevance, importance, and significance of all material studied is at once clear to both staff and students, as it derives from a clinical problem and the students chose it for its ability to contribute to the understanding and management of a clinical issue.

2. The emphasis placed on each discipline is directly related to its ability to contribute relevant, important, and significant knowledge to each problem. There is no fixed allocation of student time to disciplines.

3. Interdisciplinary collaboration is enhanced, as every discipline is preparing and implementing material related to the same problem at the same time. Additional management strategies to promote and reinforce horizontal communication and involvement have been adopted as well.

4. Students are actively involved in their own learning. They are required to accept progressively greater and greater responsibility for initiating, defining, and researching their own learning and for applying it to the patient under study.

5. Students learn how to learn and how to structure their own learning, thereby acquiring tools essential for their continuing education. Students are exposed also to the process and strategies of clinical reasoning, from the earliest point in their training through the structuring of the clinical problems.

6. Students are exposed to information in the clinical context, thus promoting conceptualization and storage of that information in the framework within which they will subsequently be retrieving it for clinical use.

7. Having learned material, students immediately have the opportunity to apply their knowledge. Such application reinforces it and gives it algorithmic association.

8. Students are exposed from the earliest point in their training to patients, to the clinical context, and to the patient care environment. This exposure enhances their enthusiasm and motivation.

An educational strategy alone, however, is inadequate to overcome all the deficiencies associated with conventional course of study. For example, to ensure a proper orientation to the community, problems are selected to represent every facet of the health care system from hospital, primary care, health center, industrial clinic, domiciliary care, and any others that are relevant. Likewise, the tutors with whom the students work are drawn from varied clinical backgrounds, including physicians, veterinarians, dentists, and others. All tutors are carefully prepared for their educational roles before every academic session, and their performance is monitored to ensure that it is consistent with the goals of the course. Student assessment is geared less to simple possession of knowledge than to demonstration of clinical competence and application of that knowledge to the patient problems. Finally, regular review of every aspect of Faculty activities is carried out by students and staff to ensure quality control, to maintain program relevance and flexibility, and to improve student and staff satisfaction. As a result of this review process, a range of deficiencies of the curriculum have been identified some of which are reviewed elsewhere.[17] This has resulted in a greatly modified and improved educational program introduced from 1985.

## Objectives

Objectives have been prepared for the course at a number of levels of detail (Fig. 9.2). They serve the aims of ensuring that (1) staff know what is and should be covered in each part of the course, and (2) students know what it is that they need to study and what their subsequent assessments will be based on. Thus to

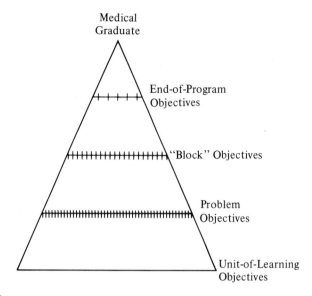

FIGURE 9.2.

the students, objectives act as learning contracts. These objectives are action-oriented. They specify skills the student should be able to demonstrate. They cover not only the propositional knowledge that is the preserve of the traditional disciplines but also propositional and algorithmic knowledge relating to process skills, attitudes, behaviors, and patient contact skills (e.g., physical examination). Each objective at a lower level (Fig. 9.2) is designed to help the student achieve a specific objective on the level above, thereby ensuring that even at the most detailed level of the learning units there is a direct relevance of the material to the goals of the program.

## Curricular Structure

Rather than the conventional curricular plan of a number of discipline-based courses running in series and in parallel, a more integrated approach to learning is required. The curriculum has therefore been divided up into a sequence of integrated units or blocks each based on a single theme. The themes have been selected to be organ–system units and/or medical specialties, each lasting for between 5 and 10 weeks. The sequence of blocks is indicated in Figure 9.3. These blocks constitute the horizontal integration within the curriculum, since the material studied within each block relates to the same functional system.

Running longitudinally through the curriculum are four main "strands" of activities, distinguished by the differing types of skills they aim to develop and the differing learning environments within which they take place. Three of these strands—working problems, professional skills, and population medicine—run

| Phase and Title | Year | Term | Outline of Content |
|---|---|---|---|
| I: Introduction | | 1 | Overview of scope of medicine<br>Introduction to problem-solving, small groups, and assessment |
| II: Problems in the adult | 1 | 2 | Acute interruption of function from traumatic and psychosocial causes |
| | | 3 | Problems relating to the renal and gastrointestinal systems |
| | | 4 | Problems relating to the respiratory and cardiovascular systems |
| | 2 | 5 | Problems relating to the musculoskeletal, hemopoietic, and endocrine systems |
| | | 6 | Problems relating to the nervous system |
| III: Problems in the adult (cont'd) | 3 | 7 | Problems relating to the skin, ear, nose, throat, and sexuality |
| | | 8 | Acute emergencies and problems relating to eyes |
| | | 9 | Multisystem disease and chronic systems failure |
| | | 10 | Elective |
| IV: Problems of growth and aging | 4 | 11 | Elective |
| | | 12 | Problems relating to reproduction and early development |
| | | 13 | Problems relating to children and adolescents |
| | | 14 | Problems relating to aging and terminal care |
| V: Integrated practice | 5 | 15 | Problems relating to all aspects of medicine (half-time) centered around a "theme of the week" |
| | | 16 | |
| | | 17 | Junior Intern on rotation of clinical attachments (half-time) |
| | | 18 | |

FIGURE 9.3.

concurrently and are coordinated, with a particularly close association between the first two. The fourth strand—elective studies—is intermittent and normally remains temporally distinct from the others.

In broad terms, the working problems strand offers the students an opportunity to develop the biomedical, pathophysiological, and psychosocial knowledge base that underpins an understanding of medical practice. This knowledge is developed within a functional structure and in the context of its application to selected clinical problems as outlined above: this is in marked contrast to the normal disciplinary structure of learning. The working problems are studied primarily in the tutorial room, in small groups of 8 students with a tutor. In years 4 and 5 of the curriculum, the knowledge base continues to be developed through problem-based learning at the bedside, as well as through a sequence of weekly seminars on integrated topics. The professional skills strand, by contrast, has as its goal the development of cognitive and psychomotor skills relating to patient contact. This includes interviewing, communication, physical examination, and professional behavior, as well as some additional clinical expertise. Professional skills activities take place largely in the various clinical environments of the health care system, hospital wards, clinics, private practices and health centers, and the students work in smaller groups of 1 to 4. The skill of clinical reasoning is shared between these strands and serves conceptually to unite their styles and activities.

The population medicine strand concentrates on development of knowledge and skills related to the community. This involves both the use of problems about community and group problems (e.g., environmental, epidemic, occupational, statistical) as well as activities in the community (e.g., surveys, interventions). Placing the problems of individuals in the community context, and understanding the epidemiological perspective and the role of risk factors. Students work mainly in groups of 8 with a tutor. The goals of elective studies are to develop the skills of the student to learn and work responsibly and independently, as well as to develop expertise in areas of special interest. Both short (1–2 weeks) and long (8–10 weeks) elective periods exist: short electives may be taken whenever the student has satisfactorily completed studies for that academic session, while long electives are scheduled twice in the latter part of the course. Each elective requires a contract stating the goals, methods, place, and anticipated outcome of the study, together with the method of assessment, and is signed jointly by supervisor and student before being approved by the electives committee.

The curriculum may be viewed as a model (Fig. 9.4) in which the vertical axis denotes the passage of time and the sequence of blocks through which the students pass. Each discipline and resource area is developed cumulatively throughout the whole 5-year program. Their individual contributions to each block are coordinated by the objectives and scope of each block, thus forming the horizontal integration of the curriculum.

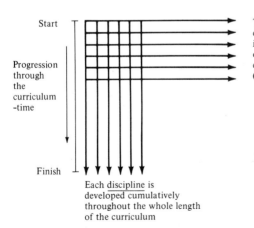

The contributions of each of the disciplines are coordinated and integrated through clinical problems organized into blocks of learning, each of which has a common theme (e.g., organ-system)

Start

Progression through the curriculum -time

Finish

Each discipline is developed cumulatively throughout the whole length of the curriculum

FIGURE 9.4.

## Using Problems for Learning

There is often confusion about the terms "problem-based learning" and "problem solving." They both may occur in the context of the same problem, or they may be separated in time and place. However, it is essential to appreciate that simple exposure of students to problems is unlikely to achieve any significant development of independent learning or clinical reasoning skills. The learning experiences have to be designed, developed and implemented with the specific intention of developing knowledge and process skills.

The process of problem-based learning can be considered as any situation where a problem gives rise to the development of knowledge and understanding. When confronted by such a clinical problem, as well as developing knowledge, the students may also be expected to find their way toward the "solution" to the problem, both to the diagnosis and to the management plan and strategy. This is termed "problem solving." Similarly, when confronted by a clinical problem which he or she is expected to "solve" the student may discover a topic about which his or her knowledge is defective. This may lead the student to learn. Problem-based learning and problem solving are, therefore, terms that express the intentions of the teacher and may result in a reordering of the priorities ascribed to the possible outcomes (Figs. 9.5 and 9.6): the purposes of such sessions must be clearly conveyed to the student if the strategy is to be educationally successful.

It is possible to develop a model for problem-based learning as illustrated in Figure 9.7. In effect, this was the model adopted in Newcastle from 1978 until 1984 (Mark 1 curriculum). Here, the sequence of trigger materials is shown on the left of the figure. Each trigger is designed to initiate certain actions and discussions in the student group (center column), and anticipates certain learning outcomes (right column). As a model for problem-based learning it was quite

| Problem-based Learning | | |
| --- | --- | --- |
| Input | Process | Outcome |
| Trigger material on patient problem | Students hypothesize, analyze, discuss, etc., using existing, often limited, knowledge base | 1. Define and undertake further learning necessary for understanding: apply to this (and other) problem(s)<br>2. Suggest next step in clinical encounter<br>3. Practice process of clinical reasoning<br>4. Practice process of structuring learning |

FIGURE 9.5.

| Problem Solving | | |
| --- | --- | --- |
| Input | Process | Outcome |
| Trigger material on patient problem | Students hypothesize, analyze, discuss, etc., using existing knowledge base and experience of clinical reasoning process | 1. Determine next question/action in clinical encounter<br>2. Define topics where knowledge is weak or inadequate<br>3. Reach diagnosis and formulate plan of management<br>4. Consolidate processes of clinical reasoning and independent learning |

FIGURE 9.6.

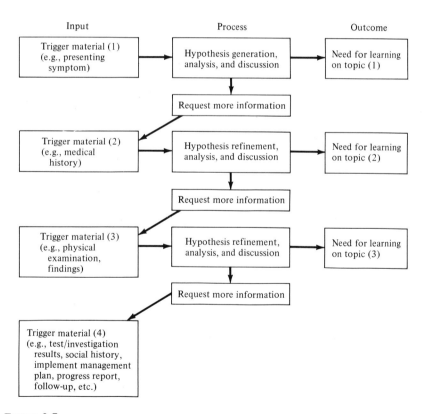

FIGURE 9.7.

acceptable. Problems were clearly structured and organized. However, in the following section, some implications of this Mark 1 problem structure for the development of process skills will be considered.

## Learning Process Skills

The Undergraduate Program Objectives specify several attributes that relate to the willingness and ability of the students to reason effectively and efficiently in the clinical context, and to take responsibility for their own learning independent of their tutors. These goals have very significant implications for the ways in which the learning experiences have to be developed and implemented: some aspects of the way in which independent learning skills are developed in the students are discussed by Neame and Powis.[18]

Clinical reasoning is viewed by the Faculty as being the central and uniting thread of the curriculum. Considerable effort has been expended in developing a functional model of the process and developing problems to conform with this model.

## The Mark 1 Curriculum

Early attempts at developing both clinical reasoning and independent learning were not as successful as had been hoped: certain of the difficulties with this Mark 1 problem structure have been outlined by Neame.[17] Two specific aspects of problem development are outlined briefly here. The first is that the early problems were of a "lock-step" structure. The materials through which the problem was developed were presented to the group as a series of handouts (or in other forms) and the order of these was predetermined. This approach is illustrated diagrammatically in Figure 9.7. The group knew that they would be getting the next handout however much or little discussion they did. Students became discouraged from taking too active a part because often the succeeding handout was inconsistent with the direction of their discussions and the perceived needs of the group. Consequently, the groups preferred to react to the handouts, rather than trying to structure the problem for themselves and think proactively about what items of information they would require in order to diagnose and manage the problem. In Figure 9.7, the boxes marked "Request for more information" were being omitted by the students.

The second main defect of the Mark 1 problem development was that the learning materials prepared by the staff to accompany each problem were extensive, amounting to a problem-based textbook prepared by the Faculty. In effect, the staff had transferred their educational input from the conventional didactic lectures and tutorials into their written equivalent. Furthermore, the students received these materials regardless of whether or not they perceived the need for them. Often, parts of the learning materials students received were unrelated to the learning objectives identified by that group. Consequently, the groups expended decreasing effort in identifying learning objectives for study as they worked through the problem and preferred to wait for the prepared materials to be handed to them.

## The Mark 2 Curriculum

Since 1985, a Mark 2 curriculum has been introduced, starting with year 1 in 1985, year 2 in 1986, and so on. The fifth and final year of the Mark 2 curriculum should commence in 1989. This Mark 2 curriculum introduces several major changes, based on experiences with the Mark 1 curriculum. The more significant of these changes are outlined as follows.

The first change relates to the nature of the "trigger" material that is used to present the problem to the students and of the hypotheses expected to result from that trigger. In the Mark 1 curriculum trigger material was often quite detailed and specific, such that few hypotheses were tenable from this early stage of the problem. The hypothesis generation stage was, therefore, restricted. In the Mark 2 curriculum, this stage, which is seen as crucial to the proper development of both reasoning and knowledge, has been expanded by deliberately limiting the detail given in the trigger material. Because of the scarcity of clinical detail, the hypotheses generated must be broad and encompassing, based on the major or pivotal components of the complaint and symptoms.

Emphasis is placed in the Mark 2 curriculum on basic mechanisms of disease at this stage. Hence, confronted by a patient with a swollen ankle, the students should generate hypotheses of the type:

Increased lymphatic pressure (e.g., lymphatic blockage)
Increased interstitial osmotic pressure due to capillary protein leakage (e.g., vas-
    culitis) or cellular constituents leakage (e.g., cellulitis, cell lysis)
Decreased plasma protein osmotic pressure (e.g., liver failure)

By contrast, in the Mark 1 curriculum for the same presentation, an hypothesis set as below might have been acceptable:

Bee sting
Sprained ankle
Neoplasm
Cardiac failure
Dietary deficiency

This leads directly to the second major difference. At this early stage in the problem, the learning that is identified as required by the group in the Mark 2 curriculum relates to basic pathophysiological and psychosocial mechanisms of disease, which is seen as one of the prime goals of medical education. By contrast, the Mark 1 curriculum tended to restrict and confine learning to the specific condition on which the problem was based.

This has been further promoted by a change in the way in which learning is specified. The Mark 1 curriculum specified traditional learning objectives. While valuable as a statement of intent, these became too prescriptive and restricting: the students began using these as the definition of the "real" curriculum, thus degrading the value of the problems as the focus and catalyst to learning. Many learning objectives seemed to have little relevance to the problem and were little more than disciplinary statements of their expectations.

The Mark 2 curriculum states the required learning in the form of "goals": these define the functional issues that must be resolved in order to progress with this problem, and so lead directly to applied and integrated learning. A learning goal, might, for example, be:

How do proteins enter and leave the interstitial fluid?
Which particles contribute most to the osmotic pressure?

In turn, this leads directly to the third major change, which relates to the nature of the learning materials provided to the students. The Mark 1 curriculum provided every student with extensive reading material giving detailed insights into the objectives identified by staff. The Mark 2 curriculum does away with this, on the basis that these learning materials constitute little more than lectures in another format and give little real learning independence to the students. The sheer quantity and complexity of the learning material presented to the students tended to ensure that its purpose and conceptual significance was lost in the wealth of detail, and that little understanding resulted.

The Mark 2 curriculum substitutes learning goal "overviews." These are designed to present, in 1 to 2 pages of typescript, a conceptual overview of that goal, with sufficient detail only to enable the student to find his/her own further reading material. Thereafter, the onus is on the student to research the area, using the available resources (library, staff, colleagues) and to generate a summary for presentation to the group on the outcomes of this research and the way it impinges upon the problem. In earlier years and problems, some suggested references may be provided: later in the course, the students are left entirely to their own devices. The quality of learning is checked in subsequent group meetings, where students report back and try to use their learning in the context of the problem. Thus, every group and every individual learns different details from different sources at different times, but the end result of this independent learning, overall, should differ by little.

Returning to the group session, the next major change relates to the way in which patient information is gathered by the students. The Mark 1 curriculum had them receiving quanta of data in a fixed sequence in the form of printed handouts. This is clearly inconsistent with any proactive model of reasoning, and the lock-step nature of this process tended to inhibit any real development of reasoning skills: the group simply waited for the next handout, and drew inferences from it, rather than trying to impose their own control on the flow and capture of patient data. The Mark 2 curriculum has no fixed order of data acquisition or prepared sequences of handouts. Patient data are available from and through the tutor, who is provided with information sheets listing all relevant details. The data are only provided to the students when the group has identified, item by item, what it thinks is required to execute its strategic enquiry about the source and nature of the patient problem. The data are released to the group as they identify a need. This places emphasis on the tutor as an information broker.

This leads directly on to the last major change introduced in the Mark 2 curriculum—relating to the role and activities of the tutor. The Mark 1 curriculum created the myth of the "nonexpert" tutor: tutors found themselves on occasion completely ignorant of the content and thus custodians solely of the process, unable to identify major conceptual errors or defects, and unable to offer specific guidance to the group. The Mark 2 curriculum recognizes that tutors must be expert in the learning process: in addition, tutors require a conceptual understanding of the problem, to be able to keep up with, and ahead of, the flow of the discussions. The tutor may assist the group in structuring their thoughts, identifying clinical contingencies (if . . . then), and formulating learning needs. The tutor controls the flow of information to the group and can subtly influence thinking by determining what data to release and when.

The tutor is expected also to be able to review critically discussions and propositions within the group and to identify major misconceptions and matters where further clarification and study is required. Thus, the tutor is expert with regard to the problem-based learning and problem-solving processes, the conceptual basis of the problem, and the general disease mechanisms that are to be studied in the course of the problem.

## The Educational Model

The Mark 2 curriculum for the first time required an explicit model of the problem-based learning and reasoning process (there was no explicit model developed for the Mark 1 curriculum). This model is shown diagrammatically in Figure 9.8: while it is not suggested that this is the only model of clinical reasoning actually used by clinicians, it is certainly a model recognized as effective by clinicians. Each problem commences with a patient presentation: from this the student is expected to extract important verbal and nonverbal cues and to develop an initial formulation (or working synopsis) of the problem. From this, the group identify "pivotal" aspects of the presentation and use these to develop a plausible set of hypotheses. The hypotheses are then organized according to the nature of the mechanisms involved in each, so that there is at this stage a relatively small number of generic causes that could have given rise to the presentation. The group identifies specific information items required to identify the cause of the problem in a step termed the strategic enquiry. This information is provided by the tutor on demand. Data so gathered are incorporated into the formulation (running synopsis), which constitutes the working conceptualization of the problem. When plausible generic hypotheses have been reduced in number, further hypotheses in the form of specific conditions may be advanced and the strategic enquiry cycle repeated.

Side by side with the gathering of patient information relevant to the problem is a simultaneous process of identifying learning deficits and thus of goals for further learning. An exactly equivalent model has been developed for the two

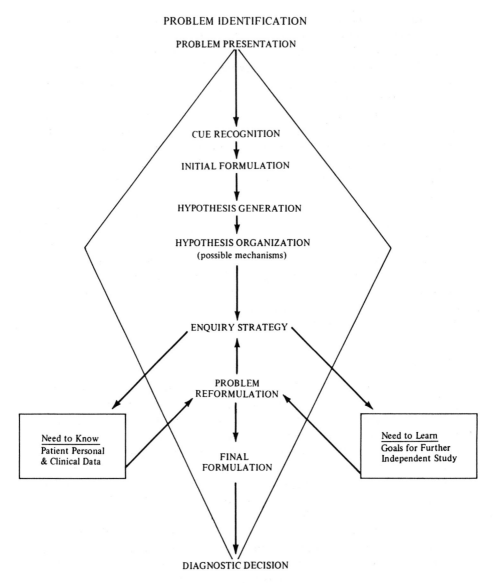

PROBLEM IDENTIFICATION

PROBLEM PRESENTATION

CUE RECOGNITION

INITIAL FORMULATION

HYPOTHESIS GENERATION

HYPOTHESIS ORGANIZATION
(possible mechanisms)

ENQUIRY STRATEGY

PROBLEM
REFORMULATION

Need to Know
Patient Personal
& Clinical Data

FINAL
FORMULATION

Need to Learn
Goals for Further
Independent Study

DIAGNOSTIC DECISION

FIGURE 9.8.

remaining major stages of the clinical reasoning process. The second stage is that of planning the patient management. This proceeds by identification of major treatment goals, options, and limitations associated with each option. Patient data are gathered to identify the best fit between these. The third major stage of the clinical reasoning process is that of assessing quality of care and outcomes. This requires that the possible patient progress pathways are identified, and a monitoring plan instituted that will provide timely and definitive data as to which

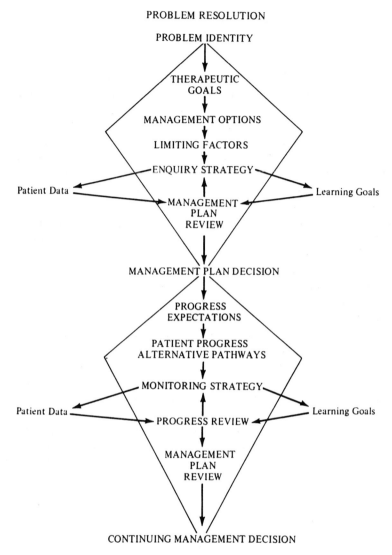

PROBLEM RESOLUTION

FIGURE 9.9.

pathway this particular patient is following. Management must be modified in the light of progress data. These are briefly outlined in Figure 9.9.

The details of these models are explained to tutors. But equally important is that they are explained to the students at the commencement of the course and at several sessions during the course. Both documents and diagrams are provided for staff and students, and these are often referred to both in and out of tutorial sessions. These models and documents have proved to be a vital part of the whole curriculum revision process.

## Staff for Problem-based Learning

The main threat to the development of clinical reasoning and independent learning skills has been found to be the staff themselves. Tutors feel that they must lead and tutor, that they must teach the students: discipline experts feel a similar need to impart their expertise and knowledge, to transfer their understanding to the students; clinicians feel the need to assert and demonstrate their expertise and clinical prowess. All staff seem to experience this pressing need to speak with authority and exhibit a powerful drive to "make sure" that the students progress along the "right" pathway and undertake the "proper" learning of "core" material that is "essential" for all doctors. In so doing, they take the initiative out of the hands of the students and deny them the opportunity to develop independence in learning and reasoning. These are complex skills and may at best be difficult for many students to master within the duration of the course of medical studies. Learning experiences must be constructed specifically for this purpose. As Popper[19] states the problem, the student must be encouraged to develop his or her "mental searchlight," rather than the teacher being permitted continually to fill the student's "mental bucket."

The need for additional effort in staff training has been recognized and accepted. From 1984, the Faculty in Newcastle has devoted substantially increased resources to staff preparation in order better to prepare them for their educational roles. The working problem tutors must be appropriately prepared for their roles, as outlined above. But at least as important is that all other tutors, and especially those who operate at the bedside and are accorded special mentor status by the students, should be similarly prepared. All tutors should subscribe to the same basic model of process skills and especially of clinical reasoning and independent learning if the skills developed initially in the working problem sessions are to be nurtured thereafter. Staff training is a lengthy and continuing task, both with regard to development of skills in newer recruits as well as to continuing improvement of the skills of the more experienced staff.

## Learning Environments

Problem-based learning activities are centered around a tutorial room where students meet in groups of eight with a tutor. Tutorial meetings occur twice a week and have a nominal duration of up to 3 hours each. Learning through group discussion and learning to work as part of a team are viewed as important, especially for those students who are less experienced or who find this new approach to learning more taxing. Students are randomly allocated to groups, the composition of which changes each year.

One role of the problem-based learning tutor is to guard the group dynamic processes and facilitate discussions. The tutor is not supposed to act as a content expert (indeed the tutor may genuinely not be an expert in the subject matter under discussion) but does possess a medical overview that is valuable in helping the students see the problem in context. The tutor is not expected to inject resource material into the discussion unless perceiving it is essential to the immediate progress of the group. The aim is to ensure that the students recognize the steps in the learning process and work through them in a logical and orderly fashion. The tutor must specifically guard against short-circuiting any of the group activities that contribute to the development of independent learning abilities.

Study of the identified resource materials is undertaken by the students alone or in groups according to their personal preferences.

Professional skills activities take place largely in health care environments. They are distributed throughout the spectrum of health care settings and utilize the skills of tutors from a parallel range of backgrounds. Population Medicine has activities based both in the tutorial room and in the field, as described. Tutors are drawn from a wide cross section of health professionals with an interest in the community.

## Learning Resources

The use of problems as a basis for study offers a vehicle through which every discipline may contribute relevant material within a clinically applied context. The frame of reference of these materials relates not so much to the discipline as to the relevant organ-system of the body. This provides the basis for interdisciplinary integration, and offers the student a functional structure for learning.

Since a principal goal of the approach adopted by Newcastle is that students should learn to learn for themselves, access to comprehensive library facilities is essential. However, the same goal can be achieved with less reliance on library resources if the students, alone or in groups, are able to take their learning topics to staff for resolution. This is the basis of the "resource" function of staff: the objective is that the students should generate the learning issues and control the information flow. This is in contrast with the more conventional lecture or tutorial format where the staff member adopts this controlling role. There are two problem formats outlined above. The first relates to the Mark 1 structure of problems prior to 1985, and the second to the Mark 2 curriculum introduced from 1985 on. These required quite different resource material support.

## Mark 1 Problem Materials

Each problem in Mark 1 curriculum required numerous trigger materials for use during the structured tutorial (Fig. 9.7). Each trigger item took the problem one logical step further, and was planned to raise one or more discussion issues and learning topics.

The Mark 1 curriculum presented students with detailed learning materials (typically 50–150 pages) for each problem. These materials were interdisciplinary in nature and included references to texts, journals, and audiovisual materials, as well as practical activities, where appropriate. These materials in effect formed an integrated framework for each problem, each system, and for the course as a whole. They required considerable staff time for preparation, and

University of Newcastle
N.S.W.
Faculty of Medicine                    Block 4A:  The Cardiovascular System

At the end of Term 4 and when confronted with a patient with one or more cardiovascular problems, the student will be able to:

1. Develop a problem list for the patient by:

    1.1  identifying in the reported history elements that suggest a cardiovascular disorder

    1.2  recognizing symptoms that suggest a cardiovascular disorder (see Appendix A)*

    1.3  suspecting, eliciting, and recognizing physical signs that suggest a cardiovascular disorder (see Appendix B)* [1]

2. Generate credible hypotheses about the cause of the problems and be able to request appropriate investigations and interpret the results in order to distinguish, support, confirm, or refute the hypotheses (see Appendix C)*

3. Develop a plan of management based on the problem list developed. Such a plan shall include:

    3.1  an explanation in appropriate terms to the patient and his family of the problem, its causation, the management options, and the prognosis

    3.2  an explanation at a more technical level for the purpose of professional communication, which will include a description of the problem, its etiology, pathology, the management options, and epidemiologically based estimate of prognosis

    3.3  a strategy for monitoring the progress and effectiveness of the adopted plan of management which also ensures the most efficient utilization of resources

    3.4  sufficient flexibility to allow for its modification in the light of feedback from 3.3 above

4. Implement, either alone under supervision or by referral to a colleague, the plan of management (see Appendix D)*

5. Be familiar with and be able to perform certain practical procedures (see Appendix E)*

In order to achieve the above objectives, the student must be able to demonstrate knowledge and understanding of the structure, function, and regulation of the components of the cardiovascular system of the normal individual.


*Each appendix contains a list of items.  For example:

Appendix A − Symptoms

| | |
|---|---|
| Faintness | Palpitations |
| Sweating | Chest pain |
| Pallor | Breathlessness on exertion |
| Collapse | Breathlessness at rest |
| Cold, clammy skin | Orthopnea |
| Muscular weakness | Cough ± pink, frothy sputum |
| Anxiety | Swollen ankles |
| Distress | |

FIGURE 9.10.


students had little need to seek further material. Objectives were specified for each problem: these were distributed at the end of the first session on that problem. System objectives were also prepared and distributed at the start of that block.

Examples of some of these materials are shown in Figures 9.10 to 9.12. Figure 9.10 shows the objectives (abbreviated) for the cardiovascular system; Figure

| Faculty of Medicine<br>University of Newcastle, N.S.W. |  |

| Block 4A | Working Problem 2 | Package A |

Contents

|  | Introduction |
| Learning Unit 1 | "A rapid, thumping heartbeat"—<br>The electrical and mechanical activity<br>in the heart |
| Learning Unit 2 | Electrocardiography |
| Learning Unit 3 | Etiology, signs, and symptoms of<br>paroxysmal tachycardia |
| Learning Unit 4 | Management of tachycardia |
| Learning Unit 5 | Medical certification |
| Learning Unit 6 | The doctor/patient relationship |

FIGURE 9.11.

9.11 lists the titles of prepared learning materials for one of the four cardiovascular problems; and Figure 9.12 shows the cover page for one of these learning materials indicating the relationship between the material and the problem, and the specific objectives of that material. Further detail about this may be obtained elsewhere.[20,21]

## Mark 2 Problem Materials

For reasons already discussed, the Mark 2 curriculum has been extensively modified. The initial trigger material presenting the patient to the group has been abbreviated. Further clinical information is available to the students only through the tutor who consults patient information sheets. These sheets are structured such that initially only history and examination items are available, but later in the session investigation items are available on request. Further handouts may be prepared for two purposes. Some may summarize the information that the group should have obtained by interrogation of the tutor: these are distributed as an aide memoire after the activity, not before. Others present patient progress monitoring data and are presented when the first round of the clinical reasoning process has been concluded: these act to initiate further clinical reasoning activity.

Similarly, the prepared materials have been drastically reduced in length. For each learning goal that the students are expected to identify, a brief overview (1–2 pages) is prepared outlining in broad terms the structure, function, or mechanism involved. Students must then seek further information and details from texts of their own choice. During the first year, some guidance may be

| Block 4A | Working Problem 2 | Learning Unit 1 |
|---|---|---|

"A rapid, thumping heartbeat"— The electrical and mechanical activity in the heart

From time to time, this patient has "palpitations" of the heart, which cause her considerable distress and leave her feeling weak and tired. During an attack, she feels her heart thumping at a very fast rate.

You have seen for yourself from the ECG record that her heart rate during an attack is greatly increased from normal.

Clearly, the normal rhythmicity of the heart, which we take for granted, can be disturbed.

In this Unit, we will consider what normally controls the rhythm of the heart, causes the heart muscle to contract, and maintains synchronization between contraction of the chambers.

When you have completed this Unit, you will be able to:

* describe the cardiac conducting components,

* describe how an impulse from the SA node spreads to all the heart muscle cells,

* describe the movements of ions in myocardial cells, pacemakers, and Purkinije cells,

* describe the ionic movements that couple electrical excitation of the myocardium and mechanical movement, and

* describe the process of muscle contraction in the heart.

Learning Resources:

Vander AJ, et al. *Human Physiology: The Mechanisms of Body Function,* 2nd edition, New York: McGraw-Hill, 1975.

Guyton AC. *Textbook of Medical Physiology,* 5th edition. Philadelphia: WB Saunders, 1975.

This Learning Unit was prepared by:
Dr. David Powis and Mr. Greg Doran,
who are also the Resource Persons.

FIGURE 9.12.

offered on references. Thereafter, both overviews and references are reduced, and many goals from the second year on come with little or no supporting material.

Examples of some of these materials are shown in Figures 9.13 to 9.16. Figure 9.13a shows a typical problem trigger. In Figure 9.13a and b is the clinical information available through the tutor. The first part (Fig. 9.13a) of this Tutor Information is available as students request it; the second part (Fig. 9.13b) is available only when the tutor judges that the group has reached an appropriate stage in the reasoning process. Figure 9.14 shows a set of learning goals for the same problem. The list draws the attention of the students to learning resource sessions associated with this problem. Figure 9.16 shows the material that is provided as the learning resource for one learning goal.

## PROBLEM PRESENTATION

Patient:        Mrs. Christine Buchanan
Age:            27 years
Occupation:     Housewife

Presentation:   Four-month history of intermittent lower abdominal pain. The pain is dull, cramping in nature, bilateral, but often worse on the left side. Each attack lasts from 1–3 days, but over the last week the pain has become almost continuous.

She has had diarrhea over the same period, worse during the attacks of pain. She passes 3–6 rather soft bowel motions daily. On occasions she has noticed mucus mixed with the bowel motions. The diarrhea has also worsened over the past week, with 5–10 motions daily. These motions have been soft to fluid, with both blood and mucus present.

## TUTOR INFORMATION SHEET

THIS INFORMATION IS TO BE MADE AVAILABLE TO THE GROUP AS EACH ITEM IS REQUESTED

Background:     She has lived all her life locally in Maitland, and never been overseas. She is married with 3 children (ages 2, 5, 7). No one in her family has had a similar problem.

She has never had a constipation problem, and never taken laxatives. She has lost 5 in weight over the last 2 months. She has had no nausea, vomiting, upper abdominal pain, jaundice, or urinary symptoms.

Her periods are regular, and the pain seems unassociated with her menstrual cycle.

She has no previous significant illnesses or hospitalizations.

Alcohol:        One glass of low-alcohol beer per day on average
Smoking:        Nil
Medications:    Oral contraceptive; occasional aspirin for headaches
Allergies:      Band-Aid sticking plasters

Examination:    Thin, anxious
Temp 37.1°C, Pulse 84 per min, Blood Press. 125/85 mmHg
Mouth normal

Abdomen soft, not distended; mild tenderness in left iliac fossa; no guarding or rebound tenderness, no hepatosplenomegaly, no masses

Rectal examination: discomfort on digital examination but no specific abnormality found. Blood and mucus noted on the glove

Office urinalysis – normal

No other abnormality noted on examination

FIGURE 9.13a.

NEXT SECTION OF INFORMATION AVAILABLE ONLY WHEN SIGNIFICANT ITEMS
ABOVE HAVE BEEN REQUESTED:

| INVESTIGATE: | Hb | 118 g/L | (115–165 g/L) |
|---|---|---|---|
| | WCC | $14 \times 10^9$/L | $(4–12 \times 10^9$/L) |
| | neutrophils | 70% | $(2.5–7.5 \times 10^9$/L) |
| | Eosinophils | 2% | $(<0.4 \times 10^9$/L) |
| | Basophils | – | $(<0.1 \times 10^9$/L) |
| | Lymphocytes | 23% | $(1.5–4.0 \times 10^9$/L) |
| | Monocytes | 5% | $(0.1–0.8 \times 10^9$/L) |
| | Platelets | $300 \times 10^9$/L | $(150–400 \times 10^9$/L) |
| | ESR | 40 mm/hr | (3–8 mm/hr) |
| | Serum electrolytes: | | |
| | Sodium | 139 mmol/L | (136–145 mmol/L) |
| | Potassium | 3.0 mmol/L | (3.5–5.0 mmol/L) |
| | Chloride | 108 mmol/L | (95–109 mmol/L) |
| | Bicarbonate | 20 mmol/L | (21–30 mmol/L) |
| | Total Protein | 60 g/L | (64–83 g/L) |
| | Albumin | 30 g/L | (37–51 g/L) |
| | Urea | 3.5 mmol/L | (2.4–7.0 mmol/L) |
| | Creatinine | 0.06 mmol/L | (0.04–0.12 mmol/L) |

*Sigmoidoscopy*: mucosa reddened, edematous, friable with contact bleeding. Loss of normal vascular patterns.

*Stool microscopy and culture*: no cysts, ova, or parasites detected. Normal fecal flora on culture.

*Biopsy*: Inflammatory infiltrate in lamina propria with mucous gland depletion and occasional crypt abscesses. [slides 1 (low power) 2 and 3 (high power) of biopsy in problem box].

*Barium enema*: loss of haustration in lower descending and sigmoid colon, with spiculation suggesting microulcers.

FIGURE 9.13b.

In both versions of the curriculum, staff members are available to students as expert content resources. Staff may be consulted as required by individuals or groups. During most weeks, sessions are scheduled at which staff are available to discuss learning difficulties with the entire student cohort. These sessions are termed fixed resource sessions. In both types of resource sessions, the aim is for the students to set the agenda and control the direction of the session.

## Problem Selection

Clearly, the choice of the problems for study is of considerable significance, as they effectively define the content of the curriculum. The Faculty has developed the concept of the "priority problem" to provide a philosophical basis for the problem selection process.

A priority problem (Fig. 9.15) is a clinical situation that a newly qualified doctor in a contemporary practice (meaning within the society in which we are working) should recognize and be able to manage alone, under supervision, or by appropriate referral. It should also be a situation in which appropriate medical

Learning Goals

1. How does the site and nature of abdominal pain assist in defining the problem?
2. What mechanisms may cause diarrhea?
3. What is inflammatory bowel disease?
4. What principles of management apply to patients with inflammatory bowel disease?

Fixed Resource Sessions

Bowel microflora
Biochemical changes in diarrhea and vomiting
Bowel obstruction and surgery
Pharmacological agents in the management of inflammatory bowel disease
Pathological appearances and mechanisms in inflammatory bowel disease

FIGURE 9.14.

"The Priority Problem"

A clinical situation which a newly qualified doctor in contemporary practice should recognize and be able to manage along, under
supervision or by appropriate referral:

1. Serious or potentially serious

2. Appropriate medical care has a significant role

3. Common in the community

4. Implications for prevention

FIGURE 9.15.

care plays a significant role. There are many situations where medically there
is very little that can be done: the term "appropriate medical care" includes
both caring for the patient as a person and caring for the disease. Finally, a
priority problem should have implications for prevention. Preventive care is
much more cost-effective than is curative medicine. This fact must be emphasized in the face of the rapidly escalating costs of medical service. These then are
the four criteria by which problems are selected for inclusion in the curriculum.
Not every problem satisfies all these criteria, but the aim is to select those that
come closest.

The above criteria make no mention of the educational desirability of the
problem. Educational expediency is clearly important. A group of problems with
a common theme (e.g., cardiovascular system) must provide the opportunity for
students to encounter all the essential fundamental concepts and principles relevant to that area. A group of cardiovascular problems concerned only with valvu-
lar disorders would clearly not provide adequate breadth of coverage or scope for
introduction of all relevant cardiovascular concepts and principles. However,
given a group of problems, each of which relies on similar underpinning concepts

and principles, a decision about which to select for inclusion in the course is based on the "priority" criteria above.

## Assessment

Three aims for assessment are certification of competence, feedback to students on their performance and achievement, and feedback to staff on the effectiveness of the course. To some extent these areas have been separated by providing self-assessment instruments as well as the formal certifying assessments. In all but the final year of the course, an ungraded pass/fail system of reporting assessment results has been adopted because it is considered that it is less likely to promote competition between students or to disrupt group learning dynamics or team-work. The assessments are criterion-referenced and directly linked to the relevant set of educational objectives. Because certifying assessment has as its aim the identification of students who have fulfilled certain criteria, there is no objection to their making multiple attempts at satisfying the assessors, particularly if this strategy helps reduce test anxiety.[22] However, a limit of about 3–4 attempts is imposed in practice for administrative convenience.

To be consistent with the aims and philosophy of the school, assessment must be based on the application of knowledge to practical clinical situations and on the ability to solve and manage clinical problems rather than on the ability to recall texts without demonstration of understanding. Possession of knowledge seems to have little correlation with clinical ability.[3,4] Likewise, success in preclinical (theoretical) examinations has little correlation with success in finals or clinical practice.[3-5,23]

The principal assessment instruments used are short-answer questions often in the form of modified essay questions,[24] objective structured clinical assessments,[25] and clinical long and short cases of the conventional type. Structured viva voce examinations are also used, especially in situations where a student may not have performed satisfactorily in a written instrument, and where a student is being reassessed. In addition, a number of special assessment instruments have been developed, including a "group task" that focuses on group problem solving and individual problem-based learning. In the later years, this instrument is replaced by a limited time period task where the individual student is allocated a learning task and has 1 or 2 days to return with a summary of the questions he or she addressed, the resources searched and the outcomes of the enquiry.

All assessments are criterion referenced. Model answers are generated in advance, together with the level of competence that is expected of the student. In the case of clinical examinations, student performance is judged by reference to itemized checklists of behaviors and activities that the student is expected to exhibit, both psychomotor (by direct observation) and cognitive (by inference and interview). Students are invited to review the criteria used for judging their performance, and the student comment on each assessment instrument and item is considered by the assessors prior to scoring. Student performance is judged by

Learning Goal 2   WHAT MECHANISMS MAY CAUSE DIARRHEA?

Definition

The word "diarrhoea" implies a change in bowel habit of the individual. This change usually means increased frequency, increased fluidity, or the presence of abnormal constituents, such as blood, mucus, or pus. However, there is considerable individual variation in the pattern of bowel movement. In health, the frequency of bowel movements may range from three times daily to three times weekly. Consistency of stools is equally subjective and variable.

Any discussion of diarrhea requires an understanding of normal patterns of intestinal absorption and secretion of electrolytes and fluid, including absorption of fats, proteins, and carbohydrates. Furthermore, these mechanisms must be understood in relation to different parts of the gastrointestinal tract, such as the jejunum, ileum, and the colon. Diarrhea can be considered as an excess of fluid in the stool due to abnormalities in fluid secretion of absorption. In many cases an understanding of the pathophysiological mechanisms helps establish the differential diagnosis early in the course of the disease and provides the basis for rational therapy.

1. Disorders of intestinal secretion

The stimuli known to increase intestinal secretion are diverse. They include bacterial enterotoxins (e.g., with infections due to cholera, staphylocci, E. coli); gastrointestinal hormones as seen with islet cell tumors of the pancreas (e.g., vasoactive intestinal polypeptide); bile acids as seen following distal ileal resection where their secretory effect is on the colon; and laxative abuse. Certain diarrheogenic viruses evoke jejunal hypersecretion. Increased cyclic AMP may be the "intracellular messenger" for the secretory process in some situations such as hormonally induced diarrhea and with certain bacterial enterotoxins.

2. Exudative diseases

Exudation of serum proteins, blood, mucus, or pus from sites of inflammatory, ulcerative, or infiltrative disease can contribute to increased fecal volume, and hence diarrhea. Such diseases include inflammatory bowel disease, villous adenomas of the rectum, and invasive bacterial infections of the intestine including shigella and parasitic infections such as giardiasis.

3. Osmotic diarrhea

This condition occurs when an excess of water-soluble molecules remain in the bowel lumen, leading to an osmotic retention of water. Certain laxatives achieve this effect, as a result of slow and incomplete absorption of the polyvalent ions of magnesium sulphate and phosphate. Diseases associated with carbohydrate malabsorption result in large amounts of carbohydrate in the lumen and water is, therefore, retained to achieve intraluminal isotonicity with the extracellular fluid.

4. Transit disorders and deranged motility

This is essentially a mechanical problem and involves inadequate mixing of the food or inadequate contact with the mucosal surface, as may occur after gastric surgery or resection of long lengths of intestine, respectively. Increased irritability and hypermotility of the bowel occurs with acute infective and inflammatory disorders, some laxatives, "irritable bowel" syndrome, thyrotoxicosis, and diabetes.

FIGURE 9.16.

140    R.L.B. Neame

5. Malabsorption

The basis for diarrhea in malabsorption states relates to several of the pathogenetic mechanisms considered above. Failure to absorb fats (steatorrhea) stimulates fluid secretion into the bowel lumen. This is often further aggravated by an associated bile acid malabsorption since bile acids stimulate mocosal secretions. An example of the multiple mechanisms operating in a single disease is seen in the inflammatory bowel disorder called Crohn's disease. Often the bowel will have been removed surgically and the remaining bowel may be diseased. Carbohydrate and fat may be incompletely absorbed, ileal disease may lead to bile acid malabsorption, and transit may be rapid. Bacterial overgrowth may result from strictured segments with proximal dilation causing local mucosal inflammation and exudation. Osmotic diarrhea secondary to the malabsorption of carbohydrates may occur, furthermore, a large amount of unabsorbed amino acids can have a similar osmotic effect.

In general, most of the clinical states of diarrhea can be explained on the basis of one or more of the mechanisms described above.

References

Elias E, Hawkins C: *Lecture Notes on Gastroenterology*, 1st ed. Oxford, Blackwell Scientific Publications, 1985.
Phillips SF: Diarrhoea: A current view of the pathophysiology. *Gastroenterology*, Vol. 63:495, 1972.
Sleisinger MH, Fordtran JS (eds): *Gastrointestinal Disease: Pathophysiology, Diagnosis, Management*, 3rd ed. Philadelphia, PA, WB Saunders Co, 1983.

FIGURE 9.16. *Continued.*

reference to these overt performance criteria. Further details on the assessment system may be found elsewhere.[26,27]

## Organization and Management of Resources

Such an innovative approach to medical education makes unusual demands on the disciplines, individuals, and management system of the Faculty. Strategies must be developed not only for determining the material to be included but also for ensuring that the necessary level of communication is achieved to promote effective interdisciplinary collaboration. Arrangements must be made for groups to take responsibility for areas of knowledge not otherwise encompassed by conventional disciplinary territories (interdisciplinary areas; process and algorithmic knowledge; behavioral, professional, and attitudinal characteristics; and so on).

### General Organization

The Faculty has established 13 conventional disciplines but has not accorded them the degree of autonomy that is typical of other schools. In parallel with the disciplines are three major committees of the Faculty Board, responsible for the areas of undergraduate education, research, and service. To each of these

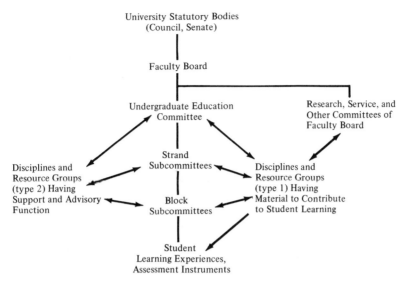

FIGURE 9.17.

committees the Faculty has delegated its authority with respect to the development of policy, philosophy, and implementation of Faculty goals.

The Faculty Board (Fig. 9.17) has established also committees responsible for advising on the utilization of Faculty resources (equipment, finance and personnel, library) and for performing special functions for the Faculty (student admissions, program evaluation). In addition, there are a number of departments and committees of the university with which the Faculty interfaces (budget, accounts, salaries, personnel, maintenance, etc.). These areas are not considered further here.

## Educational Structure

In order to achieve the Program Objectives outlined previously, four main strand of activities were required, each activity being characterized by different aims or involvements. The strands are described in a previous section of this chapter. Subcommittees responsible for the organization, development and administration of each strand have been established (Fig. 9.17).

In addition to this longitudinal division, the course is further divided sequentially into a series of "blocks" (Fig. 9.3).[21] Earlier blocks concentrate on organ systems; later blocks are more integrative and center on clinical specialty areas. Each block is developed and organized by a project group, comprising a chairman, appointed by the Undergraduate Education Committee, and an interdisciplinary membership.

In the interests of collaboration and integration and to promote group ownership of the whole course, decisions relating to any course component are made by the relevant subcommittee of the Undergraduate Education Committee in consultation with other interested groups (disciplines, other committees). It is only through the educational substructures that disciplines and resource groups may present learning materials, experiences, or activities to the students.

Certain aspects of such an innovative curriculum fall outside the scope of the normally established disciplines (e.g., clinical reasoning, problem solving, independent learning, communications, scientific method, critical appraisal, professionalization). It has been recognized that additional resource groupings are required to service these academic areas. These are formalized in one way or another by the Undergraduate Education Committee from time to time. Such groups are drawn from individuals with special interest and expertise in the appropriate area whose principal appointment is to one of the established disciplines. Within the educational domain such groups are accorded status that is essentially the same as any of the established disciplines, and are shown in Figure 9.17 as "Type 1 Resource Groups."

Also appearing in Figure 9.17 are Resource Groups identified as "Type 2." These are also formalized under the auspices of the Undergraduate Education Committee but differ from the Type 1 groups in existing primarily to support the educational system. These groups provide expertise and logistical support to other Faculty staff as regards such areas as student assessment, program evaluation and quality control, timetabling, room and student group allocation, and staff training. The Type 2 groups normally have little or no direct contact with students and do not aim to impart special content or expertise to the students.

FUNCTIONAL ORGANIZATION

Disciplines and resource groups (type 1) propose material and activities for inclusion in the curriculum, represent their views in negotiations with the various project committees, prepare and implement agreed-on educational and assessment activities, provide expert consultative and counseling services as requested by students, and make expert evaluative comment on the program. Their principal interaction is with the project groups. The chairman of each project group functions as a "generalist integrator," synthesizing proposals and opinions expressed by the experts into a practical educational package consistent with the scope of the block and the educational policy and philosophy of the school. His function is to (1) involve the experts; (2) negotiate, discuss, and achieve a consensus on the concepts, principles, skills, and activities to be incorporated; and (3) obtain suggestions and approval from the Faculty for his plans. Because the program and every component of it is "owned" by the whole Faculty, their involvement and assent is a vital part of achieving their commitment to it.

The function of the resource groups (type 2) is to provide essential support and maintenance to the Faculty in terms of advice, techniques, and logistics. Certain of the established disciplines also serve this function, notably the discipline of Medical Education.

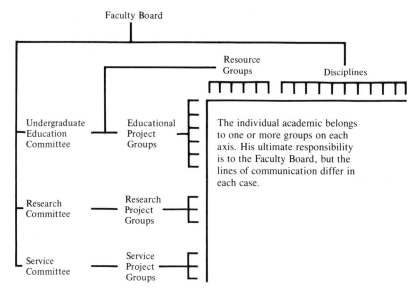

Faculty Board

Resource
Groups
Disciplines

Undergraduate
Education
Committee

Educational
Project
Groups

The individual academic belongs
to one or more groups on each
axis. His ultimate responsibility
is to the Faculty Board, but the
lines of communication differ in
each case.

Research
Committee

Research
Project
Groups

Service
Committee

Service
Project
Groups

FIGURE 9.18.

## Matrix

The conventional bureaucratic model of faculty organization with its autonomous departments is seen as inconsistent with the needs of the curriculum for horizontal communication and integration.[12] Thus, a matrix model has been adopted in which the established disciplines and the additional resource groups constitute one axis, and the educational task and project groups form the other (Fig. 9.18). The project groups include not only educational but also the research and service projects under the coordination of their respective committees of the Faculty Board.

The same academics, who are nominally allocated to disciplines, also comprise the membership of all the other resource and project groups (Fig. 9.17). The Faculty tends to place greater emphasis on the interdisciplinary projects (Fig. 9.18, ordinate) than on the disciplines, as reflected by the allocation of faculty resources.

Matrices of this type have many advantages for an institution with needs for integration, innovation, and flexibility.[28] It is difficult to see how a conventional bureaucratic model would cope with these needs in the absence of superimposed project groups. Structures of this sort exist in most institutions and can easily be added to any bureaucratic organization. However, for them to be effective it is essential that they be given resources, authority, responsibility, and status commensurate with their proposed function by the Faculty.

# Evaluation

The first students graduated from Newcastle in 1982, and at the time of writing 7 cohorts of students have graduated at yearly intervals. These graduates are being followed as part of a long-term program. Both formal and informal evaluation of their performance has been received, and this has been very positive. There has been no suggestion that these graduates are in any way less skilled or competent than their conventionally trained colleagues. In some dimensions, the Newcastle graduates seem to be more skilled than their conventionally trained counterparts, but definitive data will not be available for some time yet. Medical graduates of the University of Newcastle are accredited and recognized by the General Medical Council of the United Kingdom, and recognized by all Australian Federal and State medical registration bodies.

Student opinion about the course is invited and received on a regular and frequent basis at the end of most academic sessions. Two national surveys[29,30] have revealed evidence that the medical students at Newcastle are more satisfied with their learning environment than others in Australia. Many of the issues raised in student evaluation have resulted in action, which has resolved that problem (eg, 22). The Mark 2 curriculum that has been operational since 1985 was a consequence of student feedback combined with staff perceptions. Preliminary evaluation from staff and students has shown that this new development of the course has proved highly successful and acceptable.

Staff attitudes towards this curriculum have also been studied.[31] This again shows a high degree of satisfaction with aspects of philosophy, implementation and outcomes.

# Summary

The factors leading up to the development of an innovative approach to medical education in Newcastle, New South Wales, are reviewed. The systematic approach adapted to curriculum planning, implementation, evaluation, and review is outlined. The educational objectives of the school, developed through interaction with various external bodies, are much wider in scope than those of comparable institutions, specifying, in addition to conventional biomedical and psychosocial information, a range of process skills, attitudes, and behaviors as well as communication, interactional, and professional skills.

Student learning is centered on clinical problems, real or simulated. Through these problems and through their involvement in clinical environments, the students are exposed from the outset to the processes of clinical reasoning and independent learning. It is anticipated that students' learning within the clinical context will so organize their long-term memory that relevant information required for subsequent patient involvement will be easier for them to retrieve than for traditionally trained graduates.

The problem-based approach to learning makes additional demands on the staff. It has necessitated alternative approaches to staff management and organization. A matrix structure has been adopted. Numerous project and resource groups have been established in addition to the conventional disciplines. Evaluation by both staff and students has indicated that this course is well received, and that student knowledge, understanding and professional skills are well developed.

# References

1. Surgeon General: Healthy People. No. 79-55071. Washington, DC, United States Department of Health, Education & Welfare (PHS.), 1979.
2. Flexner A: Medical Education in the United States and Canada: A Report to the Carnegie Foundation, Bulletin No. 4. Boston, Updyke, 1910. Reprinted: New York, Arno Press and The New York Times, 1972.
3. Wingard JR, Williamson JW: Grades as predictors of physicians' career performance: an evaluative literature review. *J Med Educ* 1973;48:311–322.
4. Veloski J, Herman MW, Gonella JA, et al: Relationships between performance in medical school and first postgraduate year. *J Med Educ* 1979;54:909–916.
5. Rhoads JM, Gallemore JL, Gianturco DT, Osterhout S: Motivation, medical school admission and student performance. *J Med Educ* 1979;49:1119–1127.
6. Royal Commission on Medical Education: London, Her Majesty's Stationery Office, 1968.
7. Simpson MA: *Medical Education: A Critical Approach*. London, Butterworth, 1972.
8. Engel GL: Biomedicine's failure to achieve flexnerian standards of education. *J Med Educ* 1978;53:387–392.
9. Maddison DC: What's wrong with medical education? *Med Educ* 1978;12:97–102.
10. Sheldrake PF, Linke RD, Mensch IA, et al: Medical Education in Australia: Present Trends and Future Prospects in Australian Medical Schools. ERDC Report No. 16. Canberra, Australian Government Printing Service, 1978.
11. Neame RLB: The preclinical course of study: help or hindrance? *J Med Educ* 1984;59:699–707.
12. Neame RLB: Final Report of the Task Force on Organizational Structures. Newcastle Network of Community-Oriented Educational Institutions for Health Sciences, University of Newcastle, 1982.
13. Neame RLB: Academic Management and Organization in Medical Colleges to Fulfill the Needs of Integration and Innovation. Symposium on the Scope and Policies of College of Medicine & Medical Sciences, Arabian Gulf University, Bahrain. Bahrain, Ministry of Health, 1982, pp. 49–61.
14. Working Papers of the Faculty of Medicine, Nos. I–XVI. Newcastle, The University of Newcastle, 1975–1979.
15. Barrows HS, Tamblyn RM: *Problem-based Learning: An Approach to Medical Education*. Springer Series on *Medical Education*, Vol. 1. New York, Springer Publishing Co., 1980.
16. Barrows HS: *How to Design a Problem-based Curriculum for the Preclinical Years*. New York, Springer, 1985.

17. Neame RLB: Problem-centred Learning in Medical Education: the role of context in the development of process skills, In Schmidt HG, DeVolder ML (eds). *Tutorials in Problem-Based Learning: A New Direction in Teaching the Health Professions*. Assen, Netherlands, Van Gorcum, 1984.

18. Neame RLB, Powis DA: Toward independent learning: curricular design for assisting students to learn how to learn. *J Med Educ* 1981;56:886–893.

19. Popper KR: *Objective Knowledge: An Evolutionary Approach*. Oxford, England, Clarendon Press, 1972.

20. Neame RLB: How to construct a problem-based course. *Med Teacher* 1981;3:94–99.

21. Powis DA, Neame RLB: The way we teach the cardiovascular system. *Med Teacher* 1981;3:131–137.

22. Feletti GI, Neame RLB: Curricular strategies for reducing examination anxiety. *Higher Educ*, 1981;10:675–686.

23. Edouard LK, Harris TTC, Buckley-Sharp MD: Linear study of medical undergraduate performance. *Med Educ* 1976;10:386–397.

24. Knox JDE: The Modified Essay Question. Dundee, Association for the Study of Medical Education, 1972.

25. Harden RMcG, Stevenson M, Downie EE, Wilson GM: Assessment of clinical competence using objective structured examinations. *Br Med J* 1977;1:447–451.

26. Engel CE, Feletti GI, Leeder SR: Assessment of medical students in a new curriculum. *Assess Higher Educ* 1980;5:279–293.

27. Feletti GI, Saunders NA, Smith AJ et al: Comprehensive Assessment of Final-Year Medical Student Performance Based on Undergraduate Programme Objectives. *The Lancet* 1983;2:34–37.

28. Cleland DI, King WR: *Systems Analysis and Project Management*. New York, McGraw-Hill, 1968.

29. Feletti GI, Clarke RM: Construct validity of a learning environment survey for medical schools. *Educ Psychol Meas* 1981;41:875–882.

30. Williams C: *The Early Experiences of Students on Australian University Campuses*. Sydney, Australia, University of Sydney, 1982.

31. Neame RLB: Academic Roles and Satisfaction in a Problem-Based Medical Curriculum. *Studies in Higher Education* 1982;7:141–151.

# 10
# Toward an Emphasis on Problem Solving in Teaching and Learning: The McMaster Experience

JOHN C. SIBLEY*

The McMaster Medical School curriculum, of 3 years' duration is divided into four phases of different lengths. We enroll 100 students per year and have graduated sightly more than 1000 doctors.

## Phase I

Phase I is a multifaceted 10-week introduction to the community, faculty, learning resources, and institutions. The major objective is to develop competence in self-directed learning, problem-based learning (or learning by inquiry) as a member of a small tutorial group. Students begin exploring essential concepts in the sciences underlying medicine and begin to integrate these universal concepts of structure, function, behavior, and measurement. In this process the student develops an ability to use all learning resources—the health sciences library, audiovisual resources, faculty, clinical facilities, and laboratory. The student also begins to develop interviewing and clinical skills during this phase.

A typical phase I problem for students during the first week of medical school is entitled "Mary Cornell" (see case 1, below). The scenario focuses on a 22-month-old child who accidently sustains a 30% steam burn while playing unattended in the kitchen. The child is rushed to a burn unit and experiences the usual physiological, microbiological, and emotional trauma one might expect. The essential laboratory findings, treatment, and outcomes are presented. Each student selects some aspect of the problem, develops a hypothesis to be tested, identifies the key issues relating to that hypothesis, searches out the necessary information, begins critically to evaluate the data acquired, and attempts to integrate or synthesize this information and reach a conclusion. Individual students might use this problem to explore, for the first time, fluid and electrolyte balance, protein metabolism, gram-negative infections and shock, the epidemiology of acute childhood illness, family crisis, community health care planning, or the coping mechanisms of a disabled child.

---

*Dr. Sibley died in 1983. Since then, the structure of the M.D. program has changed, although the methods have not.

## Phase II

The 12 weeks of phase II have a general theme of reaction and adaptation of the body to stimuli and injury. In concentrates mainly on how cells, tissues, and the whole organism respond to inflammation, neoplasia, ischemia, emotional changes, and chemical agents. Again, students use a series of problems to explore underlying concepts. Two phase II problems (the Lazarus and Sally Moutarde problems) are presented in cases 2 and 3, below. These problems require students to explore and use basic concepts in temperature regulation, tissue metabolism, physiological changes with age, host resistance, immunological deficiencies, and epidemiology of congenital illnesses.

## Phase III

Phase III is a 40-week period using an integrated systems approach to deal with the major body organ systems. Clinical problems are explored in greater depth with emphasis on their underlying physical and behavioral mechanisms. Throughout the first three phases, students have ongoing sessions on interviewing and clinical skills.

## Phase IV

Clinical clerkship is the period during which each student, under supervision, begins to take clinical responsibility for patients. Blocks of time are spent in the traditional clinical disciplines: Medicine, Surgery, Family Medicine, Psychiatry, Obstetrics/Gynecology, and Pediatrics. The student now uses real patients as the problems to be solved and uses those patients again to identify fundamental concepts and apply those concepts with increasing sophistication to the resolution of clinical problems. The students have tutorials twice weekly. In 1981 we instituted regular phase IV tutorials on the critical appraisal of data relevant to each clinical discipline.[1] Students are presented with problems that stimulate them to learn how to assess evidence of efficacy and effectiveness to treatment, to measure the predictive value of diagnostic tests, to deal with evidence of causation, and to critique studies, focusing on clinical error, bias, and quality of care. Finally, 26 weeks of the curriculum are elective time, permitting students to pursue personal interests, strengthen areas of weakness, explore individual topics in depth, or have a clinical experience in community settings elsewhere in Canada or abroad.

## Curricular Objectives

It is intended that through this educational process of learning by problem-solving and self-directed learning students will achieve the following educational objectives:

1. Identify and define health problems at both an individual and a community level and to search for information to resolve or manage these problems.
2. Examine the underlying physical, biological, and behavioral mechanisms of health problems. This area includes a spectrum of phenomena from the molecular to those involving the patient's family and community.
3. Investigate community health problems and recommend efficient and effective approaches to deal with environmental, occupational, behavioral, and public policy issues.
4. Recognize, maintain, and develop the personal characteristics and attitudes required for a career in a health profession, including the following:
   a. Awareness of personal assets, limitations, and emotional reactions
   b. Responsibility and dependability
   c. Ability to relate to, and show concern for, other individuals
5. Develop the clinical skills and knowledge required to define and manage the health problems of patients, including their physical, emotional, and social aspects, within the context of effective health care.
6. Become self-directed as a learner, recognizing personal educational needs, selecting appropriate learning resources, and evaluating personal progress.
7. Assess critically professional activity related to patient care, health care delivery, and health research.
8. Function productively as a member of a small group engaged in learning, research, or health care.
9. Be aware of, and to be able to work in, a variety of health care settings.

Evaluation of a student's performance is carried out on a continuous basis, stressing, in educational jargon, a formative evaluation process with the student's peers and faculty participating in the process. (For further details, see Chap. 11.)

## Why Problem-based Learning?

The intent of our curriculum is that students learn both how to solve problems and how to use problems to explore and attain knowledge. It presents an alternative to studying blocks of classified knowledge in a predetermined, organized sequence. A student must begin to identify the issues contained within the problem, define the questions that must be answered, determine the information required, research and evaluate that information, and finally integrate and synthesize that information to arrive at a reasonable resolution of the problem and formulate appropriate management. The students thus take a clinical problem and work back to the most fundamental science. It is our belief that such an approach encourages habits of inquiry, produces an intellectual and scientific approach, and ensures relevance to the student's future professional role whether in clinical medicine, scientific research, or both. As one student expressed it, he had the advantage of the stimulation of studying medicine at an "inquiry" level. Medicine is "explored" rather than "learned." This approach produces technicians, observers, and deducers.

## Do Students Learn Science?

In the absence of formal courses in the biological sciences, concern is occasionally expressed that students may slip through a problem-solving approach to education without acquiring a sound grounding in the underlying sciences. Not unexpectedly, this idea is not infrequently expressed by basic scientists in one of the disciplines such as anatomy, pathology, microbiology, or biochemistry. This potential omission is minimized by the use of the tutorial system, which lends itself superbly to the development of a scientific attitude of mind and intellectual and scholarly challenge.

## Tutors

Much depends on the ability of the tutor. We have addressed this question by having formal tutor training workshops, which all new faculty are encouraged to attend. We stress that tutors do not lecture. Rather, their role is to stimulate, be provocative, and explore concepts and issues with the students.

## Problem Selection

The selection and design of a suitable range of problems throughout the program ensures that students explore and learn the full spectrum of scientific concepts basic to medicine. The curriculum therefore is built around the selection of appropriate problems rather than the listing of core content. The writing and development of biomedical problems does take some skill and experience. When selecting problems (cases) for analysis, our planners use the following criteria.

*Prevalence.* The problem should be relatively common.

*Treatability.* There should be sound scientific evidence that an intervention (either preventive or curative) does more good than harm. Of course, there are many conditions where the evidence is incomplete, and it is useful for students to know this. However, it is important that where there is evidence available about treatment effects, it must be available.

*Prototype value.* A problem, although infrequent and not treatable per se, may be an excellent model for study (e.g., the hemoglobinopathies) of some basic concepts.

*Interdisciplinary input.* The problem should elicit concepts from a range of disciplines.

*Length.* We have found that problems of intermediate length are the most suitable. If too long, the students become overwhelmed and lose interest. Problems that are too short do not provide sufficient challenge.

*Format.* Students prefer a problem to be presented so that the clinical story unfolds as in real life. They prefer not to have questions listed or posed by faculty because it eliminates the challenge of exploring the problem, sensing or identifying the key issues, and researching those issues that are pertinent and challenging. Learning is a resolution of tension. If we list the questions for the student, we deny him or her the challenge and the tension to be resolved. Everyone likes variety, so we have problems available in several forms: case protocols, problem boxes, card decks, and simulated patients.

In addition, we have revitalized our discipline groups in Pharmacology, Morphology, Cell Biology, Epidemiology, Measurement, and Behavior. We have developed new groups in special subject areas of Geriatrics, Nutrition, Environmental Health, and Occupational Health. Their task is to identify the major concepts in these areas that students should be able to understand and apply in the various phases of the curriculum. They work with phase planners in the design of problems that raise these issues and ensure that appropriate educational resources are in place so that students can have access to the necessary information.

Finally, these groups develop self-assessment packages that students may use to determine their progress. The discipline and special subject area groups do not plan the units or phases. They do not give lectures or courses. They do not examine students on those disciplines. They can and do supply resources (people or services) and assist the educational planners and students as required.

## Does Problem Solving Encourage Integration of Knowledge Rather Than Fragmentation?

All human beings—including medical scientists—seem to get particular satisfaction in reproducing their own kind. There is thus a tendency for enthusiastic organ system specialists, from neurologists to nephrologist, to promote and isolate their area into separate blocks of knowledge. At times, phase III has run the risk of being fragmented into specialty areas of cardiology, gastroenterology, urology, etc. Strategies to reduce this fragmentation include insisting that there be interdisciplinary planning of each of the phase III units. Cardiology, for example, is planned not only by the cardiologists but also by behavioral scientists, epidemiologists, and pharmacologists. Biomedical problems are redesigned continually so as to ensure that integration of knowledge and concepts are required for the solution of those problems.

A related problem in our system is the difficulty, at times, of maintaining a problem-based learning approach during the clinical clerkship of phase IV. Clinical clerks are quickly caught up in the excitement of making a diagnosis, prescribing treatment, and ordering tests. We are strengthening the tutorial component of phase IV so as to ensure that students are again challenged to address basic concepts, underlying mechanisms, and broader issues in health care. Our emphasis on critical appraisal of data mentioned above is an example of this approach.

## Can Community Medicine Be Taught by Problem-solving Approaches?

John Evans, the founding dean of the McMaster Faculty of Health Sciences, identified three waves in the evolution of health services that reflect the main causes of death or morbidity in developed countries over the past century. The first phase, at the end of the last century, was dominated by malnutrition and communicable disease. The second phase, now upon us, Evans labeled "the phase of chemical pathology": cancer, cardiovascular disease, diabetes, hypertension, etc. There is some evidence that mortality rates are beginning to decrease for certain of these diseases, e.g., hypertension, heart disease, and cancer. Phase three is also upon us, the "wave of social pathology": the diseases of human behavior, geriatrics, environmental hazards, toxicology, alcoholism, and drug dependency.[2] We share Evans' concern that these problems must be addressed in the mainstream of our medical program. For us that means using a problem-solving approach. Although we have addressed some of the population, epidemiological, and preventive medicine issues to some extent, we have not yet brought them into a central place in our studies.

There are several reasons for this deficiency. First, in Canada our primary care and community health services are not organized to address population and environmental problems but, rather, to address individual, isolated patient problems. We need to develop alternative health problems in order to have a legitimate and exciting educational base for students. We need the community equivalent of the institutional intensive care unit as a base for education, research, and service focusing on the environmental, social pathology, and self-induced illness problems.

We need not only "paper" problems but "real" problems for this educational base. We are currently looking at methods for eliminating this deficit in our system.

Second, the traditional separation of public health and clinical medicine has contributed to our failure to produce sufficient numbers of exciting young scientists and clinicians capable of developing an integrated approach in our faculties. At McMaster, we have been fortunate in having a strong Department of Clinical Epidemiology and Biostatistics that has profoundly influenced our clinical departments, so that the practicing physicians are acquiring the skills to address population and community problems relevant to their clinical disciplines.

Third, faculties must have the collective will and the organizational capacity to reallocate resources as necessary to develop academic strengths in the community, for psychosocial issues, and for environmental health. If students and faculty are to use a problem-solving approach to inquire about and explore these fundamental concepts, the resources for the student must then be in place.

## Can a Problem-solving Approach Be Used in Large Classes Rather Than Small Tutorial Groups?

In our system the small tutorial group is a key component in the problem-solving approach to learning. Admittedly, it is an ideal situation that permits maximum student involvement and discussion, prompt feedback to the student, and an intellectual challenge. We have often been asked if the small group tutorial approach is an essential component to problem-based learning. This question is obviously key for medical schools (often in developing countries) where the faculty/student ratio is unfavorable. Undoubtedly, some small group work is necessary. How much is the question. We have maintained that the tutor needs to be an expert not in the subject area but in tutoring. An accomplished tutor is able to stimulate and encourage students to become competent, self-directed learners. Large classes can, with care, be given problem-oriented seminars and lectures.

## Can All Faculty Effectively Use the Problem-solving Approach?

As expected, some faculty have natural skill in this regard. However, many faculty members need assistance in learning the strategy of teaching in this manner. As part of our faculty development program, we have established faculty workshops to develop faculty leadership that understands the rationale for problem-based learning and skills in problem design and educational planning (see Chap. 20).

## Conclusion

Our experience with a problem-based curriculum over twelve years at McMaster indicates that the problem-solving approach lends itself to an intellectually stimulating and rigorous educational experience. However, continuous ongoing care and attention are required to ensure that knowledge is integrated and not fragmented. The greatest safeguard, of course, is the student. Integration of knowledge takes place in the head of the student despite the faculty's tendency to fragment knowledge from time to time. Careful monitoring, periodic revision, and review of problems are necessary if we are to keep the curriculum relevant to changing health care priorities. The most powerful problems for learning are real-life clinical problems. It means we must ensure that we have relevant and appropriate health services settings in which the student can learn what might be called "modern medicine," i.e., community medicine with its related psychosocial, environmental, and self-induced health problems. Evidence is developing that students who learn by problem-solving and inquiry continue to learn in this manner after graduation. Our hope is that we have begun to produce a generation of health professionals who are, in fact, continuing learners.

## Case 1. Mary Cornell: A Typical Problem

*Part I*. Mary Cornell, age 2 years, 3 months, was playing in the kitchen while her mother prepared dinner. The phone rang, and her mother left the room to answer it. Moments later Mary wandered over to the stove and reached for a pot. Potatoes and hot water splashed over her upper right arm, face, pectoral area, and neck. The mother grabbed Mary, hot, wet clothes and all, wrapped her up in a blanket, and screamed into the phone for help.

You, the physician, receive a call from the friend to whom Mrs. Cornell was talking on the phone and meet Mrs. Cornell in the Emergency Department. She and Mary arrive by ambulance.

*Part II*. Examination shows Mary to be screaming. Her pulse is 150 and blood pressure (BP) is 80/60 mm Hg. Her airway, lungs, and abdomen are normal. She has second-degree burns to approximately 15% of her body (front and partially on the back) and an area of third-degree burns on the anterior shoulder.

*Part III*. Intravenous fluids were started, and Mary was treated with pain medication. On admission, the whole blood hemoglobin was 13 g/dl and the hematocrit 45. Twelve hours later, these values were 14.8 g/dl and 52, respectively. Forty-eight hours after the burn, Mary was able to start taking oral fluids. The intravenous fluids were discontinued at 72 hours.

*Part IV*. Contractions developed around the anterior axilla and required two surgical grafting and reconstructing procedures. Mary was discharged home after 57 days in hospital. Her mother was not available to pick her up.

## Case 2. Lazarus Problem: A Phase II Problem

This case describes a true story. A 5-year-old boy walked out on a frozen river and plunged through the ice into the water. Forty minutes later, he was recovered by scuba divers. Mouth-to-mouth ventilation and external cardiac compression was started immediately; the boy arrived in hospital 10 minutes later. There was no spontaneous respiration or circulation, his rectal temperature was 24°C, and his skin was cyanotic; i.e., he appeared dead. Despite this appearance, with appropriate therapy the boy woke up a few hours later. Three months later he was completely normal in all respects.

What factors led to his miraculous recovery?

## Case 3. Sally Moutarde: A Phase II Problem

Mrs. Moutarde, while in her eighth week of pregnancy, developed a fever and a morbilliform rash. During the next day, tender lumps appeared at the back of her neck. After 1 week, all symptoms disappeared and she felt well. During her next prenatal visit, which was 3 weeks later, she mentioned the illness to her physician, who took a blood sample for antibody analysis. Antibodies were assayed by hemagglutination inhibition, and a titer of 1:512 was obtained. Antibodies to rubella virus of the immunoglobulin (IgM) class were present. Therapeutic abortion was discussed but decided against.

The rest of her pregnancy was uneventful and a 7 pound 7 ounce girl was delivered at term without complications. No apparent abnormalities were noted at birth, and the baby did well during the first 3 months of life. However, at 4 months of age she developed pneumonia and was noted to have a scaly erythematous rash on her arms, legs, face, and trunk. Other findings included generalized lymphadenopathy, hepatosplenomegaly, cyanosis, and a systolic heart murmur. At this time she was treated with antibiotics and digoxin.

At 8 months of age the child was admitted to hospital. Over the preceding 2 months she had suffered from four mild upper respiratory tract infections and had failed to thrive, being below the third percentile in weight and 5th percentile in height. The lymphadenopathy and hepatosplenomegaly as well as the heart murmur were still present.

Lymph node biopsy showed germinal centers and medullary sinusoids replaced by sheets of pleomorphic mononuclear cells. Serum immunoglobulin levels were as follows.

| | | |
|---|---|---|
| IgG | 600 mg/dl | (expected: 725 mg/100 ml) |
| IgA | 0.5 mg/dl | (expected:  19 mg/dl) |
| IgM | 272 mg/dl | (expected: 100 mg/dl) |

Over the next year the child received various forms of supportive therapy and gradually began to gain weight. By 19 months of age, the lymph nodes and liver were of normal size, and the spleen was no longer palpable. She had experienced only occasional upper respiratory tract infections during the 6 months prior to being examined. Serum immunoglobulin levels were similar to those observed at 8 months of age.

At age 3 the child was found to have difficulty hearing and was fitted with a hearing aid. In addition, she developed milky opacities of both eyes. These were removed surgically. When last seen at 5.5 years, she was reported to be having learning difficulties in school, and serum immunoglobulin levels were as follows.

| | |
|---|---|
| IgG | 700 mg/100 ml |
| IgA | 150 mg/dl |
| IgM | 104 mg/dl |

## References

1. Sackett DL, Haynes RB, Tugwell P: Clinical Epidemiology. Boston, Little, Brown, 1985, pp. 285–321.
2. Evans J: Measurement and management in medicine and health services training needs and opportunities. In Lipkin M Jr, Lybrand WA (eds): Population-Based Medicine. New York Praeger, 1982, pp. 4–6.

# Part IV
# Evaluation in Innovative Medical Education

MARTEN W. DE VRIES

In response to the critique that medicine, in its singular emphasis on biomedical research, has grown too distant from the day-to-day concerns of community life and the illness experience of its patients, an attempt to develop innovative medical educational programs has taken place. These programs attempt to address medicine's shortcomings primarily by being community responsive and educationally relevant to the learning needs of young physicians. The institutions are thereby in no small measure attempting to change the way medical care is practiced today.

A clear need of innovative medical education programs is to demonstrate both their adequacy in the traditional medical sense and their capacity to meet the broad, newly defined objectives of a primary care curriculum. The burden of proof falls on the student evaluation process. The scope of the problem may be measured in the generosity of the challenge "health for all by the year 2000" where health is defined by WHO, somewhat broadly, "as the total physical, mental, and social well-being of an individual." These objectives have been translated into specific curriculum goals as espoused by Neufeld and Sibley (Chapter 11):

- To identify and define health problems at the individual, family and community level;
- To examine underlying physical, biological, and behavioral mechanisms of health problems including the spectrum from the molecular, to the individual and the community and to recommend effective and efficient management of such problems;
- To recognize, maintain, and develop the personal characteristics and attitudes required for a career in the health professions;
- To assess critical professional activity related to patient care delivery, health care delivery, and health research.

In addition, to assessing whether such goals have been achieved, evaluation procedures also play a crucial role in dictating and maintaining the structure of the curriculum.

Much time and energy has been spent establishing fair and purposeful evaluation systems, as the contributors to this section show. Numerous issues are brought forth. Specific programs and methods are discussed. Results of student evaluations are offered, as are plans for comparative prospective studies. The modes of evaluation introduced are unique and student oriented, modeling the humanitarian orientation of the primary care curriculum's aim of producing patient-oriented physicians.

The Emperor of China first introduced formal tests and proficiency requirements for his public officials in 2200 BC. Today's evaluation procedures stem from the achievement tests introduced by Rice in 1890 and the behavioral objectives introduced by Tyler in 1934. These developments have evolved to the systematic and multimethod approaches described here.

Basic questions about the nature, reasons, and goals of evaluation have been actively considered in these programs. What skills, knowledge resources, and attitudes need to be reassessed and for what purpose—certification, social protection, achievement, motivation, direction, or to merely help administrators with student selection? When should students be assessed, by whom, and with what methods? These concerns have been incorporated in the development of evaluation programs with the result that teaching methods take their place with pre-entrance and student selection factors in becoming important considerations of the medical faculty.

Traditionally, a criterion applied to mature academic disciplines is the recognition of the discipline in the academic sense as a body of knowledge and skills extended constantly by research and teachable to medical students and other health professionals. Do these innovative programs provide such a context for research, practice, and training in which students and program outcomes may be evaluated?

As Neufeld and Sibley's four objectives demonstrate, the primary care orientation attempts to be fair, person—not disease—oriented, and function—not diagnosis—oriented. It also seeks a more equitable distribution of practitioners in a population. Training such physicians brings with it a unique aspect of health care practice as well as unique needs for the acquisition and maintenance of skills. Continuity of care is emphasized, as is the capacity to detect psychosocial and community problems requiring knowledge of epidemiological factors and sociocultural analytic skills. The capability to manage other health care professionals, referral structures, and the capacity to function in a close relationship with other primary care services must also be realized. These are quite specific and varied demands that may be asked of the graduate of an innovative health care program over and above the accumulation of traditional medical knowledge.

The challenge for the evaluation system is to measure competence in these unique areas, and not just assess the capacity of an individual to aggregate little bits of knowledge in a variety of specialties. Innovative programs are attempting to evaluate the didactic outcome of these goals by means of measuring student performance. The preliminary data presented in the following chapters suggest that this is becoming a reality. These chapters take the first step in justifying these educational approaches.

Furthermore, a formative dimension has been added to the summative approaches, which are aimed at assessing if a graduate has the necessary competence to embark on patient care in relation to standardized measures. Attempts at formative evaluations of students are presented that seek to shape the development of cognitive and integrative skills and attitudes, and thereby seek to circumvent a test-preparation academic mentality. The evaluation systems described are broad based, examining the development and outcome of program, teacher, and student alike. These assessments are obviously intertwined. For example, teacher evaluations, although it is a difficult process, is a useful part of program evaluation for allocation resources, reward, and promotion. Student evaluation outcomes are also important outcome variables for program evaluations.

The programs discussed present innovative approaches to these problems in which the evaluation of the student and the program are generally interlaced. The reader should keep in mind that student assessment methods are often viewed and presented as direct measures of the effectiveness of the program. This is justified since graduate performance and activities are the ultimate product of the medical curriculum. Student capacity, postgraduate career choice, and comparative standing with other schools become key data for the innovative programs as well as serving a real part in the students' own evaluation process. Three unusual and key aspects of curriculum evaluation are brought forward here. First, in many of the programs the admission policies attempt to select a broader-based student population, including a larger range of student varying in academic performance and background, than is traditionally the case. Second, instructional procedures tend to transfer control of the learning process to the student and provide most teaching through a problem based educational approach, as discussed in the previous section. Third, and perhaps most importantly, the innovative evaluation programs attempt to foster a mode of logical, problem-oriented thought and to avoid hindering the cognitive development of the student by imposing test preparation learning.

In the first chapter, Neufeld and Sibley's systems model offers a balanced overview of the goals, implementation, and evaluation results of the McMaster curriculum. They discuss the McMaster selection systems, the interim activities of the teaching program and learning assessments, as well as the results of the graduate performance. In McMaster's selection procedures, previous academic ability is balanced by an assessment of personal qualities. No specified premedical course prerequisites are set. The results of these policies have been studied. In these studies, premedical grade-point averages did not predict performance as measured by in-course assessments and performance on the national Canadian licensing examination.

Furthermore, students without the natural science course prerequisites usually required in North America performed equally well as those who have these typical requirements. Although these conclusions are not firm, they are interesting and supportive results for their innovative selection method. We do need to be cautious in interpreting the admissions figures and we must realize that follow-up performance has not been fully assessed.

In medical student assessment, Neufeld and Sibley discuss two new developments that have occurred. The "triple-jump exercise" is a three-step structured oral examination that tests clinical problem solving and self-directed learning ability. Second, an increased emphasis has been placed on teaching a scientific reasoning method, the "critical appraisal of evidence." The effects of introducing these new approaches were recently tested in a controlled trial. Clinical clerks who used this educational method scored better in their ability to criticize and use clinical journals than students who received standard teaching.

Neufeld and Sibley next review the first generation of McMasters program evaluations. A survey of the first six graduating classes revealed that most of the graduates felt better prepared for internship than fellow interns from other institutions. While the aggregate pass rate of McMaster graduates on a national licensing examination is just under the national average, the performance of graduates in specialty-certifying examinations is above the national average. McMaster's graduates have also consistently obtained a higher rate of first choice internships than the national average.

Perhaps most importantly, 50% of the graduates have entered primary care careers and a high 10% have accepted full-time academic slots. In a study of performance in the first postgraduate year, clinical supervisors assessed McMasters graduates at or above a comparison group on all competencies reflected in the McMasters doctoral program.

Next, the University of Limburg program at Maastricht, The Netherlands, is presented, with its innovative rationale and approach to student evaluation. The Maastricht educational system has many similarities to the McMaster program but places a stronger emphasis on its problem-based learning curriculum. It is an examination system that tests students' *integrated* knowledge base rather than specific subject knowledge.

This base consists of a series of "progress tests" taken simultaneously by all students every 3 months. It is expected that an individual student will progressively improve performance on these tests, standards for which are set at the level of young practitioners entering independent medical practice.

The Dutch experience, and struggle, in implementing this program in a developing university curriculum is instructive. The first hurdle was reorienting the faculty to its evaluative programs. Since the faculty was initially busy establishing the general medical program, the first student evaluations were carried out with a true–false test format that resulted in producing a regressive "slip-back" to test preparation studying rather than a continuing involvement with problem-based learning. The effect on the curricular goals of the evaluation system employed was thus underlined.

This program also indirectly pointed out the labor intensive nature of an evaluation program that requires much faculty time as well as student agreement and support. During the evaluation and curriculum development period, disagreement resulted among the faculty as to the appropriate balance between assessment intended for diagnostic feedback and assessment for end-of-course decision making. The Maastricht faculty has grown to feel that the formative model has to be balanced by the summative "hurdle model" so that the school can fulfill its obligations to society by insuring that its graduates are competent. A special challenge in the practical implementation of student assessment has been the preparation of an end-program examination that reflects the goals of the program. The first exam was implemented in 1980. The Maastricht chapter openly discusses the difficulties experienced in implementing the primary care program at Maastricht, highlighting the tensions common in all innovative programs and faculties.

Neufeld follows with an overview discussion of student and program assessment experiences at McMaster and other medical schools. He asks three key questions about student evaluations.

1. Can an assessment system be designed that does not preclude the fostering of independent learning?
2. How can the "steering effect" of traditional assessment methods be minimized?
3. How can an appropriate assessment method be developed and used?

Neufeld offers guidelines for the achievement of content-valid, credible, and high-quality student testing procedures that involve the student more fully while minimizing the steering effect of the test. The second part of his discussion deals with a more difficult level of evaluation—the assessment of the program itself. He feels that the most important feature of program evaluation is the clarification of program aims and of the expected outcomes of academic activities. Neufeld thus urges the scientific investigation of programs so that allocation of resources to innovative medical schools may be justified and actively sought at both the university and national levels. Finally, Neufeld focuses on the need for further international comparative studies and provides suggestions for collaboration between institutions that employ innovative curricula. The goal of population-based educational and medical approaches and should demonstrate to colleagues and planners alike the contributions that innovative programs can make.

Next, Kraan and Crijnen and their colleagues at Maastricht present a unique interview evaluation testing program. This chapter is an innovative attempt to evaluate student progress on an important medical skill, the medical interview. In the article, the 4-year, highly structured, small-group teaching program for medical interviewing at the University of Limburg Medical School is described. The learning effects of the interview tutorials are evaluated by assessing the students' skill levels with the Maastricht History-taking and Advice Checklist (MHAC), developed by the authors. The theoretical background and psychometric characteristics of this research instrument, including the reliability data, are briefly presented.

MHAC measures interviewing skills on a number of classic medical interview dimensions such as history-taking skills, formulating of the medical problem, presenting solutions, structuring the interviews, as well as assessing communication skills and the students' capacity to elucidate and manage emotion-laden material effectively during the interview. MHAC evaluations clearly demonstrated that the interview tutorials had a positive impact on student performance. Students' interviewing skills pertaining to history taking, presenting possible solution to medical problems and to the structuring of the interview, could be effectively learned as a result of the teaching program. To a lesser extent, the same holds true for the students' interviewing skills required in exploring the emotional aspects of the patient's history. Interpersonal skills as well as communication skills also seemed improved. Interestingly, the students' acquisition of traditional medical knowledge and the increasing ability to solve medical problems during the course of their training exerted a negative influence on the maintenance of their "humanistic" skills. The growth of medical knowledge and greater interview efficiency gained throughout the medical curriculum was associated with a decrease in patient oriented approaches in the interview situation. During the clinical rotations when interview tutorials were not offered the effect was most marked, leading to the conclusion that interview skills should be taught without interruption throughout the 6-year medical education program.

Schmidt follows in Chapter 19 with a review of 15 studies that compare various educational outcomes of problem-based, community-oriented medical curricula with those of conventional programs. The data suggest that problem-based curricula provide a student-centered learning environment and encourage an inquisitive style of learning in their students as opposed to the rote memorization and short-term learning strategies induced by conventional medical education. In addition, community-oriented schools appear to influence the career preferences of their students. The few international studies available show that significantly larger proportions of graduates from these schools seek careers in primary care. Some of the studies reviewed suggest that students in conventional programs perform somewhat better on traditional measures of academic achievement than do students in problem-based curricula. However, these differences, if any, tend to be very small. Data with respect to performance on instruments measuring clinical competence are inconclusive. Finally, Schmidt discusses the difficulties involved in carrying out comparative research at the curriculum level as Neufeld discussed earlier in Chapter 13.

In the last chapter in this section, a comparative evaluation is made of the effectiveness of problem-based learning. DeVries et al. discuss a series of studies that reflect on the cognitive and motivational effects of problem-based learning on Dutch students. The chapter explores a unique facet of the Dutch medical school selection system. Student allocations occur by lottery after the register initial interest and have met the requirements for acceptance. This results in a more equal distribution of students in relation to interest and caliber over Dutch medical schools than is typically the case.

The comparison is not totally random since such aspects of the students' previous experience and attitude before testing were not recorded, interesting differences were observed across medical schools. Positive outcomes were scored for the Maastricht curriculum on the attitudes of the students toward instruction, the amount of their study load, the number of students matriculating, and in the shortest period of study to complete training time. Test scores on achievement tests, problem-solving style, and the capability to acquire and retain new information were also better. This warrants the conclusion that there is no reason to propose that problem-based curricula provides inferior training of medical students as compared with traditional curricula.

The data provided in this chapter clearly show that medical students in a problem-based curriculum do not spend less time in their studies and that their achievement is comparable to that of students of traditional schools. The same applies to problem-solving performance. Problem-based curricula also appear to provide a friendly and inviting educational climate. Students clearly judged the Maastricht curricula in this way. Moreover, this educational climate facilitates the emergence of positive attitudes toward instruction and, possibly, results in the lower dropout rate at the Maastricht Medical School.

In conclusion, the innovative student and program evaluation studies presented here demonstrate that these educational approaches work effectively as measured by the training aims of the schools as well as by the student responses to the program. The studies further clarify the key role of an evaluation system. The steering effect and link between educational and evaluational and subsequent student behavior, learning style, and career choice is strong. The chapters in Part IV make it clear that innovative programs have earned their place and, moreover, have developed new evaluation techniques in concert with their educational objectives. These techniques are useful in different medical education programs. The results of the studies support a principle goal of this book that innovative medical schools and their evaluation systems deserve a responsible role in training physicians of the future.

# 11
# Evaluation of Health Sciences Education Programs: Program and (Student) Assessment at McMaster University

VICTOR NEUFELD and JOHN C. SIBLEY

The evaluation of a health sciences education program and methods of assessment of health sciences students are so interrelated, each affecting the other, that an attempt should be made to address at least some of the major issues in one chapter.

In this chapter a simple model for program evaluation is presented; some of the issues we have attempted to address and measure in student evaluation are identified; some of the methodological problems we face when measuring the outcomes of programs are commented on; and there is a brief summary of some of the studies we are engaged in at McMaster University in program evaluation.

The central importance of evaluation was neatly summarized by Fred Katz in one of his informal homilies when he stated: "As ye evaluate, so shall ye reap!" Evaluation is central.

The effectiveness of an educational program is determined by societal expectations; the criteria and process for the selection of students and faculty; resources provided; the educational process itself, including student and faculty evaluations as well as reward systems; and finally the performance and acceptability of the product of the program, in this case the medical graduate. These interrelations have been expressed in Figure 11.1. We use this model to identify the various factors and their interactions that influence program output.

This chapter focuses primarily on in-course student evaluations and approaches to measuring program outcome. Two other factors intrinsic to the process are touched on briefly: societal expectation or "needs assessment," and the criteria and process of the student selection. The central aim of the whole educational enterprise, of course, is learning by the student. All other factors are subsidiary to this purpose. What the student is required to learn is determined by the expectations or objectives of the program. The ultimate test of the success or effectiveness of a health sciences educational program is: "How well do the graduates perform?" The definition of performance expectations or competence of a physician depends in part on who is doing the defining. From the usual academic perspective of the university, the good graduate is seen as one who had excellent marks in the various examinations throughout the program, who has been accepted into a prestigious graduate or residency training program, and

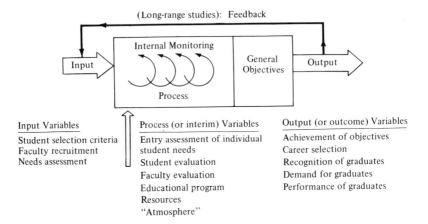

Input Variables

Student selection criteria
Faculty recruitment
Needs assessment

Process (or interim) Variables

Entry assessment of individual
student needs
Student evaluation
Faculty evaluation
Educational program
Resources
"Atmosphere"

Output (or outcome) Variables

Achievement of objectives
Career selection
Recognition of graduates
Demand for graduates
Performance of graduates

Evaluation: Defined as the precise or
approximate determination of the value,
the quantity, or the cost from which
value judgments are made in reference
to available standards. The primary
responsibility for evaluation rests
with each chairman.

FIGURE 11.1. A model for educational program evaluation, Faculty of Health Sciences,
McMaster University.

who may be clearly headed for a career as a clinical specialist, clinical scientist,
or researcher. The professor of medicine is usually reassured when he is producing one of his kind.

Those institutions in society responsible for providing health care such as ministries of health, may have quite a different definition of performance. Certainly,
they want to be assured that such a physician can provide quality care—whatever
that means. Presumably, they expect a physician to have some impact on the health
of a community and to be able to respond to the health care needs of the society
in which he or she is employed. With budgetary constraints, ministries are also
concerned with questions of efficiency and effectiveness of health care as
provided by the health professional. The patient, or consumer, may describe the
"good" physician in terms of accessibility, availability, sensitivity, and concern.

When developing a new medical school it should be possible to have the objectives of the medical education program reflect the legitimate academic concerns
of the university, the health care delivery concerns of the Ministry of Health, and
the personal concerns of the patient. Hopefully, the objectives of the educational
program reflect the social, economic, and health value systems and the cultural
realities of that particular society. If not, there is a danger of producing a medical
graduate who may be academically competent but who may not have the other
skills required for providing health care in a manner that is relevant, effective,
sensitive, and acceptable.

A poor definition of needs is reflected in a lack of clarity in program objectives and, in turn, limits the relevance of any evaluation process. As societal needs continue to evolve and our understanding of health issues improves, the objectives of the health sciences education program require rethinking and redefinition.

The educational objectives of the medical school at McMaster have been presented in detail in Chapter 10. A summary of the objectives includes the following:

1. To identify and define health problems at the individual, family, and community level
2. To examine underlying physical, biological, and behavioral mechanisms of health problems — including the spectrum from the molecular to the individual and the community — and to recommend effective and efficient management of such problems
3. To recognize, maintain, and develop the personal characteristics and attitudes required for a career in the health profession
4. To assess critically professional activity related to patient care delivery, health care delivery, and health research

## Selection of Students

It is evident that on the input side of our model the characteristics of the student population accepted in a health sciences program is a major determinant of the success of the educational program and of the outcome. The selection of medical students dealt with here primarily, though the issues are common to the other health professional programs. All programs wish to select very bright, intellectually capable people. Traditionally, we assume that this parameter is measured by the marks, or grades, the applicant has received in preliminary educational programs. Very bright students, however, may express their capabilities in ways other than examination marks. Furthermore, because the field of medicine is so broad, we thought we should not limit selection to students with a background in the biological sciences but should also admit students with academic backgrounds and interest in a variety of areas such as behavioral and social sciences, humanities, engineering, mathematics, etc. The basic criteria for eligibility is that the student must have completed 3 years of university work on entry to the medical program with at least a "B" average, i.e., a grade point average of 2.5 or higher or 70% average. Although biological science backgrounds are not essential, it is expected that the students are capable of learning science and applying it. The selection system emphasizes personal qualities and experiences in addition to academic performance. The selection process includes a review of the previous academic record, an 800-word letter written by the applicant identifying his or her reasons for desiring a medical career, and letters of reference. Approximately 20% of the students are selected for an interview by a team, which includes one medical student, one member of the faculty, a community

TABLE 11.1. Grade point average and program performance.

| Grade Point Average | Number of Students | Number of Students with no Unsatisfactories | |
|---|---|---|---|
| 2.50–2.94 | 115 | 99 | (86.1%) |
| 3.00–3.49 | 321 | 296 | (92.2%) |
| 3.59–4.00 | 186 | 166 | (90.7%) |
| | 619 | 561 | (91%) |

G.P.A is on a 4-point scale: 2.50–2.99 is approximately equivalent to a B average, or 70–80.

physician, and another member of the community. Applicants then participate in a problem-solving tutorial exercise; and finally, based on performance throughout this process, 100 students are selected.

What have we learned? First, grade point averages above 2.5 do not predict student in-course performance (Table 11.1); neither do grade point averages predict success rates on the Medical Council of Canada licensing examinations.

Second, nonscience students (those without previous courses in chemistry, biology, or physics), in general, do as well as science students if we allow for age (Table 11.2). Older students (over 30 years of age on admission) tend to perform less well both in-course and on the licensing examination. The overall rate of having one or more unsatisfactory evaluations in-course is 8.7% and the overall rate of failing the Canadian licensing examination is 8.6%. If we expelled the 79 students most at risk, i.e., those under 25 years of age with no science (26 students) and those 31 years of age or over (53 students), to get at the 17 students in that category who actually received an unsatisfactory, the overall unsatisfactory rate would have been reduced only from 8.7% to 7.0%. Finally, if we had expelled all 51 students with no science background to get at the 8 who had had an unsatisfac-

TABLE 11.2. Performance of McMaster medical students by age and by premedical science.

| Age at Entry | Premed Biology, Chemistry, or Physics | Number of Students | Number with ≥ 1 Unsatisfactory in-course | Percent with ≥ 1 Unsatisfactory in-course | Percent *not* Passing Canadian Licensing Examination |
|---|---|---|---|---|---|
| ≤ 25 | Yes | 449 | 27 | 6.0 | 4.7 |
| | No | 26 | 3 | 15.0 | 11.5 |
| 26–30 | Yes | 125 | 13 | 10.0 | 13.6 |
| | No | 12 | 1 | 8.3 | 16.7 |
| ≥ 31 | Yes | 40 | 10 | 25.0 | 25.0 |
| | No | 13 | 4 | 23.0 | 30.8 |
| All ages | All students | 665 | 58 | 8.7 | 8.6 |

tory, the overall rate of unsatisfactory would have been reduced only from 8.7% to 8.1%.

Clearly, we need to be cautious when interpreting the admission figures. We do not have adequate information as yet on the performance of our students after graduation—only on success in-course and on licensing examinations. Firm conclusions are premature. At this time we see no reason to change our policy of accepting students with backgrounds in areas other than the biological sciences and with grade point averages of 2.5 and above.

# Evaluation of Student Performance

## Principles of Evaluation

Our evaluation system has been developed on the basis of five principles.

Student performance should be measured against learning objectives. At McMaster that means that we must evaluate the students' ability to identify and define health problems at an individual and a community level. The student must be able to examine underlying physical, biological, and behavioral mechanisms of health problems including a spectrum of phenomena from the molecular, to the individual, to the family, to the community. The student must be able to recommend effective and efficient approaches to deal with environmental, occupational, and behavioral issues. Finally, he must have the ability to develop the personal characteristics and attitudes required for a career in the health profession.

Evaluation methods should be compatible with the learning objectives. Evaluation should be carried out within the framework of problem-solving in which selection, understanding, and integration of concepts from a variety of disciplines are assessed.

Evaluation information should come from a variety of relevant sources. In our system we stress self-assessment, peer assessment, and assessment by the tutor and other faculty supervisors.

Evaluation should be ongoing. Immediate feedback and ongoing evaluation permits the student to identify and therefore correct areas of weakness, thereby strengthening and reinforcing the learning process.

Evaluation is a shared responsibility. Students in a self-directed learning program share in the accountability for evaluation. It is not just an assessment imposed and controlled by faculty.

## What Do We Evaluate?

### PROBLEM-SOLVING

Because learning through problem-solving forms the basis of the McMaster approach, the student is evaluated on his or her ability to solve problems. The steps in problem-solving include the following.

*Problem identification.* Can the student identify a variety of problems in a given situation? Is a student able to describe the problem in a form that is broad enough to facilitate generation of a broad range of hypotheses? Can the student assign priorities to the problem depending on the importance of the problem and the possibility of intervening effectively in managing the problem?

*Hypothesis formation.* When faced with a problem, the student should be able to develop a variety of hypotheses and to express them in terms of basic mechanisms rather than just as disease entities.

*Hypothesis testing.* The students should show that he or she can logically describe the testing of the hypotheses and then rearrange them in order of likelihood as further information is gathered. This ability demands the gathering of data from clinical history, physical examination, laboratory results, or response to therapy.

*Integration and management strategy.* Integration of the knowledge acquired involves being able to explain the nature of the patient's illness, the mechanism of the disease, and the results of investigation. It also involves identifying those aspects of the problem that remain obscure. Finally, it demands a statement regarding the degree of confidence with which the most likely hypothesis or explanation is established. The student should then be able to form a management plan appropriate to his or her stage of learning, taking into account the risks and the benefits of treatment or no treatment, the concepts of the natural history of disease, causation, efficacy of therapy, and prognosis.

## KNOWLEDGE

Assessing the knowledge acquired through problem-solving is critical. Such assessment should include not only some sense of the amount of knowledge acquired but the relevance of the knowledge and the ability to apply that knowledge in a relevant manner.

## CRITICAL THINKING ABILITY

Critical thinking involves evaluating available information, as well as being able to understand the appropriateness of various mechanisms postulated, to determine the predictive value of investigations, and to evaluate the effectiveness of proposed therapy.

## PERSONAL CHARACTERISTICS

In addition to evaluating the student's ability to problem-solve we are also concerned about assessing the student's personal characteristics—self-appraisal ability, responsibility, and ability to relate to patients, peers, and the health care team.

## SELF-DIRECTED LEARNING

Students at McMaster must be self-directed learners. They need to identify their personal learning objectives, order their priorities when searching out information, and test their ability to use that information in a problem-solving format. Furthermore, we hope that the student will become a permanent self-directed learner. The tutor, student advisor, and student each have a role in assessing the student's capacity for learning in this manner.

## Methods of Student Evaluation

As we have no lecture courses at McMaster with the usual terminal examinations, the tutorial is the place where most of the evaluation is carried out. At the end of each tutorial the tutor gives immediate feedback to each of the students as to their performance in the relevant areas mentioned above. Peer evaluation is also encouraged as well as student self-evaluation. Students remain in a tutorial group through a unit lasting generally, 10 to 12 weeks. At the midphase of that unit, a formal written assessment is made by the tutor, discussed with the student, and forwarded to the student advisor. At the end of each tutorial unit, a detailed evaluation is carried out using a structured format that identifies the components of problem-solving, knowledge gained, and personal characteristics. The tutor discusses the evaluation with the student, and the student can add his or her comments. It then becomes part of the student's academic record. A final assessment of either "satisfactory" or "unsatisfactory" is made. Should the student be unsatisfactory, the chairman of the student assistance group meets with the student and the student's advisor to plan a remedial program. If a student should have a second unsatisfactory, a formal faculty review board chaired by the Associate Dean (Education) is established to review the student's progress and make a decision whether the student should have further remedial work or be dismissed from the program. During the past 2 years there have been six faculty review boards, and three students have been asked to leave the program, which represents an attrition rate of about 1%.

### SPECIFIC EVALUATION STRATEGIES:

There are three major student evaluation strategies: external evaluation, patient management problems, and triple-jump exercises. In an effort to avoid bias and increase the objectivity of the evaluation, most of the units now require an *independent evaluation* by one or two faculty members who have not been involved in any way with the student during that unit, or phase. Both students and faculty have expressed strong support for the introduction of this external evaluation.

### PATIENT MANAGEMENT PROBLEMS:

Students are given a synopsis of a clinical situation with appropriate clinical and laboratory information and are asked to do a written analysis of the problem, identify the issues, develop a hypothesis (or hypotheses), search out relevant information, evaluate the data, integrate the information, and test out the hypothesis. The evaluator critiques the written assignment with the student. In most tutorial groups peers are also asked to review each others' written assignments.

Triple-jump exercises are structured three-part exercises. The first part consists in giving the student a written or oral presentation of an appropriate clinical problem. The student responds to the initial presentation and elicits from the tutor, or evaluator, specific data required for an efficient and logical exploration of the problem. For example, if the patient was hypertensive, the student would probably ask if there were any changes in the optic fundi to indicate the severity of the hypertension. At the conclusion of the first part, which has probably taken 30 minutes, the student identifies the issues to be explored.

The second part consists in the student's study and exploration of these issues for a predetermined period, which may last several hours.

In part three the student returns and presents to the evaluator his progress with the problem, identifies his data source, demonstrates an understanding of the underlying concepts and their application to the solution of the problem, and submits a brief write-up with a summary of progress. The evaluator then comments on the student's performance in each part of the exercise. The triple-jump exercise allows the evaluator to probe selectively the student's understanding of basic mechanisms and to challenge the student in areas of weakness. It demonstrates the student's ability to select appropriate resources in an efficient and effective manner. The evaluator can use a structured format so as to avoid cueing the student and to ensure some consistency during the evaluation. Preliminary research studies have demonstrated the reliability of this method, and further studies are under way to test its validity and sensitivity.

The triple-jump exercise is relatively easy to develop, but its administration in its current format requires at least an hour of faculty time for each student. Student surveys confirm that it is considered one of the most useful instruments for evaluation and has a high degree of acceptability.

As students acquire clinical skills and move into phase IV (clinical clerkship) of the program, more and more of the evaluation takes place around real patient problems. Students are also evaluated specifically on clinical skills and interviewing ability.

We have systematically introduced into our clinical clerkship problems and tutorials on critical appraisal of data. To accomplish this step, we trained 42 tutors from the usual clinical departments on approaches to critical appraisal in order to assist them in developing more efficient approaches to clinical decision-making based on the application of rules of evidence to the medical literature. The educational sessions emphasize assessing quality of care studies, causation and risk factors, effectiveness of therapy, clinical error, and diagnostic tests. A controlled trial is currently under way that is attempting to measure the impact of this tutor training program on the ability of clinical clerks to critically evaluate the medical literature.

Students and faculty have clearly identified the great need for a variety of resources that students can use for self-evaluation to assess how well they can apply important concepts in the sciences basic to medicine. A start has been made in developing banks of multiple-choice questions and problems in special subject areas, e.g., clinical pharmacology, nutrition, geriatrics, and microbiology.

In general, the evaluation system has worked very well. To make such a system work, a major reorientation is required. The student must accept the fact that he is responsible for his own learning and for the self-assessment of his learning progress. The student learns that there is no satisfactory definition of core knowledge, as knowledge is always expanding. Initially, some students have considerable anxiety, but as they become skilled at learning by problem-solving and by inquiry, their confidence increases, and anxiety generally gives way to a sense of excitement and confidence. The student acquires an internal motivation for excellence that replaces the external stimulus of examination and class standing.

Faculty have required assistance in both learning how to tutor effectively and using our system for evaluation. To meet this need our program for educational development has established a series of tutorial workshops that have been attended by 260 of our faculty.

Finally, we realized early in the program that there were few readily available tools to measure the student learning progress in an educational system such as ours. As a result we have had to develop ways of measuring student learning for such objectives as problem-solving ability, the application of relevant information in problem situations, self-directed learning ability, and productive contribution to tutorial groups and health teams. It is an ongoing process, and much still needs to be done.

## Program Evaluation

Figure 11.1 summarizes the four components of program evaluation, input, process, outcome, and feedback. One can translate it into a simpler model of cause and effect. Taking this perspective, the graduate of the program is the outcome of interest or the effect, and all the components of the program are considered as the cause or the means by which the graduate's performance was produced.

In the ideal world, we would like to apply the usual principles of a rigorous experimental design to find unambiguous answers to the following questions.

1. Can we measure the efficacy and the effectiveness of our medical school program and compare it to other educational programs in other medical schools?
2. Can we isolate factors in our own educational program that have a positive or negative effect on the outcome, i.e., the cause-and-effect model?
3. Can we change or modify factors that have a negative effect on our outcomes so as to improve the effectiveness of the program?

As everyone knows, there are major problems in attempting to answer these questions, including research design problems, the definition and creation of a consensus on outcome, measurement itself, databases, and program evaluation.

The ideal design for program comparison would be a randomized controlled trial with students selected by a commonly accepted procedure and randomly allocated to medical schools with different educational programs. One need not dwell on the many reasons why such a study is impossible. We tentatively suggested such a proposal to a sister institution some years ago, and it was not greeted with any enthusiasm. Even less rigorous cohort analytical designs and case control studies are difficult and the results suspect because of the many problems of bias, nonequivalent controls, and the compounding variables inherent in the complexity of an educational environment. We are reduced, in the main, to descriptive studies with all their scientific shortcomings.

There is, however, the opportunity for randomization or cohort studies to be done with subunits in the program that might contribute significantly to the curriculum design, teaching strategies, or even selection procedures. This strategy is used in the assessment of our critical appraisal of data tutorial program for clinical clerks referred to earlier.

What is the mix of primary, secondary, and tertiary care professionals who should be produced? What are the quality-of-care attributes that should be measured—the art of care or the technical quality of care? Should the products of a "good" medical school have a measurable impact on the health of a community or on the quality of life of the individuals within that community? Is scientific development one of the program outcomes to be measured, and what are the trade-offs among basic, applied, and health care research? If program evaluation is to have meaning, institutional goals require clarification and definition.

Whereas some measures are relatively easy, e.g., career choice of graduates, demands for their services, and success rates on licensing and specialty examinations, other measurements are imprecise and require much further research and development. Measurements of quality of care, physician–patient interaction, ability to define and analyze community versus individual health problems, and the performance of graduates as continuing self-learners are a few examples.

Because of the long-term nature of education programs, evaluation data must be gathered from multiple sources with the risk of the whole process becoming cumbersome and expensive. Furthermore, many evaluation studies are retrospective rather than prospective with the inevitable problem that essential data are unavailable. When possible, program evaluations should be planned carefully, be prospective, and be as specific as possible so that a useful data base can be developed that is easily accessible, with the data retrievable, so that usable results are produced.

The questions to be addressed, the data required, and the design are influenced by the purpose of the evaluation. The common uses are evaluation for internal purposes of program modification and improvement; evaluation for efficient allocation of resources—faculty, financial, or health services; external evaluation for program approval or accreditation by government, educational, or professional authorities; research and development.

# Program Evaluation at McMaster

As seen in the following description of program evaluation activities at McMaster, we are not immune to the design, conceptual, and practical problems already discussed. Being a new school no doubt is an advantage in curriculum innovation, but it presents special problems in evaluation. First, monumental effort is required in curriculum development, faculty recruitment, student selection, development of community collaboration, and producing educational resources with relatively few faculty initially available. Second, the clarification of outcome objective evolves through experience and continuing dialogue among faculty, students, and the community. Third, it takes some years to produce a significant number of graduates practicing medicine who are available for testing and operationally defining criteria for such factors as excellence, instrument development, and feedback to the program. Fourth, we introduced two innovations at McMaster simultaneously: admissions policy and curriculum development. Furthermore, in our tutorial approach, the academic background and mix of students can have a significant impact on group learning. We attempt to select students whose learning preference matches curriculum.

Although some overlapping is inevitable, our program evaluation activities are discussed under three major headings: ongoing evaluation of the educational program by students, preparation for external evaluation and accreditation, outcome studies of our graduates.

## Ongoing Evaluation of the Educational Program by Students

On entry to the medical school, students complete an entry survey that provides background information on possible career choices and learning style, as well as demographic data not included in admission files. Just prior to graduation, students complete an exit survey that updates career choice information, outlines residency plans, and evaluates the program from the perspective of the graduating student. Students give their perceptions on the strengths and weaknesses of the program, the input of the faculty, the effectiveness of electives, and the academic rigor; they are also asked to comment on recent changes made in the program. The purpose is to give us both prompt and ongoing evaluation so that modifications may be made to increase the quality of the program.

A research team is carrying out a funded study on the graduates of our first three classes 5 years after graduation and of graduates of our fourth, fifth, and sixth classes 2 years after graduation. In addition to looking at their career pattern, we are asking them for a critical evaluation of a number of components of our program from the perspective of a graduate either in practice or in at least the third year of postgraduate training. For example, 92% of McMaster medical graduates in 1972 and 1975 responded to the survey completed during the 1977–1978 academic year. In these classes, 69 (83%) of the respondents indicated they thought they were as well or better prepared for internship than fellow interns. Eighty percent ($n = 66$) reported that the advantages of the program outweighed its disadvantages. Furthermore, the average number of advantages (1.26) reported by graduates was significantly greater than the average number of disadvantages (0.65) reported.

## External Evaluation and Accreditation

Every 5 years Canadian and American medical schools are surveyed by a joint committee from the Association of Canadian Medical Colleges and the Liaison Committee on Medical Education in the United States. In preparation for our successful accreditation in 1980, we carried out our own institutional analysis by establishing five task groups that included more than 50 faculty and students. These groups critically reviewed the evaluation system, clinical teaching, flexibility and program length, student assistance and student affairs, and the teaching of the scientific disciplines.

Recommendations were made to the Health Sciences Education Committee and the Faculty Council, and when necessary policy changes were approved and then implemented in the program. The Faculty Executive annually prepared a summary document on the issues and priorities for the next year and in this way monitors change, reallocates resources, and arranges priorities for meeting changing needs in the educational programs.

## Outcome Studies

### DATA BANK

Data generated from entry through to graduation, postgraduate training, and professional careers of alumni must be available in a manner that allows them to be linked, retrieved, and statistically treated. Initially, such data were on paper records only. After considerable debate, a computerized data bank was established. A Data Bank Board composed of three faculty members is charged with developing the system, controlling access, and ensuring security. Data incorporated into the bank are highly selective and their potential use justified. Of particular importance are data from the admissions file, entry surveys, in-course performance, some exit survey information, and annual updating information on the alumni from our alumni tracking studies. A student may have access to any information in the data base acquired about him or her. Only the chairman of the Data Bank Board and its manager have access to the system. The data bank permits rapid analysis of admission variables and outcomes, in-course performance, career choice, and random sampling of graduates for discreet studies. It has been invaluable in linking the data accumulating from various outcome studies to entry and in-course variables.

### STUDIES ON MCMASTER GRADUATES

Visitors to McMaster repeatedly ask: "Do you produce good doctors?" This global question can be broken down into a series of questions, many of which we are attempting to address. Some questions are simple: "How do your graduates score on national licensing examinations?" Others are more complex: "How well do they achieve and maintain the educational objectives of the program; for example, are they effective self-directed learners?" Still other questions are very complex and require considerable research in measures development before planned studies or comparative trials can begin. Some of these studies are presented briefly.

1. *Performance of graduates on licensing and specialty examinations.* All graduates of Canada's 16 medical schools are required to sit for the Medical Council of Canada examinations in order to obtain a license to practice anywhere in Canada. Although the Medical Council of Canada no longer gives comparative data of examination performance on graduates from each medical school, we obtain data on the performance of our graduates annually and can compare them to a national mean. Our annual pass-rates have varied from 100% to 88%, averaging about 92%.

Canadian specialty board examinations are conducted by the Royal College of Physicians and Surgeons of Canada. McMaster graduates have a first-time pass-rate of approximately 95% compared to the overall first-time pass-rate of Canadian graduates of 87%. Our first-time pass-rate in the Canadian College of Family Practice examinations in family medicine is 97%.

2. *Canadian intern matching service.* This service coordinates the matching of the graduates' choice for postgraduate internships and the various internship programs' choice of graduates. McMaster graduates have, in general, done well. In 1980, 98% of our students were matched, and 77% received their first choice, compared to 62% of other Canadian graduates.

3. *Career choices.* Consistently, 50% of our graduates have entered primary care (family medicine or general practice). Approximately 20% have gone into internal medicine, and the remaining 30% are fairly well divided among surgery, psychiatry, pediatrics, and obstetrics and gynecology; a few are scattered in other specialties. Twenty-two of our first 200 graduates have full-time faculty appointments, and another 12 at least have part-time faculty appointments at 10 universities. Ten of the first 200 graduates are still engaged in full-time research training or are completing graduate degrees at the PhD level.

4. *Performance of McMaster graduates during their first postgraduate year.* The goal of this study was to compare performance ratings of McMaster graduates during their first postgraduate year with controls from another Canadian university in the same internship program. The evaluation used a supervisor rating form. The initial approach to the control group of interns who had been selected from lists provided by program directors resulted in an unacceptably low response rate; as a result, a modified procedure was used in which the supervisor of the McMaster intern was asked to provide anonymous ratings of another intern from another Canadian medical school. This approach resulted in a total of 150 responses from McMaster graduates and 50 responses from non-McMaster residents. We are looking at such factors as professional responsi-

bility, clinical skills, knowledge base, and self-directed learning. The data are presently being analyzed.

5. *Self-directed study*. One of our objectives was to produce a graduate who would become a self-directed and continuing learner. A research study has been funded to develop a reliable and valid measure of self-directed learning. Phase I of the study, completed in the summer of 1980, focused on defining the attribute "self-directed learning," instrument development and various analyses dealing with internal consistency, and a factor structure of the items. The study is now entering the validation phase with three studies currently under way. If this research is successful, these instruments will be used to measure the performance of graduates as self-directed and continuing self-learners.

6. *Assessment of physician–patient relations*. The skill of maintaining rapport with a patient is an acknowledged prerequisite to the practice of clinical medicine and a necessary component of patient management. A patient "feedback form" to assess a physician's interpersonal skills was developed. The study involved residents in family medicine, each of whom had patient feedback forms and self-assessment forms completed on 12 to 15 patient encounters. Each resident had a supervisor observation completed on five of these encounters. Factors analyzed included response to the patient, awareness of patient concerns, instructions to patients, verbal communication, confidence, physical examination management, and professional attitudes. A reliability of 0.75 could be achieved with fewer than 10 encounters for all categories except verbal communication. It appears that the use of this patient feedback form can become a valuable adjunct for assessing interpersonal skills in the physician–patient encounter in family medicine. Further studies are under way to see if these findings can be generalizable to other clinical specialties; additional work is also required for validation.

7. *Quality of care studies*. A group at McMaster has been involved in process and outcome studies of quality of care, focusing primarily on health care ambulatory settings. Currently, research funds are being sought for a study to assess the quality of primary care provided by McMaster medical graduates in Ontario – to determine how well our graduates meet the standards for quality of care set by comparison groups of physician peers in Ontario. Measures to be used are the following.

1. Quality of care according to explicit criteria of 10 indicator conditions met commonly in ambulatory practice
2. Use of 13 drugs and drug combinations
3. Degree of physician awareness of patient concerns
4. Patient satisfaction
5. Outcome studies of specific health conditions

8. *Survey of graduates 10 years beyond graduation*. A research group is laying plans for a survey of graduates 10 years beyond graduation. If funds are obtained, this study will include interviews with a random sample of each class. Graduates, current students, and faculty will be asked to contribute to formulating the ques-

tions. Graduates participating in the survey 2 and 5 years after graduation are being asked: "What other areas do you think we should explore to better understand the long-term impact of the McMaster medical program?"

## Conclusion

A simple systems model for program evaluation has been presented as a framework for addressing some of the issues in program evaluation and student assessment. In any educational system modifying one item inevitably has an impact on others, and no factor can be considered in isolation. The type of medical students selected, for example, influence the nature of the educational program and the output.

Evaluation of an educational program focuses on the learning of the student, which in turn must be judged against predetermined objectives of the medical school program. These objectives reflect the concerns of the university, the agencies responsible for health care delivery, and the patient. Objectives require redefinition as society evolves and we have a better understanding of health care issues.

The evaluation of medical student performance should be compatible with the education objectives of the school and complement the educational approach used in that school. Innovations in medical education, e.g., a problem-based approach, requires development and testing of new measures for evaluation. Traditional measures are too often either inappropriate or inadequate.

There are major methodological problems currently limiting evaluation studies of educational programs. Nevertheless, given these limitations, further studies are needed to evaluate both the impact of the community-based medical schools on the community in which they are based as well as the effect of this approach to education on the subsequent performance of the graduates of those schools.

The exchange of such studies among the health sciences programs in the network is to be encouraged. Hopefully, collaborative studies among some of the centers can be undertaken in the future.

# 12
# The Evaluation System at the Maastricht Medical School

MAARTEN VERWIJNEN, TJAART IMBOS, HETTY SNELLEN,
BETSY STALENHOEF, MARJAN POLLEMANS,
SCHELTUS VAN LUYK, MIRJAM SPROOTEN,
YVONNE VAN LEEUWEN, and CEES VAN DER VLEUTEN

## Introduction

In 1967, the Dutch government established its eighth medical school with the goal of providing a six-year program adapted to the changing needs of the health care system in The Netherlands. Its mandate was to develop educational approaches that reflected modern educational developments. As a result, and in contrast with the other seven Dutch medical schools, the six-year program is primarily oriented toward primary health care and community medicine and the educational approach is based on the principles of "problem-based-self-directed learning".[1]

## Problem-based Learning

In this educational approach, carefully selected health care and medical problems are used as the starting point for the learning process. The problem serves as a focus for the application of problem solving or reasoning skills. It is viewed as a stimulus for an information search that facilitates the understanding of the mechanisms underlying the problem and the attempts that may be taken to resolve it. Students come together in small group tutorials to work through the presented "problems." These groups are guided by a faculty tutor, who stimulates and facilitates the learning process by questioning and reasoning rather than by lecturing. Students are encouraged to define their individual learning goals about the problem under study. Teacher-independent learning resources are available to help with this process. In addition, content experts from the various disciplines can be approached for further consultation.

In September 1974, the first class of 50 students entered the program. At that time, curriculum planning was not finished, but the changing political situation in The Netherlands required immediate initiation of the program. Detailed planning and implementation of the curriculum was carried out gradually at an ad hoc basis as the program evolved. Figure 12.1 shows an outline of the curriculum today.

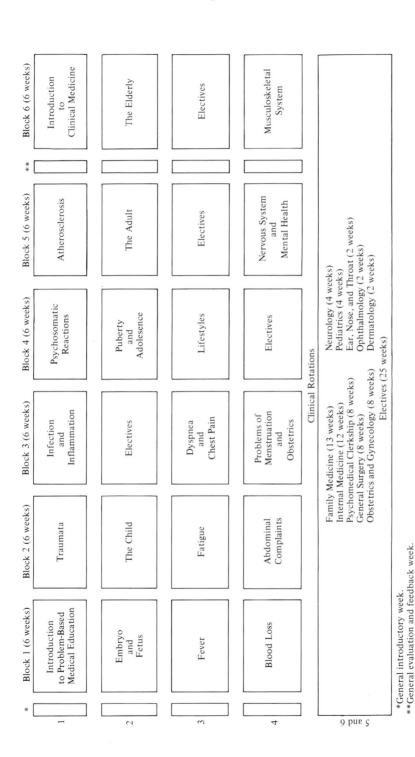

FIGURE 12.1.

Since 1974, 12 classes have enrolled. By 1982, the number of students per class has increased to 150 students per class. The admission system to medical schools in The Netherlands is based on a weighted lottery in which an applicant has a greater chance of acceptance the better his/her high school grades are. Students can indicate their preference for certain medical schools, but a national committee makes the final decision on assignment.

Each medical school in The Netherlands is responsible for the development of its own evaluation or examination system. There is no national qualifying examination board. However, each medical school has to fulfill certain broad guidelines, which are formalized in an "Academic Statute."

In the other Dutch medical schools, teaching and evaluation are the responsibility of separate departments or disciplines. In Maastricht, it is the responsibility of the faculty as a whole. Both education and research are carried out in centrally organized and directed projects by multidisciplinary groups of faculty from the various departments, a matrix–management approach.

The planning and development of the evaluation system is carried out by a multidisciplinary group of physicians, educators and psychometricians in the Project Evaluation of Study-achievements (PES).

The evaluation system is still developing. It is, in fact, a continuous process of designing, developing, evaluating, and revising to keep the educational approach and the objectives of a young developing medical school congruent with its goals. This chapter discusses this continuing process.

First, the various tests and procedures that are being developed within the program are described. Next, the counseling and certifying procedures are briefly reviewed.

## The Evaluation Program

The objective of the evaluation project (PES) is to develop a facultywide, integrated, and comprehensive evaluation program employing the following general guidelines:

1. The evaluation program should yield information that has to direct and support further learning and enable educational counseling for both students and faculty (formative evaluation). Second, the information has to enable administrative decision making and certification (summative evaluation).
2. In addition to specific strictly program-unit or block-related assessments, the evaluation program should also focus on the assessment of progress toward the final overall curriculum objectives.
3. Finally, the evaluation program should enable the assessment of *all* competency domains relevant to medicine (i.e., knowledge, skills, attitudes, and clinical competence) in *all* phases of the curriculum.

At the moment the following more or less well-established elements of the program can be identified:

1. Block tests
2. Progress tests
3. Skills tests
4. Structured orals and simulated clinical encounters
5. Clinical ratings
6. Self-assessment units

## Block Tests

Since 1974, at the end of each program unit (block), students are offered a multiple-choice "Block" test. It consists of 100 to 200 items relating to the block theme. Generally the items are in the true–false format or multiple true–false format.[2-4] A question mark or "I don't know" option is always included. The block tests are constructed by a multidisciplinary planning group of faculty responsible for planning and realization of the particular program unit.

The items are produced by the content experts involved with that specific block. After completion of the test, students are allowed to take their copy and an answer key with them. After computation of the scores, the results are provided to both students and the planning group of that block. In addition to their own scores, students also receive the overall results (means and standard deviations) of their peers for comparison. The individual scores are also put into a personal "Student File." Sometimes, postassessment sessions are held with the students to review the questions and results more thoroughly.

Students are also asked to complete a questionnaire concerning the quality of the block program. The questionnaire data together with the block test data are reviewed by the planning group of the particular block to find out whether, and if so which, adjustments to the program have to be made.

## Progress Tests

All students enrolled in the program will take a progress test four times a year. A progress test is a 250-item sample of an item bank of questions designed to measure the factual information in all areas of medical science considered necessary to graduate in medicine. At the moment, the item bank contains approximately 13,000 questions and is constantly growing. Efforts to computerize the item bank have resulted in the development of a comprehensive medical subject heading thesaurus, by which a side variety of entrances into the bank are made possible. Furthermore sophisticated software packages are developed for database management and automated test construction. Items are again in the T/F or M–T/F format, including a question mark option.

Progress tests are designed to provide a longitudinal assessment of the progress toward the final curricular objectives. The approach is very similar to that of the "Quarterly Profile Examination" (QPE), developed at the University of Missouri.[5-7] Both the progress test and QPE have been independently developed. As the tests are administered four times a year to all students, each student will take a number of 24 tests before graduation.

In addition to our students, approximately 60 residents in family medicine (all graduates from other medical schools in The Netherlands) participate in the examination to serve as a reference group. The family medicine program takes approximately one year, so that each resident will complete no more than four tests.

Each progress test is produced by a "Progress Test Review Committee" (PTRC), consisting of representatives of the basic, clinical, and social sciences, in cooperation with members of PES. To secure content equivalence of successive tests, construction is based on a predefined blueprint of content domains, paralleling the International Classification of Diseases (ICD) categories. The blueprint categories are presented in Figure 12.2. A random item-selection procedure is employed within each category.

The items are produced by the various departments. All questions are carefully reviewed by the PTRC correctness of content, format, and wording and for relevance before they are admitted to a particular progress test. Despite continuous faculty development in item writing, the experience within the PTRC over the years shows that a more or less constant percentage of 65% of the original drafts appear to be unacceptable for inclusion in the progress test due to controversial content, ambiguous wording, and/or disputable relevance. This finding emphasizes the necessity of independent item review in test construction. After completion of a test, students are invited to take home and study their

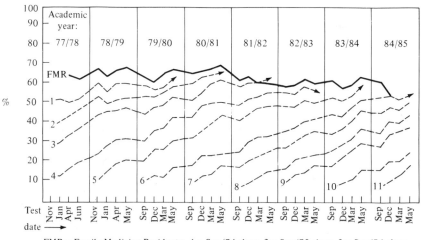

FMR = Family Medicine Residents; 1 = Sep '74-class; 2 = Sep '75-class; 3 = Sep '76-class; 4 = Sep '77-class; 5 = Sep '78-class; 6 = Sep '79-class; 7 = Sep '80-class; 8 = Sep '81-class, 9 = Sep '82-class; 10 = Sep '83-class; 11 = Sep '84-class.

FIGURE 12.2.

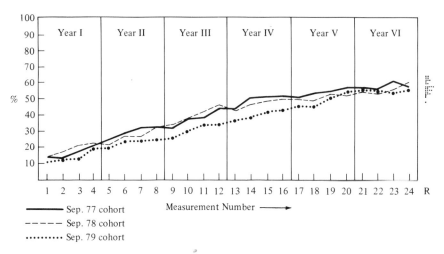

FIGURE 12.3.

copy and answer key. A detailed literature reference is added to each item, while content experts in the various subject areas are also listed in each copy for further consultation.

Overall test results (M + SD) per year class and residents group are reported to individual students, the departments, the Educational Committee, and the Student Certification Committee. Individual scores are reported to the students and their personal counselor, and the scores are also added to the personal Student File.

Students and residents are stimulated to comment on the items and the test as a whole. Standard item statistics (difficulty index, discrimination index, and item–test correlation) are routinely computed. Both comments and item statistics are scrutinized by the Progress Test Review Committee in order to identify possible ambiguous and faulty items. After consultation of the original author and/or other content experts, these items may be eliminated before the final scores are computed. Items are never eliminated on the basis of statistical indices alone. Approximately 5% of the items need to be eliminated before computation of the final results due to flaws that were not detected during preadministration review. A valid explanation as regards content, wording, or relevance has to be available. Finally, the item statistics and comments of candidates, together with specific considerations and recommendations of the PTRC, are reported back to the original authors of the items. Progress tests have been administered since the beginning of 1977.

Figure 12.3 and 12.4 present some of the progress test data that have been collected so far. Figure 12.3 graphically displays the mean results (percentage correct) of the various year groups and the Family Medicine Residents group (FMR) on the subsequent progress tests, administered since June 1977. The scores of

| Categories | % of Items |
|---|---|
| Respiratory tract | 11 |
| Hematology and lymphatics | 6 |
| Musculoskeletal system | 7 |
| Reproductive system | 7 |
| Endocrinology and metabolism | 7 |
| Cardiovascular system | 11 |
| Skin and appendages | 5 |
| Digestive tract | 10 |
| Urinary tract | 7 |
| Nervous system | 8 |
| Mental and social health/community medicine | 15 |
| Miscellaneous | 6 |

FIGURE 12.4.

three cohorts (77, 78, and 79) are presented in Figure 12.4. These graphs depict the scores by the curriculum years at the time the tests were administered. The accumulated FMR data are graphed providing a learning curve of performance throughout the curriculum.

## Skills Tests

An integrated part of the educational program is the training in basic physical-diagnostic, interviewing, laboratory, and therapeutic skills. For this purpose, a "skills laboratory" has been developed. It provides a wide variety of more or less teacher-independent training programs, using written protocols, audiovisual aids, dummies, and simulated patients.

Since the beginning of 1980, skills tests are administered to all students enrolled in the program. One test for each year group is constructed. It is intended to assess mastery of psychomotor skills. An integrated skills test providing a longitudinal assessment of progress in the skills learning (cf. progress tests), is being developed. They are being developed according to the organization model of the "Objective Structured Clinical Examination" (OSCE) introduced by Harden.[8]

The skills test consists of students rotating through stations where they are required to perform a variety of tasks. They may be asked to test urine samples, perform a cardiorespiratory resuscitation on a dummy, interview a simulated patient, apply a bandage on a sprained ankle, or perform a neurological examination of the lower extremities on a simulated patient simulating a peripheral neuropathy.

Performance is rated by trained observers on standardized checklists. Figure 12.5 gives an examples of such a checklist. A skills test will generally consist of

Station No. 5

Examination of the Peripheral Circulation
of the Upper Extremities

\*\*\*

| Criteria | Performance | | | | |
|---|---|---|---|---|---|
| | Correct | Incomplete | Incorrect | Not Perf- ormed | Unassessable |
| 1  Inspection | | | | | |
| 1.1. The skin colors of the left and right arm/hand are compared | 0 | 0 | 0 | 0 | 0 |
| 1.2. The temperatures of the left and right arm/hand are compared | 0 | 0 | 0 | 0 | 0 |
| 2  Palpation | | | | | |
| 2.1. The carotid arteries are palpated on both sides | 0 | 0 | 0 | 0 | 0 |
| 2.2. The brachial arteries are palpated on both sides | 0 | 0 | 0 | 0 | 0 |
| 2.3. The radial arteries are palpated on both sides | 0 | 0 | 0 | 0 | 0 |
| 2.4. The ulnar arteries are palpated on both sides | 0 | 0 | 0 | 0 | 0 |
| 3  Auscultation | | | | | |
| 3.1. The carotid arteries are auscultated on both sides | 0 | 0 | 0 | 0 | 0 |
| 3.2. The fossae supraclaviculares are auscultated on both sides | 0 | 0 | 0 | 0 | 0 |
| 4  The blood pressure is measured on both sides (for performance criteria, see enclosed copy) | 0 | 0 | 0 | 0 | 0 |
| 5  The student comes to the right conclusions about the status of the peripheral circulation (see data about the patient being examined) | 0 | 0 | 0 | 0 | 0 |

General impression: Good/average/bad

Remarks:

FIGURE 12.5.

about 15 stations, each station taking 10 minutes. The stations are constructed by a multidisciplinary group of faculty responsible for the development of the self-containing learning units. Each skills test is produced by a multidisciplinary "Skills-test Review Committee" (STRC). This committee reviews the stations before they are accepted for inclusion in a test and is responsible for the training and selection of examiners. After test administration, the committee will study the item-analysis data to determine whether there are any undue examiner or other confounding effects. In concert with the faculty involved, the data are corrected for those effects before the final results are computed.

Individual station and the total test scores are reported to the students who also receive a copy of the completed checklist that include examiners comments. These data will also be put into the personal Student File. Finally, overall results (M + SD) are reported to both students and faculty.

## Structured Orals (SO) and Simulated Patient Encounters (SPE)

The last two years of the program are devoted to clinical rotations. During these years, students take several examinations. Most of these examinations are strictly related to the clinical disciplines they are rotating through, some are patient-problem oriented, integrating the contribution of several clinical, basic and/or social sciences. Most of the examinations are designed on the basis of actual clinical cases. The intention is to develop each encounter between student and examiner as a structured role play simulation of a case history.

However, most of the encounters at the moment take the format of an unstructured traditional clinical viva, in which after examining a selected patient, the candidate is interrogated about this case by the examiner. Some encounters are more structured, the candidate being questioned about a specifically prepared clinical case presented by the examiner. The answers are scored by the examiner on a checklist. Cases, questions, and checklists are constructed a priori by groups of faculty from one or more disciplines. These groups are also responsible for the training and selection of examiners. All the activities are coordinated and controlled by a Clinical Test Committee. This committee reviews all cases before they are administered to students.

Although the clinical examinations should be designed to test clinical competence, most of the actual exams are focused more on "clinical knowledge" than on the assessment of "clinical problem solving abilities" or "clinical competence."

The Simulated Clinical Encounter, on the other hand, runs on the basis of a written database, which presents all the critical information about the patient that could be obtained in a real health care setting, including the way the patient will respond to various procedures. Next, a detailed script or scenario is developed which captures the sequential unfolding of the real clinical problem being simulated. It includes such considerations as how the problem is introduced, actions the student can take, resulting reactions from the patient, alternative courses of action (both correct and incorrect), real-world decisions, actions, or procedures and their consequences.

Finally, critical action checklists and rating scales are developed on which the examiner has to register and score the student's performance. The simulation is administered by a trained examiner who has access to all the data. When questioned, the examiner answers for the patient using the database to ensure that verbal responses accurately represent the background, symptoms, signs, and pathology of the patient being simulated. Abnormal pathology might be represented by photographs, X-rays, microscopic slides, lab sheets, electrocardiograms (ECGs) or described verbally by the examiner. The examiner will respond to actions taken by the student, using the scenario as a guide. The development of this type of examination is based on the approach introduced by Maatsch and his colleagues for use in the American College of Emergency Physicians Certification Examination[9,10] and adapted for use in basic medial education.

According to Maatsch et al.'s findings, the Certification Examination offers the basis for a more insightful, valid, and standardized assessment of the student's capabilities in managing clinical problems. Our experiences are still limited, and most cases that have been developed are far from perfect. In general, however, the acceptance by both students and teachers is positive. Major drawbacks are the enormous time investments in the construction of cases, preparation of examiners, and handling the logistics of large numbers of students.

## Clinical Ratings

Since 1980, standardized rating scales have been introduced to assess student performance during the clerkships. At the moment, the experiences with these rating scales are still very limited and most of the initial problems of implementing such an evaluation method (ie, predominantly standardizing rater variability) are still to be overcome. Nevertheless, the rating forms are being used and the results are recorded in the personal Student File. The rating form currently aims to assess the characteristics presented in Figure 12.6.

The rating scales are completed only by the clinical supervisor. In the future, it is intended to realize independent completion by more than one clinical preceptor, and if possible by peers and nursing staff as well. The ratings should be discussed with the students before final reports are made up for inclusion in the Student File. Finally, it is our intention to introduce similar observational ratings in other curricular phases. For instance, during small-group tutorials, electives, Skills-Lab training sessions and simulated patient sessions.

## Self-assessment Units

In addition to the foregoing evaluation methods, which certainly provide some self-assessment possibilities to students, a variety of instruments are used for self-assessment purposes only. Because of practical problems with production, development, and administration, as well as theoretical issues of validity and reliability of scoring techniques, these instruments are not yet included in the standard testing procedures of the evaluation program. As the experience with these methods grows, future implementation may however be considered. Self-

| | |
|---|---|
| 1. Professional competence | |
| 1.1. Collection of data | • History-taking<br>• Physical examination |
| 1.2. Interpretation of data | • Definition of problem(s)<br>• Analysis of problem aspects<br>• Establishment of diagnostic plans<br>• Establishment of therapeutic plans |
| 1.3. Presentation of data | • Records are clear<br>• Records are complete and systematic |
| 2. Personal characteristics | |
| 2.1. Attention to health care activities | • Presence (punctuality)<br>• Participation and involvement |
| 2.2. Relation with health care personnel | • Colleagues<br>• Paramedical staff |
| 2.3. Relation with patients | • Proper behavior<br>• Empathy<br>• Respect for needs and expectations |
| 2.4. Insight into own abilities | • Recognition of strengths, weaknesses, and limits<br>• Sense of duty |
| 2.5. Attention to educational activities | • Active participation<br>• Preparation |

FIGURE 12.6.

assessment units are made available to students for use at all times, but most of them are produced in connection with specific blocks or program units.

Although a variety of problems, cases, questions, assignments and the like are presented to students as self-assessment exercises, the self-assessment units will mostly take one of the following formats:

1. Patient Management Problems (PMP)
2. Modified Essay Questions (MEQ)
3. Problem Boxes (PB)
4. Portable Patient Problem Packs (P4)
5. Triple Jump Exercises (TJE)

## Patient Management Problems (PMP)

In this format, pioneered first by Rimoldi[11] and McGuire and Solomon,[12] the student is asked to choose from a list of possibilities, the action he/she would take, given an initial case presentation. The results of the choices are then revealed by the use of invisible ink, made visible by a felt marker.

Each PMP includes action and management sections as well as database sections (ie, history, physical examination, paramedical tests, etc.). Students gradually reveal the information needed and select appropriate actions to be performed on the basis of this information. Thus, the course of a case history, including the effects on the student's action and management, may be simulated, gradually unfolding the patient's problem. The student is able to see the consequences of his or her own decisions and can follow the problem until it has either been successfully or unsuccessfully managed. Complex situations, including complications that may arise which the student has to manage as they occur, can be simulated using branching techniques.

The PMP is designed to offer the student a possibility to demonstrate his/her skill in dealing with a particular patient problem in a written format. For assessment purposes, scores such as proficiency or efficiency in data gathering and management can be computed, provided that all available options are given numerical weights (e.g., $+2$ to $-2$) according to their positive or negative contribution to the management of the problem. The validity of these scoring techniques however, has been seriously questioned in the literature.[13-15]

Students are invited to discuss their approach with fellow-students and content experts. Sometimes also written protocols, recorded by expert physicians dealing with the case, are included to provide a more qualitative feedback.

## Modified Essay Questions (MEQ)

The Modified Essay Question, originally designed by the Royal College of General Practitioners[16] and further explored by Knox,[17] is a structured free-response series of questions about a developing biomedical problem. The information about the case or problem the candidate is confronted with, is presented in a sequentional manner. The student is provided with additional information at successive stages. The candidate is invited to respond to several open-ended questions is a given stage of the MEQ before proceeding to the next phase. The questions are structured in such a way that concise answers are required.

A question may run as follows: "List three items of information you would seek in order to confirm the suspected diagnosis of bacterial tonsillitis." In contrast with PMPs, the progression through a MEQ is not dependent on the decisions made by the candidate, nor is responding to subsequent questions dependent on answers given to previous ones. Scoring is done by hand on the basis of key answers provided by content experts.

## Problem Boxes (PB)

The Problem Box, originally developed by Barrows and Mitchell[18] as a learning tool in problem-based learning, could be described as a more realistic modification of the MEQ, to involve students with a variety of biomedical problems. As is suggested by the name of the format, all the relevant material is packed in a box. A variety of audiovisual materials are used to present realistically the problem to the students. Generally, the problem is introduced by an audio-tape that allows the student to hear the actual initial interview of the patient by the attending physician. Photographs and slides are available to demonstrate the patient's actual appearance. In addition, X-rays, fundoscopic appearances, microscopic slides, gross appearances of tissues or lesions, graphs and laboratory results, copies of letters exchanged between consulting physicians, etc. are all included.

The problem is gradually unfolded by the student working through the problem box. At several stages, open-ended questions are raised, which have to be answered before proceeding to the next stage. A separate feedback unit is one item included in the box. It is constructed in such a way that it can be consulted at any point in the workup of the case without revealing all the information at once. Thus, progression through the problem is still possible even if a student may be at a loss somewhere during his/her workup. The feedback unit also includes scoring sheets, reference material, written protocols of experts working with the problem box, etc., to assist students in evaluating their own performance.

## Portable Patient Problem Pack (P4-Deck)

The P4-deck originally developed by Barrows and Tamblyn[19] consists of a deck of several hundred cards in a variety of colors, including photographs cards of the same size. The colors represent the action categories that might be taken with a patient (ie, history, physical examination, laboratory tests, consultancies, treatments/interventions, etc.). The assembled unit of cards represents all possible or conceivable actions the student might want to take with any patient problem, not just those that may be relevant to the case at hand. Only a small percentage of the cards, however, is necessary in working effectively with the patient problem presented in a specific deck. Thus, the cueing effect of the presented options, demonstrated in objective examinations and PMPs[14-20] is minimized.

On front of each card, next to the title, a number of (standard) questions is included to stimulate the student's clinical reasoning process (eg, problem formulation at that point, hypotheses, what further actions etc.). On the back of the cards, responses of the patient or others to the actions indicated by the front title are presented along with answers to questions, physical examination findings, results of investigations, opinions of consultants, and results of treatments or interventions. In contrast with the PMP, this format allows the student to take any action possible with a real patient, in any sequence felt appropriate.

A "situation card" presenting the "opening scene" initiates the student's work with the unit and a "closure card" can be drawn whenever the student feels he or she has finished the encounter with the patient. Similar scores as in the PMP format can be computed provided each card is given a numerical weight. Promising data about parallelism in the performances between the student's use of a P4 deck and encounters with similar simulated patients have been reported.[21] Reference material, P4 sequences chosen by experts who have worked with the P4 unit, and patients writeups, done by a variety of experts or costudents, is made available to assist the student in evaluating his/her own clinical reasoning.

## Triple Jump Exercise (TJE)

Some departments offer the student the possibility of doing a "Triple Jump Exercise" during electives or clinical clerkships. The TJE is a three-part structured oral examination developed at McMasters Medical School, Hamilton, Canada.[22] It assesses problem-solving abilities such as problem identification, hypothesis formulation, information gathering, evaluation of data, self-directed learning and integration, and application of prior knowledge. It is claimed to be an instrument tailor made to a problem-based, self-directed learning program.

In short, the assessment procedure is as follows:

Part 1:         Present the problem.
(20 min.)   Discuss with the evaluator to define the major issues, formulate and pursue hypotheses, and identify appropriate key issues for the student to study in depth.
Part 2:         Individual study, adequately using the learning resources available.
(2 hrs)      able.
Part 3:         Present and discuss a precis of the issues studied.
(20 min.)   Evaluation and counseling by the evaluator.

Evaluators are provided with a list of key issues, questions to prompt the students, key references, and faculty resources as well as a standardized rating form to assess the student's performance. In addition to the development of self-assessment units or exercises, the TJE is also intended to actively involve the students in giving an integrative personal assessment of their learning progress on the basis of the data available in their personal Student File. This will be further discussed in the next section dealing with the procedures employed in graduation or certification of students.

## Education Counseling and Graduation

How should the elements of the evaluation program be used in the process of counseling? Since the foundation of our school, this issue had received minimal attention, but in 1980 students succeeded in bringing about fundamental discussion about how this could be done. The critique was that the existing method was not congruent with the educational philosophy of the school. Students felt that a one-sided emphasis was put on summative decision making with little or no attention to the formative or supportive role of evaluation. Furthermore, the fact that students are given a lot of responsibility in directing their own learning activities within the educational program was not reflected in the evaluation system. Students felt they were passive candidates instead of actively involved participants in the evaluation process. They felt that the evaluation system had evolved into too much of an "hurdle" and not enough of a "help" (cf. Leeder, et al.[23]); more of an imposition than a joint venture of students and faculty.

In response, the faculty council, representing both students and faculty, decided to take the following new approach. From the beginning of their training, students are assigned to a "Personal Student Counselor" (PSC), who supervises, guides, and supports the student for the complete duration of the study. Student counselors are regular faculty members. each counselor is assigned to 15 to 20 students. Student and counselor meet at regular intervals to discuss the learning progress and future learning activities on the basis of an assessment of the data included in the personal Student File. This Student File includes all the results of the tests and examinations administered within the evaluation program. In addition, students may add other information they feel necessary for a valid and comprehensive judgment of their learning progress. Finally, written reports of the counseling sessions between students and counselor, including comments, considerations, advice, and plans, are made up to be included in the Student File. Student profiles are be constructed on the basis of the information available in this file.

In addition to the counseling sessions, separate meetings between student and counselor are organized to consider graduation to a next phase of the curriculum. These meetings are to held at the end of years 1, 4, and 6, to determine if the student is ready for graduation. These times coincide with the three phases of university education introduced by a new higher education law.

The "graduation sessions" between students and counselor are based on an assessment of the information available in the Student File and a set of general guidelines and directives prepared by the Certification Committee. Student and counselor draw up an educational contract, stating the final learning and evaluation activities that will be undertaken in the next three months. Fulfillment of the contract leads to graduation by the Certification Committee. These are the basic elements of the new approach. A comprehensive set of guidelines, rules, regulations, and directives have been worked out to ensure an adequate balance between completely arbitrary decision making on the one hand and completely automated decision-making on the other.

## Conclusion

Although we have not yet reached the ultimate goal of a fully developed, facultywide, integrated, and comprehensive evaluation system, the Maastricht program provides an exciting stage for collaborative work between medical teachers, educational experts, and students in developing research into the innovative assessments in medical education.

## References

1. Barrows HS, Tamblyn RM: *Problem-based Learning—An Approach to Medical Education*. New York, Springer Publishing Company, 1980.
2. Ebel RL: *Essentials of Educational Measurement*. Englewood Cliffs, NJ, Prentice-Halls Inc, 1972.
3. Anderson J: *The Multiple Choice Question in Medicine*. London, Pitman Medical, 1976.

4. Harden RM: Constructing multiple choice questions of the multiple true/false type. *Med Ed 1979;13:305*-312.

5. Willoughby TL, Dimond EG, Smull NW: Correlation of Quarterly Profile Examination and National Board of Medical Examiner scores. *Ed Psych Meas* 1977;37:445–449.

6. Willoughby, TL, Hutcheson SJ: Edumetric validity of the Quarterly Profile Examination. *Ed Psych Meas* 1978;38:1057–1061.

7. Willoughby TL: Quarterly Profile Examination. *R.I.M.E. Exhibition Handout*; Annual meeting of the Association of American Medical Colleges, Washington, DC, 1980.

8. Harden RMcG, Stevenson M, Downie WW, Wilson GM: Assessment of clinical competence using objective structured clinical examinations. *Brit Med J* 1975;1:447.

9. Maatsch JL: *An Introduction to Patient Games: Some fundamentals of Clinical Instruction*. Michigan State University, East Lansing, Office of Medical Education Research and Development, 1974.

10. Maatsch JL: Towards a testable theory of physician competence: An experimental analysis of a criterion-referenced specialty certification test library. New Orleans, LA, *RIME Conference*, 1978.

11. Rimoldi HJA: The test of diagnostic skills. *J MED ED* 1961;30:73.

12. McGuire CH, Solomon CM: *Construction and Use of Written Simulations*. Chicago, IL, The Psychological Corporation, 1976.

13. Page GG, Fielding DW: Performance on PMP's and performance in practice: Are they related? *J Med Ed* 1980;55:529.

14. Norman GR, Feightner JW: A comparison of behavior on simulated patients an patient management problems. *Med Ed* 1981;15:26–32.

15. Newble DI, Hoare J, Baxter A: Patient management problems, issues of validity. *Med Ed* 1982;16:137–142.

16. Royal College of General Practitioners: The Modified Essay Question. *JR Coll Gen Pract* 1971;21:373.

17. Knox JD: *The Modified Essay Question*. Dundee Scotland, Association for the Study of Medical Education, 1976.

18. Barrows HS, Mitchell DLM: An innovative course in undergraduate neuroscience (an experiment in problem-based learning with "Problem-Boxes"). *Brit J Med Ed* 1975;9(4):223–230.

19. Barrows HS, Tamblyn RM: The Portable Patient Problem Pack (P4), A problem-based learning unit. *J Med Ed* 1977;52(12):1002–1004.

20. McCarthy WH: An assessment of the influence of cueing items in objective examinations. *J Med Ed* 1966;41:263.

21. Tamblyn RM, Barrows HS, Gliva G: An initial evaluation of learning-units to facilitate problem solving and self-directed study (portable patient problem pack). *Med Ed* 1980;14:394–400.

22. Coates G: Problem based methods of evaluation: the McMaster experience, in Metz JCM, Moll J, Walton HJ (eds): *Examination in Medical Education, A Necessary Evil? Proceedings of the 1980 Annual Conference of the Association for Medical Education in Europe*. Utrecht, Bunge, Scientific Publications, 1981.

23. Leeder SR, Felleti GI, Engle CE: Assessment—Help or hurdle? *Programmed Learning and Educational Technology* 1979;16:308–315.

# 13
# Issues and Guidelines for Student and Program Evaluation

Victor Neufeld

## Student Assessment

Three general questions that are of relevance to student assessment in innovative programs adopting community- and problem-oriented approaches arise from the foregoing chapters.

1. Can an assessment system be designed that does not preclude the fostering of independent learning?
2. How can the "steering effect" of traditional assessment methods be minimized?
3. How can appropriate assessment methods be developed and used?

### Assessment and Independent Learning

Integral to most or all of the programs represented in this volume is the idea that students should become independent learners and develop habits of learning that can be used for "lifetime learning." This concept is an inevitable counterpart of the approach that promotes learning based on problem situations – of individuals or populations. Achieving this goal of fostering independent learning requires major conceptual and practical adjustments. The faculty must "behave" differently as educators (hence the change in terminology from "teaching" to "facilitating of learning"); learning materials and events must be presented differently; and the assessment system must be altered.

The specific challenge of assessment is finding an appropriate balance between helping the students become independent and ensuring that the goals of the program are achieved (or, stated in another way, assuring society that graduates are "safe"). This dilemma is exemplified in the Maastricht chapter, using the contrast between the "help" model and the "hurdle" model. In fact, the two models are not incompatible. They can be incorporated into the same system.

Several analogies are helpful here. Any parent of teenagers recognizes that, in the process of helping children mature and become independent, parents need to set expectations and limits. The way in which these concepts are applied certainly varies from child to child, even in the same family. Using another comparison, the coach of a swimming club has quite clear ideas of the standards he wishes the swimmers to attain. The standards can be national, "club," age-specific, event-specific, or individual (and any combinations of these). A good coach creates an environment in which swimmers achieve specified goals while at the same time he helps them to have fun, gain self-confidence, and become progressively independent.

When applying these analogies to medical education, it is important to make distinctions between the entity to be assessed (i.e., the objective), the expected level of competence (the standard, or criterion), and the source of evidence on which the assessment is based. For example, a written assessment exercise can focus on a patient with hypertension. This "package" can specify the objectives to be tested (e.g., the most appropriate diagnostic work-up and management plan for the case) and the expected level of performance (e.g., which investigations should or should not be ordered). In a program that emphasizes self-directed learning, it would be quite appropriate for the same assessment package to be used for "formative" and "summative" purposes. A procedure could be developed whereby the student assesses his own performance (in relation to the criteria); the faculty tutor can review both the performance and the student's self-assessment of that performance. A decision can then be made about both objectives (the knowledge required to manage the case and the student's self-assessment ability).

It is apparent that as time goes on there should be a transition from faculty-dominated assessment activities to student-controlled activities. Given initial training and help to become independent learners, students can improve their ability to state appropriate objectives for themselves, set realistic standards, and assess their own actual performance. The challenge lies in having faculty members take the time and have the insight to develop such a system and in helping their colleagues (students and faculty) to use it appropriately.

## "Steering Effect" of Assessment

It is axiomatic that students in any program quickly discover what they need to do to "pass" and then behave accordingly. As Katz said: "As ye evaluate, so shall ye reap." Any student recognizes that the "real" objectives of a program are those reflected in the assessment system. These objectives frequently do not match the statements of intent found on the first page of a program brochure.

A common example of this principle is the observation that students do study to pass a written test, even if there are other attractive stimuli to help them learn, e.g., problem-based learning resources. If the assessment tool fails to test stated goals, or if only one of several goals is tested, a program is in danger of not achieving many of the stated intents. How can this situation be avoided or minimized? Two general suggestions are offered, both of which are quite familiar. The first has to do with matching the objectives with the test; the second revolves around the fashion in which the test is conducted.

For the first suggestion, an example from Sibley's chapter might be useful. A few years ago at McMaster University it was recognized that an assessment exercise was required that would test the abilities of students individually (in contrast to assessing performance in a group tutorial setting). Furthermore, it was thought that several important objectives could be tested in the same exercise. These objectives included problem-solving ability, independent learning, self-assessment ability, and to some extent the understanding of concepts. To achieve these objectives, a three-part structured oral examination (called the "triple-jump exercise") was designed. (1) A student "thinks aloud" through a given problem in the presence of an assessor, displaying his clinical reasoning ability (stating hypotheses and requesting confirming or disconfirming clinical data). As the discussion proceeds, it becomes apparent that the student's knowledge base is incomplete; specific questions for further study are then identified. (2) The student then explores these questions, usually for about 2 hours in a library. (3) The student returns for a final discussion with the assessor, describing how he spent the time and incorporating new knowledge gained into a cogent synthesis of the problem. The student is also asked to assess his own performance. Studies are under way to ensure that this tool is sufficiently reliable and valid.

The steering effect of assessment is also reflected in the fashion in which assessments are conducted. A "take home" or "open book" examination has a different effect on students than a comprehensive test conducted in an examination room with a time limit. The latter is, of course, easier to standardize (all students are given the same challenge under the same circumstances), but this procedure has the disadvantage of being very different from the practice setting in which students eventually have to function independently. Each institution has to wrestle with the most appropriate balance between "standardization."

## Designing Appropriate Assessment Tools

Any institution that makes a serious attempt to pioneer new approaches to education soon realizes that commonly available assessment tools have serious drawbacks. These limitations are varied. For example, common approaches to testing knowledge (multiple-choice questions, true–false items) do not usually test the understanding of broad concepts; standard oral examinations, unless accompanied by careful training of examiners and construction of assessment protocols, tend to be unreliable. It soon becomes apparent that a decision needs to be made about where an institution's efforts should be directed. Should existing methods be used and possibly adopted, or should new assessment tools be constructed?

Several institutions have adopted a combined approach, using some readily available methods but also designing some new ones. Examples of the latter are the "structured oral performance" (SOP) developed at Maastricht for the end-of-program examination, the hypothetical organism test (HOT) at Beer-Sheva to test hypothesis-generating ability, the modified essay question at Newcastle, and the triple-jump exercise at McMaster. The following guidelines are proposed.

1. The most important consideration is whether the new test is "on target"; that is, does it match the stated objective. This test attribute is sometimes called "content validity" or "credibility." The latter is probably a better term. Unless a new

test is seen by its users (students and faculty) to be credible, to accurately reflect a stated objective, there is not much point in proceeding to further methodological development.

As an example, a survey of McMaster students about the use of the triple-jump exercise revealed that an overwhelming majority stated that the test was credible. It matched the stated objectives of the program; it was very similar to the pattern of study activities most students pursue.

2. There must be a commitment to sound and high quality developmental research. The field of medical education (and education generally) is strewn with new assessment methods that have been introduced and advertised but whose development is incomplete with respect to reliability, validity, and feasibility. This commitment to producing a high quality test involves time and finances. It also takes time and patience. The researchers involved in test development must now prematurely introduce a new test for regular use. The potential users must avoid uncritical acceptance of the new test.

3. Orientation of users is an important component of test development. Both students and faculty should be included. With respect to students, efforts to provide an orientation for students are then well rewarded: Students can contribute ideas to aspects of test development; student acceptance is higher if they are involved early; and with student acceptance the performance in the new test is a more accurate reflection of actual ability. Similarly, efforts to "pilot test" a new method with faculty colleagues yields certain benefits. Early faculty involvement gives them time to adapt to the idea of something new; they develop a sense of "ownership" because they contributed to a new approach in its evolutionary state.

## Issues in Program Evaluation

Program evaluation is a more difficult activity to discuss than student assessment. It may be because program evaluation is seen by some to be optional, whereas student assessment is unavoidable. Indeed, it can be said that many medical schools around the world have no program evaluation at all. More innovative institutions, however, have indicated that some form of program evaluation is important. It is apparent, on reading the foregoing chapters, that there is considerable variation among institutions in carrying out this activity. Some institutions have made only a statement of intent; others have been collecting information for some years.

For this discussion, we consider some basic elements of program evaluation. Each institution needs to consider them when planning for program evaluation. These elements are clarifying aims, defining outcomes, designing data collection methods, and allocating resources. Each of these components is now considered. Again, examples from various institutional reports are used.

### Clarification of Aims

Why conduct program evaluation? It is evident that no institution should spend time, money, and energy on program evaluation until this question has been adequately considered. It is worth taking the trouble to discuss the question widely and thoroughly in order to arrive at some agreement and clarity about it. If a consensus can be reached, there a greater chance that students, graduates, and faculty will support and contribute to the effort.

There are various reasons why innovative institutions have embarked on program evaluation activities. They can be grouped under three headings.

1. *To modify the program*. The most common aim of program evaluation, it can be achieved through short-range activities, e.g., questionnaires or surveys at the end of a curriculum block or unit. It can also be done on a long-range basis. An example is the long-range follow-up study of the careers of McMaster graduates done by an "annual update" survey.

2. *To "validate" innovative curricula*. Although this aim may be related to the first aim listed above, it is worth stating separately, as it applies particularly to the new programs. These programs are under a great deal of scrutiny in their own countries and around the world. It has been said that any program, old or new, innovative or established, should be required to validate its curriculum. Although in theory this idea may be reasonable, the fact is that in many countries there is no system to ensure that it happens. Even in North America, where there is an accreditation system, the periodic scrutiny of medical schools does not generally include a validation of the teaching method used. Institutions are not clearly asked: "What is the evidence that your program is achieving its stated aims or producing the kinds of graduates the country needs?" The fact that innovative institutions are taking initiatives to carry out program evaluations should lead not to paranoia but to a sense of purpose and confidence.

3. *To contribute new knowledge*. In addition to the two more practical and "mission-oriented" aims above, program evaluation activities can also have intrinsic value. They represent systematic efforts by researchers to ask questions, collect information, and draw research. Although there is a considerable body of knowledge on program evaluation in the general education literature, there is remarkably little in medical education. Research reports on program evaluations in medical education are important and very much needed.

## Definition of Outcomes

When listening to the stories about how the new programs began, one can usually sense that there is a particular reason, or perhaps several reasons, why the program was started. Most commonly this reason has to do with physician performance. There may have been dissatisfaction with aspects of existing physician activity; hence statements are made about the intended professional abilities of graduates of the new program. Sometimes the reason is not so much how graduates perform but where they will practice and what their specialty will be. Alternatively, the reason may be unrelated to graduate performance; rather, it may be to provide a curricular approach that is more efficient or more relevant to national manpower needs.

Whatever the reason, it is important to translate the original main intent into measurable end-points. Some are relatively easy to define from a methodological perspective. For example, the Beer-Sheva program stated the intention that a significant number of graduates should practice in a primary care setting in the Negev. This outcome is clearly defined and can be easily measured.

Other outcomes are more difficult to define. As an example, one of the stated performance outcomes at McMaster, mentioned in the chapter by Sibley, is the ability to be an effective, self-directed learner. When researchers at McMaster began to search for an instrument to measure this specific attribute, they were unable to find a satisfactory tool. As a result, they had to deploy efforts to "tool-making" in order to create an acceptable measure of effective learning by physicians that could be applied in a practice setting. Part of this project involved not only the creation of a tool but the further definition of the attribute itself. It became clear that self-directed learning had both motivational and technical components. This situation is an example of where efforts to define an outcome measure led to greater clarity of the attribute of interest.

As a corollary to defining the outcome to be measured, it is important also to state what is *not* measured. There are some intended performance characteristics for which no tools are readily available. It also may not be feasible for a given institution to put its efforts into measuring several parameters. For whatever reason, it is important to be realistic and not to promise more than can be realistically done.

In addition to defining outcomes that are clear and realistic, an institution must select those outcomes that are most appropriate to the socioeconomic and cultural climate of the country.

## Design of Research Projects

Having clarified the general purpose of program evaluation and having defined outcomes that are clear, realistic, and appropriate, specific projects must be designed. It is important that these areas are viewed as research projects, where there is an attempt to design a method of data collection that is most likely to provide clear and credible answers to the stated question. Such opportunities vary from one country to another. Each institution encounters difficulties that may be unique to its own setting.

In Canada, for example, each institution has its own selection system. It would be impossible to randomly allocate students to an "innovative" program and to an "established" comparison program, although it would be the best research design. However, this design may be possible in countries where there is a nationally coordinated selection system and where selection is largely by lottery. Such an opportunity should be actively explored and should be possible in the Maastricht program, for example. A related program is the challenge of obtaining comparative data. The difficulty is not so much methodological as "political." For example, to make arrangements for measuring an outcome of interest in graduates of both an innovative and established program requires careful prior negotiation.

This negotiation involves discussion about the aim of the project, the outcome measure of interest, the methods of obtaining data, and perhaps most important the anticipated conclusions and publication of results. There may be various ways to handle this difficult situation. The deans of the institutions involved may need to establish safegaurds for collecting the research data and publishing the results.

There are other ways in which the design of program evaluation projects can be credible and of high quality. Some institutions conduct surveys of their graduates. The general principles of good survey design can be applied to such projects. A survey "instrument" must be carefully designed and pretested; in surveys where the same instrument is applied several times, the instrument must be stable and not changed from one application to another. There should be careful and persistent efforts to ensure a high response rate.

Even when the research design is well conceived, there may be unanticipated events that significantly influence the results. For example, the founders of the Maastricht program had definite ideas that many University of Limburg graduates should practice high quality primary care, and a good proportion should be in South Netherlands. In recent years, at about the time the first classes were graduating, there has been an increasing manpower overproduction problem in Holland and in Western Europe. Partly because of the Common Market there is much easier migration of physicians from one country to another. Dutch nationals are trained elsewhere in Europe and are coming back to Holland. As a result, some Maastricht graduates are having difficulty finding desired practice locations. Clearly, any surveys of where Maastricht graduates are practicing and what they are doing would be significantly affected by this factor—a situation over which the institution itself may have little control.

To summarize, it is important to select the best possible scientific design to answer the question of interest. To do this may require negotiations at the national or multiinstitutional level. Whatever the eventual research design, the "rules" of rigorous research must be applied.

## Allocation of Resources

It may be too obvious to mention, but a program evaluation project (no matter how rigorous the research design or how precise the measures) is useless unless there are available resources to conduct the study. The resources required are not only finances but people with the interest, ability, and time to carry them out.

Some institutions, although stating clear intentions to carry out program evaluation studies, have not yet begun any definite work. Others have project groups that had begun but for a variety of reasons had not produced any definite plans or results. The lesson appears to be that if an institution is serious about program evaluation there must be a definite commitment to it. This commitment must be expressed in appropriate "institutional behavior." For some institutions it might mean setting up a high profile committee, allocating a proportion of institutional research funds, or some other appropriate activity.

One other lesson has to do with establishing a "data base" and doing it quite early in the life of a program. At McMaster, for example, it took several years before it was realized that a systematic profile of entering classes would be required for program evaluation purposes. Fortunately, time and effort were devoted to this question sufficiently early that this institution was able to "catch up" on the initial classes. The result is that researchers at McMaster have established an "educational data base" that is accurate, quite comprehensive, and relatively easy to update and maintain. In addition to serving as the basis for several research projects, it is also used for other purposes, such as providing a mailing list for an active alumni organization.

In sum, each institution needs to carefully consider at the outset, and periodically review, the reasons for program evaluation and the specific outcomes anticipated. The projects to be carried out must be carefully and scientifically designed. Adequate resources, maintained over a considerable period of time, must be committed and available.

## Assessment of Innovative Institutions

Should comparative studies be done? Should there be other collaborative projects? Although the discussion on these two questions overlaps to some extent, it is worthwhile to consider them separately.

### Comparative Studies

It has been proposed from time to time that certain aspects of the educational experience of innovative institutions be compared. For example, because several programs emphasize problem-solving ability, could there not be a study that would compare the problem-solving ability of students or graduates of several institutions?

There are major obstacles to conducting such comparative studies. These difficulties are both scientific (methodological) and practical. From a methodological perspective, there are major differences between institutions that would be quite difficult to control in any comparative study. These differences include aspects of the selection system, the student body profile, the teaching/learning methods themselves, and the institutional and national setting. For example, McMaster University has a comprehensive institution-based system, in contrast to a national, primarily lottery system in The Netherlands. Students in North America have had several years of university experience before entering medical school, in contrast to most other countries where students enter longer medical programs usually in their late teens. An exception is Israel, where most medical students complete military training before entering medical school. Again, the North American setting is exceptional in terms of a standard examination that must be taken by all medical graduates in order to be licensed. These are some examples of the large differences that would create major methodological difficulties in any comparative study.

There are also obvious practical difficulties. Comparative studies are difficult enough when two or more institutions are within 100 km of each other, and where the individuals are fluent in the same language. The geographic spread and language differences to be surmounted in a cross-national comparative study would be even more difficult. Added to this are financial considerations. Perhaps the practical question: "What would we do differently when the study results are available?" might help to put such an adventure in perspective. Although comparative studies seem to have large impediments, collaborative projects most certainly can be done.

## Collaborative Projects

A number of collaborative activities are already in progress in areas other than student assessment and program evaluation. Some beginnings have also been made to collaborate in the area of assessment and evaluation. Summarized below are several possible ways in which collaboration may be expanded.

1. *Exchange of expertise in evaluation*. It has already occurred to some extent. Individuals in innovative institutions have been invited to other institutions to provide consultation regarding assessment systems or the design of specific instruments. It is hoped that it can continue.

2. *Provision of training opportunities*. It has begun as well; some individuals from newer institutions have spent time in more established innovative schools to learn about principles and practices of assessment and evaluation. With careful planning and adequate resources, it can be a mutually useful experience.

3. *Sharing measurement tools*. This area may be less practical because of institutional and cultural differences. However, provided the original designers of an instrument have no objection, a tool can be adapted to the needs of a given institution. When the tool is being considered for a new setting, there needs to be rigorous and careful pretesting. It is rarely possible, for example, to simply translate a survey instrument and expect to use it directly.

4. *Sharing ideas about arrangements for research*. Each institution has its own administrative style and peculiarities. The actual arrangements for conducting student assessment and program evaluation vary considerably across institutions. However, there may be some principles and lessons from a given institution that are useful to others. Including aspects of funding, training of personnel, conducting studies, and publishing results.

To summarize, comparative studies may be almost impossible to conduct at this stage of development. The reasons are both methodological and practical. There are, however, several ways in which sharing can occur. Some specific suggestions from collaborative projects are offered.

# Comment

In closing, this chapter considered some general issues in program evaluation and student assessment brought up by the previous chapters and discussed some guidelines and problems with interinstitution research. This ongoing collaboration is vital, as the evaluation of programs and students is central to the life and future of innovative medical programs.

# 14
# Teaching and Measuring Interviewing Skills in the Maastricht Medical Curriculum

HERRO F. KRAAN, ALFONS A.M. CRIJNEN, JAAP ZUIDWEG, CEES VAN DER VLEUTEN, and TJAART IMBOS

The medical interview is the basic clinical medium in primary care.[1,2] Over the last decade, studies have demonstrated the positive influence of adequate interviewing on the physician–patient relationship including patient satisfaction and compliance with medical requirements as well as other aspects of medical competence.[3] In large measure, interviewing skills determine what physical and mental problems are presented during the medical consultation.[4] Accurate data collecting and diagnosis are therefore closely related to the physicians' interviewing skills.[5,6]

Further, patient-centered interviewing[7,8] and negotiation between physician and patient about problem definitions and treatment plans[9] are important aspects of the hallmarks of the primary care consultations[4] that depend on the physicians' interviewing skills.

In this chapter, we describe the teaching and evaluation program of medical interviewing and related psychosocial skills at the University of Limburg, Medical School in Maastricht, the Netherlands. We introduce the Maastricht History-taking and Advice Checklist (MAAS) as an interview evaluation method and demonstrate its use in testing. Reliability and validity data are also presented and the effectiveness of the Maastricht teaching program, as measured with MAAS is explored.

## The Teaching Program in Medical Interviewing

The principles incorporated in the design of the Maastricht interview training program have been most clearly formulated by Carroll and Monroe.[10] They identified several key principles for designing teaching programs in interviewing skills.

1. Direct observation and feedback of students' interview behavior by instructors or peers of simulated patient is fundamental to the design of instruction. Seemingly an educational platitude, it is nevertheless a common situation in clinical teaching that interviewing students/residents are not directly observed and instructed by their supervisors. In training programs, feedback by video is a

useful device, but the use of this technology may also add complications. During videotape replay, students tend to limit attention to aspects of the consultation such as problem-solving aspects, peculiarities of the presented case, or their own physical appearance on the screen.

2. Standardized presentations of illustrative patient interviews may be more effective than live demonstrations of unselected patient interviews. A "spontaneous" interview may fail to exhibit expected interview behaviors, therefore such demonstration interviews may exhibit only a limited range of relevant interviewing skills.

3. Teaching programs should include explicit (behavioral) statements of the interviewing skills to be learned, and these should be integrated into a highly structured and programmatic instruction.

At the Maastricht Medical School, the Netherlands, a substantial part of the 6-year medical curriculum is devoted to the training of medical interviewing skills.* Training takes place in small groups of maximally 8 students guided by a physician and a behavioral scientist. During the first 4 years of the medical curriculum, the small groups meet about 15 times a year for 2 hours. During the fifth and sixth year there is no formal training in interviewing skills. Several different teaching methods are combined during this training program of 4 years duration.

1. *Structured training courses in interviewing skills.* The skills are taught according to a hierarchy in complexity. In the first year, basic interviewing skills are stressed, such as asking open- and closed- ended questions, discussing emotional topics, empathizing, summarizing, etc. Moreover, students learn to explore patients' reasons for an encounter. In the second year, more attention is paid to medical history-taking skills and to obtaining information about psychosocial issues. The third-year program focuses on presenting solutions to patients, including the provision of information and negotiation about the treatment proposal. In the fourth year, students learn to manage interviews in "difficult" situations such as with aggressive patients, dying patients, patients with sexual problems, etc. The teaching format is a highly structured program in which videotapes, which show each skill separately and in context, are used. Courses further employ role-playing exercises on videotapes in which "critical incidents" in demonstration interviews are presented.

2. *Interviews with simulated patients.* Here, students act as "physicians" and as "critical observer." Several students will interview the same patient in such a way that the videotaped interviews can be compared. These interviews are reviewed by peers, students, and experts. Not only the interviewing behavior but also other aspects of competence (diagnostics, treatment plan) are discussed.

3. *Clinical experiences in health care throughout the curriculum.* Experiences with actual patients may be subject of discussion within the small group. The emotional impact on the students by the patient and his or her problem gets

---

*Maastrichts skills job director: Jan van Dalen.

attention. Problematic interviews caused by deficient skills or countertransference get attention. When a student has mastered an adequate interview technique, as has shown in the past with simulated patients, the difference between a problematic interview with a "real" patient and his or her usual interviews with simulated patients may be a strong learning experience.[11]

4. *Attitude development*. Students' experience in health care practice, in interviews with simulated patients as well as with colleagues and educators, are further explored in the training group. Attention is paid to the students' attitudes underlying norms and values towards patients and the health care system. Proponents of "confluent education" and "experiential learning"[12] stress this integration in learning processes. The attitude of the physician toward patients and their problems determines his or her interviewing skills. Nevertheless, some critical remarks should be made. Ajzen and Fishbein[13] extensively studied the relationship between an individual's attitude and behavior. They conclude that the prediction of an individual's social behavior (like interviewing skills) from his or her attitudes has a low to moderate reliability. Situational factors (like time restrictions, external pressures, unexpected incidents during the consultation hour) and external norms (for instance, the influence of the belief that prestigious colleagues would or would not perform a certain behavior) lower the degree to which behavior is determined by attitudes. Nevertheless, in training programs attention should be paid to the exploration of the students' attitudes. Furthermore, during "attitude development," the interviewing behavior of the student can be analyzed with models of Leary[14] to clarify underlying interaction patterns (dominance, submission, controversy, cooperation). Underlying values and norms are brought into awareness by techniques of value clarification.[15]

The evaluation program is closely connected to these educational and training goals in order to assess the effectiveness of the entire training program and to assess the progress of individual students.

## Method

### Construction of the Maastricht History-taking and Advice Checklist (MAAS)

The format and item choice of the MAAS has been largely determined by the following options:

1. *Focus on skill measurement during initial interviews*. Medical consultations in Dutch primary care are characterized by an undifferentiated mixture of somatic and psychosocial complaints, often strongly interwoven with the life circumstances of the patient. Presented problems are a mix of acute severe disorders, chronic disabilities, nonserious and self-limiting diseases, and nonmedical problems in living. For practical and didactic reasons, the research group chose to measure the initial interview, since an initial interview is carried out in about 60% of the consultations in Holland.

2. *Focus on "trainable" interviewing skills.* The objective is to provide feedback on the level of the individuals' interviewing behavior by means of the MAAS. Interviewing skills, that are deemed to reliably influence by training such as non-verbal communication, are not covered by the MAAS. This restriction has two methodological consequences. First, the items will be dominated by verbal interviewing behaviors. Second, the focus of the MAAS focuses mainly on the measurement of process aspects of the interview shaped by the physician. The patient's contribution evaluated by the MAAS are responses to the physicians' questions and questions initiated by the patient during the interview.

3. *Focus on "instrumental utility".* According to the Dutch psychometrician, de Groot,[16] the instrumental utility is high when the balance between practicability on the one hand and reliability and validity on the other hand is optimal in terms of a cost-benefit ratio. Practicability depends on the instruments construction but also on the ease of scoring, time investment in observer training, test length, comprehensiveness of the observers manual, etc. The instrumental utility decreases when the content validity is heightened by increasing the items that tap more detailed interviewing skills and content topics.

These criteria have strongly determined the content and goal of the MAAS. Approximately 20 instruments measuring behavioral (process) aspects of medical interviewing skills were reviewed to established the MAAS unit of analysis.* The methods reviewed did not directly satisfy our criteria, but the approaches taken, guided the construction of our instrument and resulted in three categories of questions in the MAAS.

- Items describing interviewing skills as simple, single-act behaviors. *Example*: uses close-ended questions properly.
- Items combining simple interviewing behavior with medical content aspects. *Example*: Asks for the localization of the complaint (directive question for the patient to be specific about the localization of the complaint).

---

*These instruments used the following modes of analysis:

- Categorical systems resembling the Interaction Process Analysis of Bales.[17] These systems, used by Korsch et al.,[18] Roter,[19] and McDonald and Templeton,[20] consist of a restricted number of mutual exclusive behavioral classifications applicable to both physician and patient.
  Systems with these "molecular" elements yield long profiles of sequenced physicians' and patients' behaviors during the interview. However, they lack specificity as to the characteristic interviewing process skills in primary health care. Moreover, their scoring is time consuming.
- Categorical systems, built up with "molar" interviewing skills specific for primary health care.[21-23] These instruments often allow direct feedback to individuals during training because of their concreteness in describing the interviewing skills of the physician.
- Categorical systems, measuring global dimensions in the physician's interviewing style. Their unit of analysis can be considered as the whole interview or major parts of it. Examples are found in the instruments of Hollifield et al.,[24] Hess,[25] Jarrett et al.,[26] and Mumford et al.[27] Often, these systems are too abstract to provide feedback to students on the skill level.

• Items describing multiple act interviewing behavior, related to more complex interviewing skills. *Example*: makes proper confrontations when necessary.

## Description of the MAAS

The foregoing criteria resulted in the construction of a 68-item observation instrument. The MAAS is divided in 5 segments or subscales. The first 3 subscales called "exploration of the reasons for encounter," history-taking," and "presenting solutions," respectively, contain possible interviewing skills, that the physician may display during the three typical phases of the initial interview.[28] This type of initial interview follows the primary care consultation model described by several authors like Katon and Kleinman[7] and Pendleton et al.[1] These models incorporate the biopsychosocial model[29] and are characterized by patient centeredness by attention to illness behavior and by negotiation between physician and patient about major "conflicting" issues during the consultation. The fourth and fifth subscales, called "structuring the interview" and "basic interviewing skills" mainly represent the physicians' process skills in performing an initial interview. These five subscales are described in detail.

1. *Exploration of the reasons for encounter.* The function of this phase of the interview is to collect information about the patients' frame of reference and the prepatient phase of seeking help.[30] The physician provides the patient an opportunity to express his or her complaints and symptoms in the patient's own words, to expand on the causes and consequences of the complaints and the events that triggered the visit to the physician as well as what solution the patient or his family have attempted. This has been shown as important for the "affective" satisfaction of the patient.[31] The 8 items of this subscale have the following format: "Asks for (one of the prior mentioned topics)" or "Explores (one of the prior mentioned topics"). The aspects of process in this phase are open questions, probes within the patients' frame of reference, active listening, emotional reflections, and stimulating summarizations. These process skills are assessed in the subscale "basic interviewing skills" (e.g., one item is "Explores the influence of the complaints on daily life").

2. *Medical history taking.* During this phase the patient is questioned from a medical frame of reference about the character of the complaints, localizations, course and intensity, past illnesses and treatments, medication and intoxications, etc. Further items pertaining to the search for factors that trigger, aggravate, maintain, and alleviate the complaints have been included. This search for cues is necessary for the physicians' clinical reasoning.[5] This subscale also contains items about psychosocial issues: interpersonal relations, family life, professional and leisure time functioning, important biographical life events, vulnerability and risk factors, etc. The appropriate skills during this phase is—in its typical form—the so-called "open-to-close-cone" questioning[4]: some important cue is given during the interview. Next, the physician proceeds with more probing, directive questions and may end with direct falsifiable questions to acquire

accurate factual information. Although the types of questions differ, the item format resembles that of the previous subscale: "Asks for (medical topic)" or "explores (medical topic)." (e.g., this subscale includes 22 items, "Asks for the localization of the complaint").

3. *Presenting solutions.* This phase follows both previous phases and — if carried out — the physical examination. The physician informs the patient about his or her illness condition or problems, its causes and its prognosis. Next the doctor proceeds with an exploration of the patients' feelings, evoked by this information. A negotiation about the problem definition between physician and patient may ensue. Next, the physician makes a proposal for further follow-up: further exploration or investigations, referral, treatment, preventive advices. Alternative proposals may be given by the physician and again negotiation may ensue. Finally, the physician gives concrete advice based on the outcome of the negotiation process. This negotiation for consensus has been shown effective in relation to outcome measures, like satisfaction, compliance, therapeutic outcomes.[32,33] The physician concludes with appointments for follow-up. The editing of the 12 items describing the skills during this phase may take various formats: "gives information about (medical information)"; "discusses (medical information)"; "explains the effects of (medical information)"; "explains why (medical information)" (e.g., one item: "Gives information about the prognosis of the complaint").

4. *Structuring the interview.* This subscale includes 8 items and measures the skills by which the physician opens and closes the interview and how well he or she links the aforementioned three phases. For example: does the doctor begin the "presenting solutions" phase with the providing of information about the problem definition or diagnosis (e.g., one item: "Begins 'presenting solutions' with a diagnosis or problems definition").

5. *Basic interviewing skills.* According to Hess,[25] basic interviewing skills can be divided into interpersonal and communicative skills. Interpersonal skills refer to interviewing behavior that contributes to establishing patient rapport, trust and acceptance. They are found to be important for patient compliance and satisfaction.[18,34] These effects are attributed to several interviewing skills: showing empathy, warmth, and concern; active listening; facilitative behavior; instillation of positive expectations; self-disclosure. Communicative skills promote the information flow between physician and patient. These skills are related to the use of appropriate techniques of questioning, providing information and giving advice.[35] The 17 items of this subscale are scored on a three-point scale (yes, indifferent, no), allowing a qualitative rating (according to the criteria of the observers manual) of an item that checks whether the patient understood the information.

## Measurement of the Patients' Contribution to the Interview: The Subscales "Obtained Information"

In the first 2 subscales of the MAAS (exploration of the reasons for encounter and history-taking) the physician collects information from the patient. Parallel to both 2 other subscales called "obtained information" have been constructed, reflecting the same content aspects as the comparable (physicians') subscales. For example, the item: "Asks how the patient attempted to solve the problem" becomes "attempted solutions" in the "obtained information" subscale. In interviewing research with simulated patients, the items in the "obtained information" subscales can be edited more specifically according to the "program" of the simulated patient. Using the same example, "attempted solutions" becomes more specific, for instance, "I went to bed after drinking a glass of warm milk" (in case of a duodenal ulcer). These subscales can have a function as product evaluation when the quantity and quality of the obtained information is used as an outcome measure of the medical interview.

## Protocol and Psychometric Properties of the MAAS

The foregoing version of the MAAS has been tested for reliability over the last 2 years as a medical evaluation instrument. Reasonable reliability is only attained after substantial training of observers. At the start, medically trained observers have a slight advantage in comparison to nonmedical observers. After training this difference disappears. The initial training consists in reading the manual for observers that contains an introduction to the MAAS a list of definitions of interviewing skills, and a list of criteria for scoring each individual item. Two training sessions of 2 to 3 hours are devoted to step-by-step scoring of test videotapes. The observers' training groups discusses the score on each item, especially differences from appropriate scores in order to learn the criteria for scoring.

Refresher training sessions of 1 to 2 hours are necessary when observers have not scored the MAAS for several months. In the teaching program at Maastricht, the MAAS is used as a guide or inventory of interviewing skills for staff and students in order to provide individual feedback during training sessions. When the MAAS is used as a test, for instance, in summative evaluation, further comments should be made. Judging the quality of the physician's interviewing skills has to encompass both the physician's interviewing behavior (scores on the MAAS subscales) as well as the patient's contribution to the interview (scores on the subscales "obtained information"). In this way, process aspects of the physician's interviewing and product aspects (quantity and quality of the information given in response to the physician's questions) are measured. The judgment is more complete when other aspects, like patient satisfaction, comprehension, reassurance, intention to comply, etc. are also taken into account. Such a judgment by the patient can be accomplished with the Patient Satisfaction with Communication Checklist (PSCC), a patient rating scale, derived from the MAAS.[28]

When the MAAS is used as a test, a wide array of process and product aspects of interviewing skills can be included, but the purposes of testing ultimately determine which subscales or items are selected for a given test, for instance, to manufacture a shorter test. A reduced number of items can be randomly selected from the whole item domain of the subscales. When the MAAS is scored in test situations by moderately trained observers, their percentage agreement varies from 0.70 to 0.90 over the 5 subscales. Further reliability studies have been carried out using an analysis of variance and by applying the Rasch model.[36] The internal consistency of the scales was satisfactory.

### Evaluating Undergraduate Students with the MAAS

Once a year, all students have to demonstrate their ability in performing a medical interview as part of a more comprehensive examination of several physicial-diagnostic and medical technical skills.[37] In 1984, we observed all 563 medical students at Maastricht Medical School. The students task in the interview was to explore the reason for encounter, to clarify the patient's complaints. To take the medical history, and to present solutions to the patient. The time available was 15 minutes. The simulated patients presented complaints that are common in general practice. A simulated patient had been selected from a large pool of lay-people, who are trained to present medical complaints to students for educational purposes. While students interviewed the patients, experienced observers rated students interview behavior with the MAAS. The observers had to complete the checklist within 5 minutes after the interview. The organization of this examination of medical interviewing skills is rather complex. Because all students in one year group had to be examined within one day, 6 to 12 observers and 12 to 18 simulated patients were needed to examine a year group.

## Results

### Growth in Interviewing Skills

Because all medical students (with the exception of the fifth-year group) were observed nearly at the same time, the test results of the year groups on the 5 sub-scales of the MAAS can be compared. This cross-sectional design enables us to establish growth patterns of students medical interviewing skills in the course of the curriculum. Of course, conclusions can only be drawn under the assumption that the educational program has been kept constant over the last 6 years that students were not assigned to the year groups on the basis of their interviewing skills and that instrument reactivity effects are unlikely.[38] We can argue that these assumptions are reasonably fulfilled. At the end of the first year, students are well able to "explore the reasons for encounter." Figure 14.1 shows that in the second year this ability declines significantly. During the third and fourth year, this ability inclines toward the first-year level. During students' clinical rotation, the ability declines significantly again. From the first to the sixth year, a significant decline in exploring reasons for encounter takes places.

The decrease in the ability to explore reasons for encounter agrees with often-heard remarks that students increasingly neglect to ask information about the patient's life in the course of the medical curriculum. This is partly due to the student's preoccupation with medical problem-solving process and partly due to clinical preceptors urging students to obtain detailed factual information about the medical problem. The incline in the third and fourth year demonstrates the

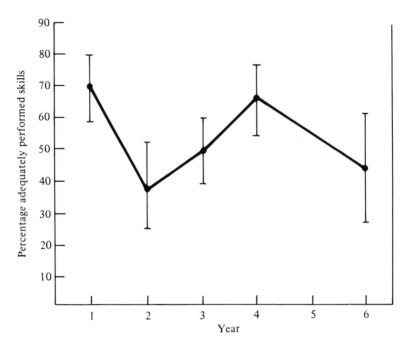

FIGURE 14.1. Percentages and standard deviations of adequately performed interviewing skills in "exploring reasons for encounter" over year groups. The differences from year to year and the decrease from the first to the sixth year are significant ($p < .001$).

acquisition of these skills as a result of training. Obviously, the skill in "exploring reasons for encounter" is easily neglected but can be learned when trained. It appears to be rather susceptible to disturbing influences. At the end of the second year, "history taking" skills declined significantly when compared to the first year results are seen in Figure 14.2. From the second to the fourth year, this skill significantly grows. A small, not significant, decline between fourth and sixth year performance takes place. We concluded that all students become skillful in asking questions that enable them to describe patients' complaints in medical explanatory terms. Students learned this skill in a developmental process, because in the second year the insufficient integration of knowledge, problem-solving strategies, and interview behavior hindered the students performing this skill well. During students' clinical rotations they learn to use this skill more efficiently. The skill in "presenting solutions" increases strongly to the fourth year. From the fourth to the sixth year, a significant decline takes place (see Fig. 14.3).

Obviously, interviewing skills pertaining to present solutions improve as a result of the ongoing interviewing course. Students' loss of competence during their clinical rotation was attributed to the absence of interviewing courses and the socializing influences of clinical perceptors. In Figure 14.4 it can be seen that students' ability in "structuring the interview" increases significantly in the course of the curriculum and is maintained at that level after the fourth year. At the end of the fourth year, almost all students have learned this skill. Toward the

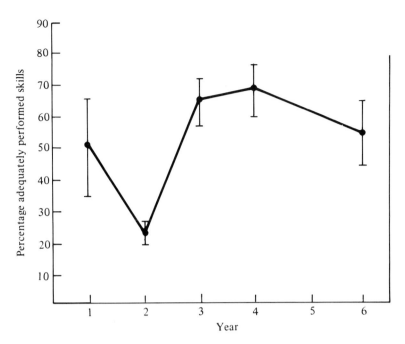

FIGURE 14.2. Percentages and standard deviations of adequately performed interviewing skills in "history taking" over year groups. The differences from year to year are significant ($p < .001$), except the increase from the third to the fourth year (n.s.). The net increase from the first to the sixth year is not significant.

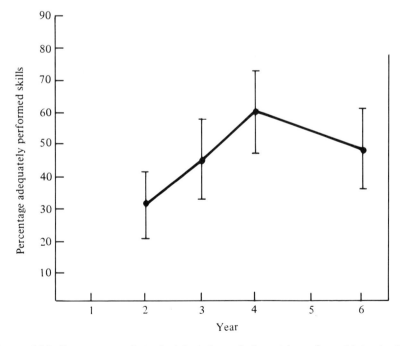

FIGURE 14.3. Percentages and standard deviations of adequately performed interviewing skills in "presenting solutions" over year groups. The differences from year to year and the increase from the first to the sixth year are significant (range: $p < .02$ to $p < .001$).

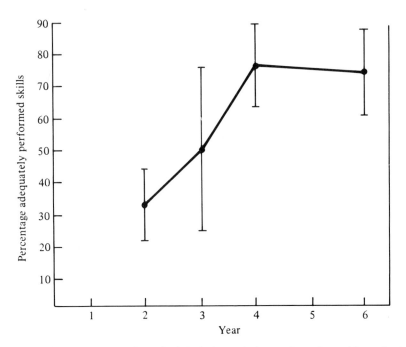

FIGURE 14.4. Percentages and standard deviations of adequately performed interviewing skills in "structuring the medical interview" over year groups. The differences from year to year are significant ($p < .001$) except the decrease from the fourth to the sixth year (n.s.).

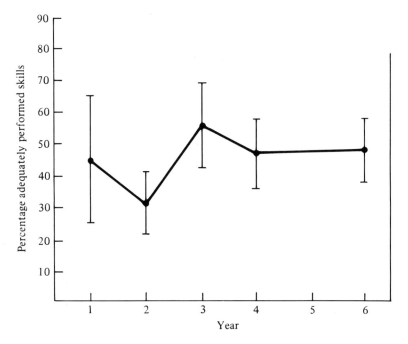

FIGURE 14.5. Percentages and standard deviations of adequately performed "basic interviewing skills" over year groups. The differences from year to year are significant ($p < .001$) except between the fourth and sixth year (n.s.). The net increase from the first to the sixth year is not significant.

sixth year, this skills does not increase further; it is not clear whether this fact is to be ascribed to a ceiling effect in the scoring or to the lack of training during the last curriculum years.

No increase or decrease of students competence in performing "basic interviewing skills" was found (see Figure 14.5). According to Scott[39] and Helfer[40] basic interviewing skills can be expected to diminish in the course of a medical curriculum. When no interviewing training is given, students use open-ended questions less often and will demonstrate reassurance, empathy and support less frequently. The results suggest that the gain of our interviewing training program is that basic interviewing skills did not undergo this decline. Yet, even with the 4-year training program, no net increase in these skills could be observed – just the counteracting of a natural decline. These finding require closer investigation in more experimental designs. We need to answer such questions as: Will different skill types (for instance, interpersonal or communicative skills) differently be influenced by our integrated training program? Which parts of our program are effective to which types of skills?

## Discussion

In this chapter, a fairly homogeneous continuous, 4-year educational program with a small-group teaching format is described that has proved to be effective in teaching medical interviewing skills. Several teaching methods integrating behavioral cognitive and attitudinal elements make up this program: expert and peer review of videotaped interviews with simulated patients, structured videotaped presentations of relevant interviewing skills (separate and in context), follow-up discussions after "real patient" interviews in health care, exploration of students' underlying attutides, values and norms.

To evaluate student performance in this innovative system, the Maastricht History-taking and Advice Checklist has been constructed. It is a 68-item observation instrument for measuring physicians and students interviewing skills in primary care. Three of its 5 segments or subscales pertain to the characteristic phases of initial medical interviews: "exploration of the reasons for encounter," "history taking," and "presenting solutions." In the two remaining subscales, the skills "structure the interview" and "basic interviewing skills" are the matter of concern.

The practicability of the MAAS is high, whereas reliability figures, like percentage agreement between observers, internal consistency, and the coefficients of generalizability are reasonable. More important: the MAAS can be reduced to 49 items, divided over 6 Rasch homogeneous subscales. These subscales allow a reliable discrimination of competent from less competent interviewers, based on "population" referenced criteria. The MAAS is used in evaluating the Maastricht training program, which has proved effective in enhancing students' skills pertaining to history taking, presenting solutions, and structuring the interview. The skills in "exploring reasons for encounter" can also be lear ned but appear easily susceptible to disturbing influences from concurrent experiences during the medical curriculum. Since these expected growth patterns in interviewing skills are reliably recorded by the MAAS, these findings are also supportive to the construct validity of the instrument.

The impact of the training program on "basic interviewing skills" turned out to be limited, not withstanding the attention paid to affective and issues in education. More research is necessary, because these skills are of prime importance in establishing rapport and in stimulating an effective exchange of information between patient and physician. The decline in test scores during clinical clerkships suggest the importance of maintaining the training program during the clinical rotations as well.*

## References

1. Pendleton D, Schofield T, Tate P et al.: *The Consultation: An Approach to Learning and Teaching.* Oxford, England, Oxford University Press, 1984.
2. Lipkin M Jr, Quill TE, Napodano RJ: The medical interview: a core curriculum for residences in internal medicine. *Ann Intern Med* 1984;100:277–284.
3. DiMatteo MR, DiNicola DD: *Achieving Patient Compliant. The Psychology of the Medical Practitioners' Role.* New York, Pergamon Press, 1982.
4. Goldberg D, Huxley P: *Mental Illness in the Community; A Pathway to Psychiatric Care.* New York, Tavistock, 1980.
5. Elstein AS, Shulman LS, Sprafka SA: *Medical Problem Solving. An Analysis of Clinical Reasoning.* Cambridge, Mass., Harvard University Press, 1978.
6. Rutter M, Cox A: Psychiatric interviewing techniques: I. Methods and measures. *Br J Psychiat* 1981;138:273–382.
7. Katon W, Kleinman A: Doctor-patient negotiation and other social science strategies in patient care, in Eisenberg, L, Kleinman, A (eds): *The Relevance of Social Science for Medicine.* Dordrecht, Reidel Publish. Cie, 1980.
8. Byrne PS, Long BEL: *Doctors Talking to Patients. Her Majesty's Stationery Office, 1976.*
9. Lazare A, Eisenthal S, Wasserman L: *The customer approach to patienthood. Arch Gen Psychiatry* 175;32:553–558.
10. Carroll JG, Monroe J: Teaching clinical interviewing in the health professions; a review of empirical research. *Evaluation and the Health Professions* 1980;3:21–45.
11. Smith RC: Teaching interviewing skills to medical students; The issue of 'counter transference'. *J Med Educ* 1984;59:582–588.
12. Rogers C: *Freedom to Learn.* Ohio; Columbus, 1969.
13. Ajzen I, Fishbein M: *Understanding Attitudes and Predicting Social Behavior.* Englewood Cliffs, N.J., Prentice-Hall, 1980.
14. Leary T: *Interpersonal Diagnosis of Personality.* New York, Ronald Press, 1957.
15. Simon SB, Howe LW, Kirschenbaum H: *Clarification of Values. A Handbook of Practical Strategies for Teachers and Students.* New York, Hart Publish. Cie., 1978
16. De Groot AD: *Methodologie. Grondslagen van onderzoek en denken in de gedragswetenschappen. 's-Gravenhage, Mouton, 1962.*
17. Bales RF: *Interaction Process Analysis.* Cambridge, Mass. Addison Wesley, 1950.
18. Korsch BM, Gozzi EK, Francis V: Gaps in doctor–patient communication: 1. Doctor–patient interaction and patient satisfaction. *Pediatrics* 1968;42(5):855–871.

*For further information about the MAAS contact Dr. H.F. Kraan, Dept. of Social Psychiatry, University of Limburg, P.O. Box 616, 6200 MD Maastricht, The Netherlands.

19. Roter D: Patient participation in the patient-provider interaction: The effect of patient question-asking on the quality of interaction, satisfaction and compliance. *Health Educ Monogr* 1977;5:281–315.
20. McDonald M, Templeton B: *Interaction Analysis System for Interview evaluation (ISIE-81)*. National Board of Medicine Examiners, Philadelphia, 1981.
21. Brockway BS: Evaluation physician competency: What difference does it make? *Evaluation and Program Planning* 1978;1:211–220.
22. Stillman P: Arizona clinical interview medical rating scale. *Med Teach* 1980:2:248–251.
23. Barsky AJ, Kazis LE, Freiden RB et al.: Evaluating the interview in primary care medicine. *Soc Sci Med* 1980;14:653–658.
24. Hollifield G, Rousell CT, Bachrach AJ et al.: A method of evaluating student–patient interviews. *J Med Educ* 1957;32:853–858.
25. Hess JW: A comparison of methods for evaluating medical student skill in relating to patients. *J Med Educ* 1969;44:934–938.
26. Jarrett FJ, Waldron JJ, Burra P et al.: Measuring interviewing skills; The Queen's University interviewing rating scale (Quirs). *Can Psychiat Ass J* 1972;17:183–188.
27. Mumford E, Anderson D, Cuerdon T et al.: Performance based evaluation of medical students interviewing skills. *J Med Educ* 1984;59:133–135.
28. Kraan HF, Crijnen AAM: *Reliability and validity studies with the Maastricht History-taking and Advice Checklist [Dissertation]*. Amsterdam, Lundbeck, 1987.
29. Engel GL: The need for a new medical model: A challenge for biomedicine. *Science* 1977;196:129–136.
30. Freidson E: *Professional Dominance: The Social Structure of Medical Care*. New York, Atherton, 1970.
31. Stiles WB, Putman SM, Wolf MH et al.: Interaction exchange structure and patient satisfaction with medical interviews. *Med Care* 1979;17:667–681.
32. Stimson GV, Webb B: *Going to see the doctor: The consultation process in general practice*. London: Routeledge and Kegan Paul, 1975.
33. Eisenthal S, Koopman C, Lazare A: Process Analysis of Two Dimensions of the Negotiated Approach in Relation to Satisfaction in the Initial Interview. *J Nerv Ment Dis* 1983;171(1):49–54.
34. Hulka BS, Cassel JC, Kupper LL et al.: Communication, compliance and concordance between physicians and patients with prescribed medications. *Am J Public Health* 1976;66(9):847–853.
35. Ley P: Patients' understanding and recall in clinical communication failure, in Pendleton D, Hasler J (eds): *Doctor–Patient communication*. New York, Academic Press, 1983.
36. Wright BD, Stone MH: *Best Test Design*. Chicago, Mesa Press, 1979.
37. Van Luijk SJ, Van der Vleuten CPM, Peet DGM: Evaluating undergraduate training in medical skills. *Proceedings of the International Conference on Newer Developments in Assessing Clinical Competence*. Ottawa, Canada, 1985.
38. Cook TD, Campbell DT: *Quasi-Experimentation: A Design and Analysis for Field Settings*. Chicago, Rand McNally, 1979.
39. Scott NC, Donnelly MB, Hess JW: Changes in interviewing styles of medical students.. *J Med Educ* 1975;50:1124–1126.
40. Helfer RE: An objective comparison of the pediatric interviewing skills of freshman and senior medical students. *Pediatrics* 1970;45:623–627.

# 15
## How Effective Are Problem-based, Community-oriented Curricula: Experienced Evidence*

HENK G. SCHMIDT

This chapter reviews and comments on a number of studies that have compared the results of problem-based programs with those of conventional curricula. The review concentrates on studies concerning the educational outcomes of the curricula of an international group of medical schools known as the "Network of Community-oriented Educational Institutions for the Health Sciences." The Network consists of approximately 80 schools, from industrialized as well as developing countries.[1] The more well-known schools include the medical faculties of the University of New Mexico in the United States, the University of Limburg in the Netherlands, McMaster University in Canada, Suez Canal University in Egypt, and the University of Newcastle, Australia.

In the next sections, data are presented on five outcomes of interest: students' academic achievement, clinical competence, career preferences, perceptions of their educational environment, and learning styles. These attributes have been selected because they encompass the areas in which differences are to be expected between conventional and problem-based curricula.

## Academic Achievement

One of the implicit assumptions underlying the structure of many curricula is that students have a limited amount of time available to study the core content of medicine. Consequently, if emphasis is put on topics or activities not considered to be part of this core, the amount of attention that could be spent on core content can be expected to decrease, causing a drop in achievement on these topics. The studies addressed in this section ask whether curricular changes of the kind described herein can be considered to be associated with a decrease in academic achievement.

---

*This chapter is partly based on an article "Comparing the efforts of problem-based and conventional curricula in an international sample," published in *J Med Edu* 1987;62: 305–315. Reprinted with permission.

Perhaps the most exhaustive attempts to compare the academic achievement of students in an problem-based school to those in conventional medical education have been made by a group of investigators at the Maastricht Faculty of Medicine of the University of Limburg, the Netherlands, in close collaboration with investigators from other medical schools in the country.[2,3] All Dutch medical schools have a 6-year curriculum and similar admission procedures. Unlike other schools, however, the Maastricht Medical School uses problem-based, self-directed learning and community-oriented educational objectives.

In order to compare academic achievement in different schools, Verwijnen and his collaborators[3] employed an instrument called the progress test to measure academic achievement. This achievement test consists of about 250 true–false items, representing medicine as a whole, selected in a stratified random fashion from a large item bank. Different, but psychometrically equivalent, versions of this test are administered four times a year to all six groups of Maastricht medical students for the purpose of assessment and remediation. This test assesses differences between individual students, between different classes within a school, and even between different curricula. In one investigation, the achievement of the six classes of Maastricht medical students on this test was compared with that of other medical schools in the Netherlands. The Maastricht group contained the whole population of 565 students. Two other schools supplied 1067 volunteers, with a third school allowing the investigators to draw a random sample of 167 students. As could be expected, growth in medical knowledge over the years is gradual, although one of the conventional schools showed significantly less progress than the other schools in its second year and more progress in its fourth year. Although some statistically significant differences between schools showed up at certain points in time, these differences tended to be small and non-systematic. The achievement scores of the Maastricht students were somewhat lower than those of two of the other schools at three measuring points, but by the sixth year these differences had disappeared.

Equivalent results have been found by Baca et al.[4] while comparing the performance of different groups of medical students from the University of New Mexico at the National Board of Medical Examiners (NBME). The University of New Mexico Medical Faculty runs two separate but parallel tracks: a conventional and problem-based program, so comparisons are relatively easy to make. According to Baca and her associates, experimental track students tend to score slightly lower on the comprehensive basic science examination, given at the end of the second year, than students of the conventional track,* but the scores on the clinical science examination, given during the fourth year, are similar.

Saunders et al[5] administered an 80-item multiple choice test to final year students at the University of Sydney in Australia and a comparable group of students

---

*However, in a personal communication, Dr. Stewart P. Mennin of the University of New Mexico School of Medicine informed us that in more recent follow-up studies these differences have disappeared.

at the University of Newcastle, the latter having the same characteristics as the other problem-based schools discussed here. The questions were largely confined to internal medicine. There were 243 University of Sydney students and 45 University of Newcastle students who participated in the experiment (a participation rate of more than 90% for both schools). The difference in achievement between the two schools on the test was very small (although statistically significant): Sydney 71% correct, Newcastle 67% correct.

For more than 10 years, Woodward[6] monitored the achievement of McMaster University graduates in comparison with those of all the other medical schools in Canada on the Medical Council Qualifying Examination. Her data show that, on the average, McMaster graduates score slightly below the national average on the multiple choice part of the examination, although results vary from time to time.

The studies reviewed here seem to indicate that, in some cases, students from problem-based programs slightly underachieve on traditional measures of medical knowledge when compared with their colleagues of conventional schools, but differences, if any, are marginal.

## Clinical Competence and Internship Performance

The ability to care for patients and solve their problems is the major objective of medical education for many people. The acquisition of knowledge is, in this view, only useful to the extent that it facilitates medical problem solving. A major proponent of this perspective puts it this way: "Doctors with encyclopedic information are useless, if not unsafe, if they do not have the problem-solving skills necessary to accurately and efficiently use that information in the care of their patients."[7] If the acquisition of clinical competence is a vital objective of the innovation, the extent to which students from these problem-based schools master this skill in comparison to students from conventional medical education, becomes an important question. Data available on this topic are limited however, possibly because of disagreement on the issues of what to measure and how to measure clinical competence.

A study was carried out by Saunders and his associates[6] on a group of Sydney and Newcastle final-year students. These students were presented with two Modified Essay Questions, which were intended to measure clinical competence. No differences emerged, although Newcastle students performed slightly better when items were marked pass-fail, as opposed to ordinal differences between students.

Woodward,[6] however, found that McMaster graduates consistently score above national average on the patient management part of the Medical Council Qualifying Examination.

Christel A. Woodward and colleagues[8] of McMaster University, in a presentation at the 1983 Conference of Research in Medical Education of the Association of American Medical Colleges, reported the results of a study that used reports from supervisors on the performance of graduates from Canadian medical schools in their first postgraduate year. They were able to show that 26.1% of the McMaster graduates were judged as performing much better than the average fellow intern from other schools, 38.3% as better, 28.7% as about the same and 6.9% as weaker. The ratings of the other interns, as compared with the McMaster group, were 10.9% much better, 34.8% better, 43.5% the same, and 10.9% weaker. However, both comparison groups were quite small.

Finally, Claessen and Boshuizen[9] compared the performance of students from the medical schools of the universities of Limburg and Utrecht in the Netherlands on a problem-solving-like cognitive task. Their subjects included small samples of second-, third-, fourth-, and fifth-year medical students. The subjects were presented with two cases, each consisting of about 50 cards. Each card contained one piece of information about the patient. The subjects were asked to go through the sets of card, reading each card aloud. Subsequently, they were asked to recall as much of the patient information as possible. The amount and the quality of information recalled is generally seen as a sensitive measure of differences in the cognitive structures underlying problem solving.[10] Taken together, the students of the problem-based school were able to recall more information. These data suggest that these students have cognitive structures available that enable them to process patient data in a somewhat better fashion than students of the more conventional school. Claessen and Boshuizen appear to attribute this phenomenon to the earlier confrontation with patient problems taking place in the problem-based curriculum.

In conclusion, there is weak evidence that students from problem-based programs perform somewhat better on tasks related to clinical competence, but this evidence is limited in scope. The differences are small, perhaps with the exception of some of the data provided by Woodward and colleagues in 1983.[8]

## Career Preference and Career Choice

The career preferences of medical students tend to be quite stable in the course of their curriculum. If there is any change between the moment of enrollment and graduation, it tends to be a shift from a preference for primary care to non-primary care specialties.[11,12] This state of affairs presents a challenge for the community-oriented schools, because their goal is to produce doctors with an awareness of the importance of primary care for the well-being of the population at large. Do they succeed in influencing the preference pattern of medical students? Two studies address the impact of the new curricula on the career preferences of their students.

The first has been carried out at the universities of Kuopio and Tampere in Finland, two relatively new medical schools. Isokoski et al.[13] investigated the type of medical practice for all physicians registered in Finland between 1978 and 1982. A total of 2917 physicians were registered during that period. Utilizing the register of the Finnish Medical Association, data concerning the school of graduation were obtained for 93.4% of the physicians. Information about the nature of the practice (primary care, hospital-based service, other) was gathered by means of a questionnaire, returned with a response rate of 78%. Subsequently, Isokoski and his colleagues computed for each medical school, for five consecutive years, a ratio between the observed frequency of choosing a career in primary care and an expected frequency under the assumption that each medical school graduated the same proportion of physicians pursuing a career in primary care. Their data show that, on the whole, a significantly larger proportion of graduates from the two new schools sought a future in one of Finland's primary care health centers. Their report unfortunately does not contain information about the (regional) manpower needs during the study period. Thus it is impossible to assess the extent to which the career choice pattern resulted from genuine curricular influences or from geographical limitations as to the type of positions available during that period. In addition, it is unclear to what extent students enrolling in the new and the old schools differ in their career preferences from the start.

Research carried out at the university of New Mexico Medical School however, suggests that the structure and aims of a curriculum may indeed influence the professional preferences of its students. Upon entering medical school, students of both the experimental and the conventional track express preference for primary care specialties to the same extent. By graduation, the students in the experimental track were shown to retain their initial interest in family medicine, whereas their conventional track colleagues to some extent have changed their career preferences toward internal medicine. According to Baca et al,[4] this difference emerges because students in the experimental curriculum had substantially more role modeling in primary care, family medicine, and rural practice.

## Perceptions of Students of Their Curriculum

The way students perceive the content of the curriculum and the instructional philosophy underlying it may have an influence on their emotional well-being and motivation to learn. Medical faculties clearly differ in their responsiveness to these needs of students. At the University of New Mexico, for instance, experimental track students perceive their learning environment as definitively more flexible, more meaningful, encouraging student interaction, and having a better emotional climate than the students of the conventional track.[4]

Many medical schools do not appear to be ideal environments for the fostering of motivated learning. Bender[14] asked a sample of more than 300 medical students from a large Dutch university to state their opinion about the quality of the (preclinical) instruction they received. The predominant evaluative responses were "dull," "tough," "irrelevant," and "hardly adapted to the needs of practice." Schmidt and Moust[15] replicated Bender's study at the University of Limburg. They asked 45 randomly selected students to write a short essay on their experiences in medical school. Subsequently, they extracted all positive and negative evaluative remarks from these essays. Of 147 evaluative comments, 117 evaluations (i.e., 80%) turned out to be positive for the problem-based program. Many of these remarks had to do with early exposure to health care practice as fostered by the school, on small-group tutorials, and on self-directed learning. Negative judgments pertained to the student assessment system and, surprisingly, to small-group tutorials. These data partly corroborate the findings of Woodward and Ferrier,[16] who asked graduated classes to describe the strengths and weaknesses of the McMaster program. They mentioned, in order of importance, (1) problem-based learning, (2) electives, (3) self-directed learning, (4) independent study, and (5) small-group tutorials. Student assessment and clinical skills teaching were considered weaknesses.

An interesting comparative study of perceived strengths and weaknesses in the content of various curricula has been done by Post and Drop.[17] They were interested in the question whether differences could be found in the perceptions of graduates of different medical schools with respect to the amount of emphasis put on various subjects in the medical curriculum. In order to investigate this question, they administered a 45-item questionnaire to all 1982–1984 graduates of the University of Limburg medical school and the 1983 graduates of all other medical schools in the Netherlands. Subjects were asked to indicate their perception of the amount of attention given to a particular subject on a 5-point scale ranging from "too much" to "too little." Response was reasonably high for the Maastricht graduates, but rather low for those from other schools (65 versus 38%, respectively; the number of forms returned by the graduates from the other schools – 498 – and the homogeneity of their responses however, make some conclusions possible). Differences in knowledge and skills were perceived as largest in the areas of primary care, mental health, multidisciplinary cooperation, human behavior, social skills, preparation for postgraduate education, and ethical issues. These topics were rated as having been given less attention by the conventional schools. Hospital-based medicine and biomedical science were the subjects that received less emphasis in the new school as compared with conventional education. It should be noticed however, that some graduates from the conventional schools felt that too much attention has been given to biomedical science and hospital-based medicine.

## Learning Styles

Recently, considerable emphasis has been put on research into the ways university students process information. According to Marton, Hounsell, and Entwistle,[18] students appear to develop a preferred "style" of studying. These different styles or approaches to learning show (moderate) correlations with achievement. Individual students have been observed to favor one of three different broad approaches to the study of subject matter: a "surface," a "deep-level," or a "strategic" approach. The surface-level approach is largely characterized by a rote learning tendency, aimed at a literal reproduction of the material, and the use of extensive memorization procedures. Students using a deep-level approach attempt to integrate what they learn with what they already know, aim at understanding the "message" underlying a test, and look for explanations rather than facts. The strategic mode is descriptive of the behavior of those who try to be successful in higher education with a minimum amount of effort. They do only what is required by a course and their depth of understanding of the subject matter is largely based on the amount of external pressure provided by the instructor.

In part, these approaches to learning are embedded in personality traits of the students, but they also may be influenced by the educational context or mode of instruction. An example, relevant to the purpose of this article, is provided by Newble and Clarke.[19] They administered the Lancaster Approaches to Studying Inventory (a 64-item questionnaire designed to measure these three modes of learning) to first-, third-, and final-year medical students of the universities of Adelaide and Newcastle in Australia, the latter being the problem-based school. Their results indicate that fairly large differences exist between the learning approaches that students from these two institutions employ and that these differences already exist by the end of the first curriculum year. Newcastle students rate themselves as having an orientation toward the pursuit of meaning in the material they learn: they utilize a deep-level approach, they are low on the reproduction tendency and study less with the strategic goal in mind just to pass the examination, whereas Adelaide students show a reverse tendency.

Of course, several explanations, other than the causal influence of the different educational environments involved, are possible. Because a self-rating scale was used, the results might not so much mirror actual differences in study approach, but might be attributed to social desirability ("everybody wants to be considered a deep-level processor"). If this is the case, however, it is difficult to understand why Adelaide students were less inclined to give socially desirable answers.

Another alternative explanation would be to ascribe the outcomes to specific characteristics of the populations studied. The groups compared may have been different from the start because of different admission procedures. Indeed, the Newcastle school admits students in part based on previous academic achievement, but also takes into account nonacademic previous experiences and personality characteristics. However, this explanation is unlikely, because Coles[20] has found the same effect in two quite different populations—first-year students of the universities of Southampton and that of Limburg. In addition, Coles showed that these differences do not exist so much on entry to medical school, but that the educational environment provided by the conventional school appears to induce a surface memorization approach in its students and actually discourages the use of a deep-level processing strategy. One may agree with Newble and Clarke,[19] who state that: "The attributes for which we would hope in a university graduate are very much those embodied in the deep approach. Disturbingly, the . . . evidence we have, suggests that not only are these attributes unlikely to be achieved by some students but they might be actively inhibited from doing so by our curriculum structures and our teaching and examining methods."

## Discussion

The studies reviewed in this contribution illustrate how difficult it is to compare, at the curriculum level, the effects of different educational approaches on the learning, and attitudes of students. Two fundamental problems are involved. First, the subjects, whose behavior is to be compared, are generally not randomly assigned to the treatments, so a major requirement for "true" experimental comparisons cannot be met. At best, comparisons of this kind can be considered "quasi-experimental."[21] Second, the period over which the treatments are supposed to do their work is so extended that it becomes difficult, if not impossible, to control for extraneous variables that might affect the outcomes but are not in itself subject of investigation. In the studies cited these uncontrolled or even uncontrollable variables include (1) differences in admission procedures that may make the populations to be investigated different from the start,[6,19] (2) differential attrition of students in the course of the program,[3] (3) unforeseen and undocumented changes in a program that affect its outcomes, (4) the use of volunteers,[3,8,17] (5) difficulty in composing adequate comparison groups, resulting in the tendency to use "whoever is available," (6) low response rates,[16] and in particular, (7) differential exposure to the instrument used to measure curriculum effects.[3,6] For instance, a more detailed assessment of the Saunders et al study[5] reveals that the students of the problem-based Newcastle curriculum had never encountered multiple choice questions before in their undergraduate course, while the University of Sydney students had no experience with modified essay questions. The differential exposure to these evaluation instruments may explain the marginal differences between both schools.

In addition, even if a difference can be trusted to represent a true curriculum effect, it is still difficult to point at those curriculum elements that produced the difference. For instance, are the primary care career preferences of students the result of actual *exposure* to primary health care delivery, or is the focus on primary care problems in the theoretical part of the curriculum a sufficient condition for transmitting this preference?

A further difficulty is that although the curricula involved are described in the same general terminology (they all are considered "community oriented" and use problem-based learning in small-group tutorial sessions as their method of instruction, emphasizing self-directed study), in reality relatively large differences among these programs can be observed. In a survey of 10 of these schools, Richards and Fülöp[22] for instance, found that three of them offered their students hardly any exposure to community-experiences, such as making home visits or conducting epidemiological studies in rural areas, and only five utilized problem-based learning as the main instructional approach (although all of them employed it to some extent). So, the generalizability of some of the results presented may be doubtful.

It will be clear from these considerations that the following conclusions should be looked upon with some caution.

1. Although differences in knowledge gains favoring the conventional medical schools involved are very small or virtually absent, some data have been presented that appear to imply that problem-based schools are not always successful in inducing their students to attain levels of academic achievement comparable to those of conventional medical education. However, the problem-based

schools have never advanced specific claims with respect to the knowledge to be acquired by their students; their particular expectation was, and is, that their students would excel in clinical competence. Since the data available in this last area are generally inconclusive, the future challenge to these schools might be to show their students to be superior in clinical competence.

2. The new schools were founded in response to the changing health needs of the various societies. It was felt that the advancement of primary care would help in alleviating at least some of the health problems of a majority of the world population. The scarce information available on the career preferences and actual career choices of students from these schools supports the notion that an emphasis on primary care may influence the professional perspectives of students; that is, problem-based schools seem to be successful in their attempts to produce physicians with a community orientation.

3. Problem-based programs also seem to be successful in providing an environment that is more adapted to the learning needs of medical students than conventional schools generally are. Apparently, the open character of problem- based instruction, emphasizing independent, self-directed learning, fosters in students an inquisitive style of learning, as opposed to the learning strategies that characterize students in conventional programs.

## References

1. Greep J, and Schmidt, HG: The network. *World Health Forum* 1984;18–21.
2. Verwijnen GM, et al: The evaluation system at the Medical School of Maastricht. *Assessment and Evaluation in Higher Education* 1982;7:235–244.
3. Verwijnen GM, Van der Vleuten C, Imbos T: A comparison of an innovative medical school with traditional schools: An analysis in the cognitive domain, Nooman Z, Schmidt HG, Ezzat E (eds): in *Innovation in Medical Education; An Evaluation of Its Present Status*. New York, Springer Publishing (in press).
4. Baca E, Mennin SP, Kaufman A, Moore-West M: A comparison between a problem-based, community-oriented track and a traditional track within one medical school, Nooman Z, Schmidt HG, Ezzat E, (eds): in *Innovation in Medical Education; An Evaluation of Its Present Status*. New York, Springer Publishing (in press).
5. Saunders NA et al: A programme of outcome evaluation studies: experiences at the University of Newcastle. Nooman Z, Schmidt HG, Ezzat E (eds): in *Innovation in Medical Education; an evaluation of its present status*. New York, Springer Publishing (in press).
6. Woodward CA: *Summary of McMaster medical graduates performance on the Medical Council of Canada examination*. Hamilton, Canada: McMaster University, Faculty of Health Sciences, 1984.
7. Barrows HS: A specific, problem-based, self-directed learning method designed to teach medical problem-solving skills, self-learning skills and enhance knowledge retention and recall, Schmidt HG, de Volder ML (eds): in *Tutorials in problem-based learning*. Assen, the Netherlands, Van Gorcum, 1984, p 20.
8. Woodward CA, McAuley RG: Can the academic background of medical graduates be detected during internship? *Can Med Ass J* 1983;129:567–569.

9. Claessen HFA, Boshuizen, HPA: Recall of medical information by students and doctors. *Med Educ* 1985;19:61–67.
10. Patel VL, Groen GJ: Knowledge-based solution strategies in medical reasoning. *Cognitive Science* 1986;10:91–116.
11. Rothman AI: Statements on career intentions as predictors of career choices. *J Med Educ* 1985;60:511–516.
12. Glasser M, Sarnowski AA, Sheth B: Career choices from medical school to practice: Finding from a regional clinical education site. *J Med Educ* 1982;57:442–448.
13. Isokoski M et al: Innovative curriculum leads young doctors to primary health care, Nooman Z, Schmidt HG, Ezzat E (eds): in *Innovation in Medical Education; An Evaluation of Its Present Status* New York, Springer Publishing (in press).
14. Bender W: Kritisch momenten in de medische studie: Enkele recente onderzoeksgegevens (Critical moments in medical education: Some recent data). *Medisch Contact* 1979;47:402–403.
15. Schmidt HG, Moust JHC: Studiebeleving van Maastrichtse medische studenten (Study perceptions of Maastricht medical students). *Medisch Contact* 1981;49:1515–1518.
16. Woodward CA, Ferrier BM: Perspectives of graduates two to five years after graduation from a three-year medical school. *J Med Educ* 1982;57:294–303.
17. Post GJ, Drop MJ: Perceptions of the content of the medical curriculum at the medical faculty in Maastricht, Nooman Z, Schmidt HG, Ezzat E (eds): in *Innovation in Medical Education; An Evaluation of Its Present Status*. New York, Springer Publishing (in press).
18. Marton F, Hounsell DJ, Entwistle NJ (eds): *The Experience of Learning*. Edinburgh, United Kingdom, Scottish Academic Press, 1984.
19. Newble DI, Clarke, R: A comparison of the approaches to learning of students in a traditional and an innovative medical school. *Med Educ* (in press).
20. Coles CR: Differences between conventional and problem-based curricula in their students' approaches to studying. *Med Educ* 1985;19:308–310.
21. Cook TD, Campbell DT: *Quasi-experimentation*. New York; Rand McNally, 1979.
22.. Richards RW, Fülöp T: *Innovative Schools for Health Personnel*. Geneva, Switzerland, World Health Organization, 1987.

# 16
# Dutch Comparisons: Cognitive and Motivational Effects of Problem-based Learning on Medical Students

MARTEN W. DE VRIES, HENK G. SCHMIDT,
and ERIK DE GRAAFF

This chapter reviews evaluation research findings from a continuing program of evaluation research carried out by the department of educational development and research at the University of Limburg. The research program attempts to clarify to what extent problem-based learning is an effective and efficient approach to medical education and if so why. We present data on the principle components of this research having to do with a medical student's attitude toward instruction, student achievements in terms of test scores measuring medical knowledge, and problem-solving capabilities acquired by students. Specific data on study duration, dropout rates, and study load are also presented.

  In this discussion, we capitalize on a unique aspect of the Dutch medical student selection system—the lottery. This process allocates students to medical schools after baseline requirements are met by the students, by chance not merit or other considerations. The student bodies of various medical schools are thereby more similar than is typically the case in Europe or in the United States. This is a boon for comparative evaluation research of the kind reported here. However, since selection of the students in this study is not entirely random, the comparisons—although scientifically justified—need to be interpreted with some caution.

## Brief Overview of the Medical Curriculum at the University of Limburg

The Maastricht medical curriculum is a 6-year program. The first 2 years are devoted to understanding pathophysiologic mechanisms underlying disease and the final 2 years are focused on clinical training. Each curriculum year is comprised of a number of 6-week "blocks" or units. During each block, students meet twice a week for a two-hour, small-group tutorial in which problems are analyzed and learning goals are formulated. These groups are guided by tutors drawn from the faculty and staff whose role it is to facilitate the learning process of the students. Each block includes a skill-training program in which students are taught diagnostic and therapeutic skills. Their newly acquired diagnostic skills are tested in encounters with subjects who simulate patients.

Each year, the blocks are organized around one central theme. The first year's theme is: Reactions of the body to physical and psychological stress, such as physical reactions to accident, infection and the body defenses meant to cope with these. The second-year theme is: The human being from conception to death. It deals with characteristic health problems around conception and birth, childhood, adolescence, adulthood, and the elderly individual. For the third and fourth years, the faculty has chosen health problems crucial in terms of prevalence and severity of various diseases in Dutch society. Problems such as pain in the chest, fatigue, and blood loss comprise the block themes. Electives encompassing a variety of research and clinical experiences may also be chosen as part of the curriculum.

Problem-based learning is the instructional method employed in this curriculum period, described briefly as follows. Students meeting in tutorial groups are confronted with the following sort problem, which essentially contains the description of complaints and symptoms of individual patients.

You have played a game of tennis during a warm Sunday afternoon. You have lost your game with 6-0, 6-0. When you walk back to the changing room for a shower, you suddenly notice that you are wet all over your body and your skin has turned scarlet. How can these phenomena be explained?

The introduction of such problems leads to a discussion and manufacturing of an outline of relevant questions with which students formulate learning goals. Students can achieve these learning goals with the help of videotapes, bibliographies, academic consultation, or other available learning sources. In the follow-up sessions, students confront each other with their findings and synthesize the information required in terms of describing the underlying processes and developing a plan for clinical management. Problems like the foregoing are collected in "block" books that guide students learning activities. In addition to medical problems, the block book contains references, audiovisual resources, a list of resource persons that can be contacted, and a timetable.

The curriculum components just sketched—problem-based learning, small-group tutorials, and a self-study emphasis—differentiates the Maastricht curriculum from the traditional Dutch medical schools with which it will now be compared.

## Review of Research Results

### Student Attitudes toward Instruction

In a study carried out in Groningen[1] students were asked to write a letter answering the following question: "What do you think of your instruction?" The returned letters depicted one general trend. Medical students generally experienced their instruction as boring, irrelevant, and sometimes anxiety provoking. Of course, there were exceptions, individual teachers or programs were genuinely enjoyed and contributed to the students, motivation to become a doctor. But, in general

TABLE 16.1. Positive and negative evaluations of Maastricht medical students on aspects of their curriculum.

| Aspects of curriculum | Positive | Negative |
|---|---|---|
| Attachments, clinical activities | 30 | 2 |
| Small-group tutorials | 13 | 10 |
| Self-organized study activities | 15 | |
| Self-directed learning | 10 | 4 |
| Skills training | 11 | |
| Educational approach in general | 9 | 1 |
| Resource persons | 8 | 2 |
| Progress test | | 10 |
| Holistic approach to human beings | 9 | |
| Use of simulated patients | 7 | |
| Electives | 3 | |
| Blockbooks/problems | 2 | |
| Total | 117 | 29 |

medical education did not appear to be an enriching experience. Schmidt and Moust[2] replicated Bender's study. They randomly selected 50 students from the Maastricht problem-based curriculum, 10 from each class, and asked them to write a similar letter about their curriculum. Ninety-two percent of the students responded. The authors extracted positive and negative evaluative remarks from the letter, coded the answers into a number of categories, and tallied frequencies (see Table 16.1).

For example, if a student wrote that he or she enjoyed a particular contact with general practitioners in the first year, that answer was coded as a positive evaluation in the "attachment, clinical activity" category that may be found on the top of Table 16.1. Schmidt and Moust scored 147 evaluative remarks by the Maastricht medical students on aspects of their curriculum. Of these remarks, 117 were positive, indicating that the Maastricht medical students had a positive attitude toward their curriculum on the whole.

A closer look at the student responses is instructive. For example, the tutorial groups in addition to being praised could also be a source of discontent. One student wrote:

During tutorial groups students behave rather uninterested or do not react at all. If the tutorial does not work the way it should or if a group doesn't click they merely shrug their shoulders, even though the tutorial group is the key to the entire study. Your relation to people is what it is all about, now and in the future. And if that is not feasible (not even in a tutorial group) then what is? One of my characteristics is that I feel very dependent on others to keep my motivation up. In this self-directing approach, the others are my stimulus.

In contrast, the small-group tutorials and study activities that were organized by the students themselves were highly valued. One of the more interesting findings was that first-year students expressed difficulties with self-directed learning.

They seem to need at least 6 months to adapt to this new learning expectation environment in which they are responsible themselves for what to study and how to study. One of them wrote:

Since we are unfamiliar with a self-directed study program we are confronted with a totally new educational system in the first year. This is strange: because we have to discover how to study by ourselves: no certainties; hardly any guidelines, but after a year's hard work it turns out to be less difficult.

Opportunities for gaining acceptance with the medical care system and patient care were most frequently positively rated. The conclusion that early and frequent involvement of medical students with a health care provider is of developmental importance to the students should be drawn. This is particularly so as a source of motivation, as one student wrote:

I gained the most insights into my studies during my electives with physicians and in the hospital. Only then I realized how little I knew. After each of those rotations I experienced a considerable increase in my study activity. For me, the confrontation with practice is a very important and positive asset in the curriculum of the Maastricht Medical Faculty. Because of this practice you get a very good—be it a rather broad—insight into the health care system. It gives you a good impression on what you're studying.

These representative qualitative descriptions provide a candid and generally positive reaction to the Maastricht curriculum by the random sample of students selected in 1980.

## Study Load

In investigating study load, Weggeman and Moen[3] took a skeptical point of departure—they asked whether the positive student attitude expressed in the Schmidt and Moust[2] study was merely an indication that students were satisfied with the Maastricht curriculum because it did not demand too much academic effort. Weggeman and Moen asked: "Does an emphasis on independent learning with a de-emphasis on summative test assessments merely produce easygoing students"? To answer this, they used a comparative approach and surveyed the study load of first- and fourth-year Maastricht medical students during one randomly selected week of the program. They calculated from this a study-load-per-year figure. The authors then compared the study-load estimates with those from various other Dutch university curricula (Table 16.2). The results of this comparison make it clear that there is no reason to suppose that stressing independent learning in the absence of the external pressure of summative evaluation create students who put less effort into their study.

## Graduation and Dropouts

Post et al.[4] investigated the relative efficiency of the Maastricht curriculum in terms of producing graduates and limiting dropouts. These are important data

TABLE 16.2. Estimate of study load per year in hours.

| University | Field of study | Year load |
|---|---|---|
| Amsterdam | Economics 1st year | 850 |
| Delft | Chemistry 1st year | 1300 |
| Groningen | Biology 1st year | 1156 |
| Groningen | Medicine 2nd year | 800 |
| Leiden | Law 1st year | 535 |
| Utrecht | Chemistry 1st year | 1070 |
| Groningen | Dental surgery 1st year | 1240 |
| Limburg | Medicine 1st year | 1378 |
| Limburg | Medicine 4th year | 1573 |

since in the early 1980s the mean dropout rate of Dutch universities was 52%. Study duration and dropout rates of the first five Maastricht classes were compared with statistics from other Dutch medical schools (see Fig. 16.1). Figure 16.1 clearly demonstrates that the efficiency of the Maastricht medical school exceeds the results of the other Dutch medical schools. A majority of the Maastricht students graduate in 6 years. Median study duration at the other medical schools ranges from 7 to over 8 years. The final height of the curves, indicating the percentage of graduating students amounts to 85% for Maastricht and falls between 64% and 71% for the other medical schools. The Maastricht curriculum then produces relatively more graduates in less time. Since there has been no selection of students, the aforementioned positive motivational effects of problem-based learning seem to be the most likely explanation for the higher efficiency of the Maastricht curriculum.

## Achievements

The dropout rates are described in a positive light as an achievement of the medical curriculum. One could, however, look at these data from a more critical perspective. Perhaps the Maastricht medical curriculum is graduating students that would not have made it in other schools. To answer this question, Imbos and Verwijnen[5] asked this question: "To what extent is test performance of the student's, in a problem based curriculum comparable to students in a traditional school?" The two investigators compared the achievement of the Maastricht medical student with students of two traditional medical curricula and a reference group consisting of graduates from various medical schools. For each group in the comparison, all levels of medical expertise were represented and all groups from first year to the sixth year took the same test. The test administered consisted of 200 items covering medical knowledge as a whole. In Fig. 16.2 the test score percentages by year for the three comparison groups are illustrated. The different curves indicate the performance of students of different levels of expertise from the three different schools. For instance, first-year students of the other medical school acquired a mean score on the test of about 15%, while first-year Maastricht students acquired a score of about 23%. The dot indicated with an "R"

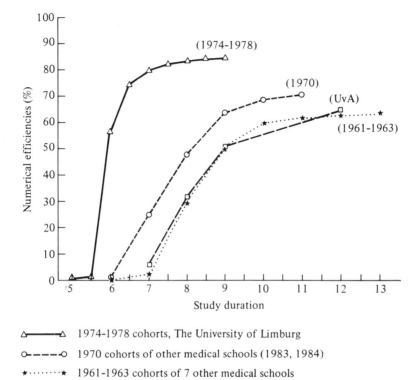

FIGURE 16.1. Cumulative numerical efficiencies.

shows the performance of the reference group of graduate physicians that had a mean score of about 70%. The main conclusion that can be drawn is that whatever difference there are, they are small at all levels of expertise. These findings, then, do not support the assertion that lower dropout rates are associated with poorer performance and less pressured scrutiny by the Maastricht medical school.

## Problem-solving Performance

A number of authors have asserted that problem-based learning promotes clinical reasoning skills.[6,7] In order to test this hypothesis, Boshuizen and Claessen[8] used an experimental procedure well known in the field of problem-solving research. It is a procedure borrowed from the work of de Groot[9] (1965) on problem solving in chess. Boshuizen and Claessen proceeded as follows: Subjects known to have a different level of expertise in medical problem-solving (eg, second-, fourth-, and fifth-year medical students, physicians) were asked to process patient-related information. They had to work through a patient case consisting of about 40 small cards that contained information about the condition of that patient (eg,

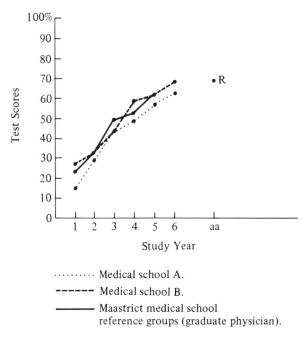

FIGURE 16.2. Comparisons of medical knowledge achievement scores between three medical schools by study year.

information about temperature, blood pressure, blood test results, complaints, etc.). After processing these items, the students were asked to recall as much of that information as they could. This method presupposes that novices and experts have different cognitive structures with respect to solving the problems at hand. The more integrated, the better organized, the more specific their cognition, the better their performance will be on this task. Boshuizen and Claessen compared the performance of University of Limburg and University of Utrecht students on this cognitive task. The dependent variable was the number of items recalled correctly, divided by the amount of time needed to process the information. Figure 16.3 shows the results of their investigation.

As you can see, the Maastricht medical students are consistently—although not always significantly—better on this cognitive task. We conclude that the data—although it is interestingly supportive—are inconclusive with respect to testing the assertion that problem-based learning stimulates medical problem solving. The result could be a measure of the continuous exposure and confrontation of students in a problem-based curriculum to patient-related information and not the result of superior cognitive functioning as such. However, support for this effect has been shown experimentally by Schmidt in 1982[10] and Barrows and Tamblyn in 1980.[6] These experimental studies showed that problem-based learning did stimulate further learning and that this process, therefore, deserves further consideration by medical educators.

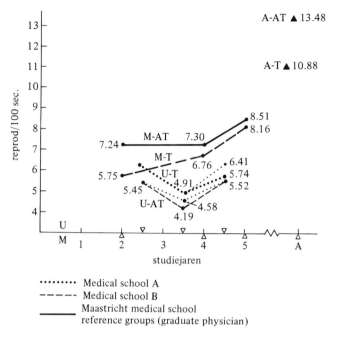

FIGURE 16.3. Problem solving and recall skills on a cognitive task for three medical schools by study year.

## Conclusion

The studies presented here have presented global comparisons of Dutch universities at the curricula level. The studies are very suggestive but their quasi-experimental nature do not allow us to conclude that the differences observed are purely the result of the differences in curriculum. The studies were outcome oriented and all take the risk of being unduly influenced by sampling shortcomings. The comparisons may also have been influenced by differences in attitudes of medical students toward their own education. Such differences could be the result of differences in instructional approaches but could also be attributed to differences that already existed by the time these students entered medical school. The outcome-oriented studies presented here, although justifiably presenting a positive reaction, have been more qualitative and associative in nature and did not deal with research shortcomings in detail.

However, these data do illustrate that there is no reason to propose that problem-based curricula provide inferior training to medical students as compared with traditional curricula. The data provided in this chapter clearly demonstrate some "bottom-line" results: medical students in a problem-based curriculum do not spend less time on their study, and their achievement is comparable to that of students of traditional schools. The same result applies to problem-solving performance. Second, problem-based curricula do appear to provide a friendlier and more inviting educational climate; the response of students in their instruction evaluation letter clearly demonstrates this feature. Such an educational climate facilitates the emergence of positive attitudes toward study and possibly create the lower dropout rate. Finally, there is growing evidence that problem-based learning approaches and problem analysis in a small-group tutorial may be an effective facilitator of the processing and retention of new information. It is a learning skill of high value for tomorrow's physician.

## References

1. Bender W: (1979). Kritische momenten in de medische studie: enkele recente onderzoeksgegevens. *Medisch Contact* 13:402–403.
2. Schmidt HG, Moust JHC: Studiebeleving van Maastrichtse medische studenten. *Medisch Contact* 1981;49:1515–1518.
3. Weggeman M, Moen J: Een onderzoek naar de studiebelasting van studenten aan de faculteit der geneeskunde, Rijksuniversiteit Limburg, in Schmidt HG (ed): *Probleemgestuurd Onderwijs*. Harlingen, Flevodruk, 1982.
4. Post GJ, DeGraaff E, Drop MJ: *Duur and numeriek rendement van de opleiding tot basisarts in Maastricht* (Study duration and numerical efficiency of the Maastricht medical school), Nederlands Tijdschrift voor Geneeskunde, 1986;130(42):1903–1905.
5. Imbos T, Verwijnen M: Voortgaanstoetsing aan de medische faculteit Maastricht, in Schmidt HG (ed): *Probleemgestuurd Onderwijs*. Harlingen, Flevodruk, 1982.
6. Barrows HS, Tamblyn RM: *Problem-based Learning*. New York, Springer, 1980.
7. Schmidt HG and DeVolder ML (eds.) *Tutorials in Problem-based Learning*. Assen, Van Gorcum, 1984.
8. Boshuizen HPA, Claessen HFA: Cognitieve verwerking en onthouden van patientgegevens; een onderzoek bij studenten in Utrecht en Maastricht, in Schmidt HG (ed): *Probleemgestuurd Onderwijs*. Harlingen, The Netherlands, Flevodruk, 1982.
9. Groot AD de: *Thought and Choice in Chess*. Gravenhage, The Netherlands, Mouton, 1965.
10. Schmidt HG: *Activatie van voorkennis, intrinsieke motivatie en de verwerking van tekst*. Apeldoorn, Van Walraven, 1982.

# Part V
# Faculty Development

HENK G. SCHMIDT

Innovative medical education puts extremely high demands on teachers who are instrumental in its implementation, a conclusion drawn from the abundant literature on this topic. Not only do those involved in the renewal of instruction have to acquire new teaching skills, they also have to discard a number of *beliefs*, pertaining to learning and instruction, that are widely shared among teachers. The chapter 17, by Schmidt, Bouhuijs, Khattab, and Makladi, provides several examples of these beliefs, for instance: "An essential body of knowledge must first be acquired by students before they can fruitfully engage in working on patient problems," "The primary function of a teacher is to impart knowledge." "Medical students are generally not capable of discerning what should or should not be taught in a medical school." "Students do their best work when they are told what to do at every step." Convictions like these are often obstacles to change because they encourage teachers to stick with approaches that bear no risk because they rely on procedures known for ages, but on the other hand, never will contribute to the *improvement* of medical education either.

Faculty development, however, involves offering opportunities for the acquisition of new *skills* relevant to the institution's educational objectives. Because many institutions for higher education tenure staff on excellence only in research, no formal requirements are set for teaching. Hence, many teachers, although experienced scientists, lack essential skills necessary for effective teaching.

In problem-based, community-oriented curricula, this problem is even more pressing because in these curricula, instructional qualities are required that are even uncommon to unusually talented teachers among the staff. In these curricula, the faculty is asked to direct small-group tutorial sessions in which problems are analyzed, to construct these problems, to produce learning resources adapted to the needs of individual students, to formulate strategies for involving the community in the teaching, or to act as a resource person without interfering with the student's self-directed learning. Chapter 18 by Benor and Mahler and Chapter 19 by Moust and Schmidt discuss several of these skills and outline ways in which faculty could be assisted in their development.

Schmidt, Bouhuijs, Khattab, and Makladi report attitudinal changes among medical teachers participating in a workshop on small-group tutorials. The workshop was aimed at the introduction of newly appointed faculty of an innovative medical school in the Suez Canal area, in Egypt, and at the educational principles underlying its curriculum. The authors investigated changes in beliefs among participants concerning educational issues using a 20-item questionnaire. Changes in the predicted direction were found particularly on issues that were addressed directly during the workshop (eg, the ability or inability of students to take responsibility for their own learning and the role of the teacher in enhancing student-centered instruction).

Benor and Mahler review a number of important problems facing teacher-training programs and challenging those who wish to renew medical education: lack of motivation with respect to education among faculty, low quality of instruction because of absence of relevant knowledge and skills, and lack of opportunities for personal development of teachers in existing curricula. In response to these problems, they suggest that teacher-training programs should comprise two dimensions. One dimension is a timewise hierarchical structure of the programs, which would enable gradual acquisition of instructional skills, progressing from generic to specific. The second dimension is that of the different mental domains: teacher-training programs should focus both on knowledge, skills, and attitudes of teachers. This two-dimensional model is illustrated by a description of the faculty-development approach at Ben Gurion University, Beersheva, Israel.

Moust and Schmidt describe the in-service training programs of the University of Limburg, Maastricht, the Netherlands, and provide data on participants that have been going through those programs since 1979. An outstanding characteristic of these programs is that the focus is as much *on students* as it is on teachers. Maastricht students participate in a number of activities that prepare them for studying the curriculum. The rationale behind this attempt is that problem-based learning is as new to students as it is to teachers. Hence, both groups should receive assistance in order to cope with the new situation.

Finally, Newble asks whether innovative problem-based learning approaches require the massive faculty reorientation suggested by the new developing schools. He describes the 10-year successful introduction of small-group approaches and problem-based learning into the medical-surgical rotation of the conventional curriculum the University of Adelaide in Australia. The chapter suggests that the first steps taken to change the conventional educational approaches in established faculties may not be as difficult as often feared.

The synthesis of new ideas and traditional educational methods may not be as straightforward, however. A tension between approaches naturally exists. Some fear that what is good in old methods will be lost. This process is easily observed in the controversy between lectures and group-teaching formats in the new curricula. This is summed up nicely by Spence[1] in a discussion of teaching methods: "The decrying of the wholesale use of lectures is probably justified. The wholesale decrying of lecturing is just as certainly not justified."

# Reference

1. Spence RB: Lecture and class discussion in teaching educational psychology. J Educ Psychol 1978;19:454.

# 17
# Attitude Change Among Medical Teachers: Effects of a Workshop on Tutorials

HENK G. SCHMIDT, PETER A.J. BOUHUIJS,
TYMOOR KHATTAB, and FATHI MAKLADI

In 1977 The Suez Canal University in Ismailia, Egypt, took the first steps toward the development of a new medical school (see Chap. 5). Although Egypt produces enough doctors to cover the health manpower needs in a quantitative sense, there exists a clear lack of primary care physicians. The new faculty has set five institutional goals in this respect: (1) to qualify physicians whose primary objective is to provide health care in a combined hospital–community system with major emphasis on primary care; (2) to relate medical education to the needs of the society so that the physicians are able to diagnose the community's health problems; (3) to develop and implement, together with the Ministry of Public Health and other health care delivery bodies, an integrated system for comprehensive health care delivery and health manpower development in the Suez Canal area and Sinai; (4) to develop and provide programs for postgraduate training and continuing education for health personnel; and (5) to develop research programs that primarily address actual health needs of the community.[1]

In order to implement these institutional goals in the undergraduate educational program the faculty decided to opt for an approach in which preclinical and clinical sciences are integrated. For the first year subject matter is organized around stages of human development from conception to death, and for the second and third years the curriculum is organized around the body systems. The faculty puts a strong emphasis on small-group tutorials as the main instructional method in order to promote problem-based, self-directed learning in students.[2] Students are confronted with preventive and curative health care from their first weeks of medical education on. They spend 1 day a week in rural communities.

In September 1981 the faculty started with the first batch of students. At that time about 20 senior staff and 100 junior staff were appointed to the faculty. An important task for a new faculty that adopts a nontraditional approach to medical education is to acquaint new staff members with the educational philosophy of the school and, more important, to enable staff to develop skills and attitudes necessary to implement the educational program. The acquisition of new attitudes is especially important because medical schools in Egypt have rather rigid curricula that have not been changed for many years. (The officially approved curriculum has existed since 1930.) The staff of the new school is for the most part trained in this traditional context.

During the past few years, a number of teacher-training activities took place. Initially, there was a high input from external education consultants. Gradually the faculty members themselves took more responsibility in developing teacher-training workshops on the new educational roles of teachers in this school. This chapter describes the program of a 3-day teacher-training workshop for newly appointed faculty. Data are presented on attitude change of teachers participating in the workshop.

## Workshop

In December 1981 a 3-day educational workshop was held. Participants were 10 newly appointed staff, 7 clinicians, and 3 basic scientists. The goals of the workshop were to provide an introduction to the philosophy of the curriculum of the medical faculty of the Suez Canal University (MF/SCU) and to train staff in executing tutorials. The program consisted in seminars and practical exercises.

The *seminars* dealt with the following topics: community-oriented approach to medical education, problem-based learning, principles of curriculum design. They generally included a short introduction by one of the workshop coordinators, presentation of concrete examples, and discussion among participants. The main themes of these discussions were the role of the basic sciences in an integrated medical curriculum, self-directed versus teacher-dependent learning, the future role of the physician in Egypt, and the relation between the medical faculty educational program and the regional health care system. The participants also had an opportunity to talk with students. The goal of this informal meeting was to clarify whether the doubts that some participants had concerning the suitability of the new educational approach for Egyptian students (in view of their prior education) was justified.

The *exercises* consisted of simulations of a small-group tutorial. Three types of simulations were used. First, the participants simulated a session of a group of medical students working through a problem. They analyzed an obstetrical problem, formulated learning goals, spent some time on independent study in the library fulfilling the objectives set by the group, and synthesized the newly acquired information.[3] One of the coordinators played the role of the tutor. Second, the participants practiced the role of the tutor themselves leading a group discussion. Third, participants were confronted with small-group problem situations they had to solve (e.g., quarrels among group members, how to handle an extremely withdrawn student).

## Workshop Evaluation: Instrument and Procedure

An attempt was made to evaluate the effects of the workshop on the attitudes of the participants toward medical education. For that purpose a questionnaire devised by Joorabchi and Chawhan[4] was used. This attitude scale measures opinions with respect to specific issues in medical education. The issues addressed in

TABLE 17.1. Items measuring attitude toward aspects of medical education

| Item | $t$ Observed | Chance probability |
|---|---|---|
| 1. A teacher is born, not made. | 0.19 | –* |
| *2. Most teachers in our medical school do a good job of facilitating student learning. | 2.45 | < 0.025 |
| *3. In general, medical students learn most from teachers who offer a large body of information. | −3.79 | < 0.005 |
| *4. The primary function of a teacher is to impart knowledge. | −1.15 | – |
| *5. Medical students can generallly not be relied on to study on their own. | −0.80 | – |
| 6. The public at large should have a role in determining what the objectives of medical education should be. | 1.17 | – |
| 7. Good research scholars generally make good teachers because they have a vast fund of knowledge. | 1.00 | – |
| *8. Medical students are generally not capable of discerning what should or should not be taught in a medical school. | 1.96 | < 0.05 |
| 9. The medical faculty should ask students to evaluate their courses. | −0.29 | – |
| 10. The students should be told at the beginning of each course what is expected of them at the end. | 0.00 | – |
| 11. In general, students cannot be expected to provide responsible and objective evaluation of the quality of teaching they receive. | −1.62 | < 0.10 |
| 12. If a professor wishes to be effective in his or her teaching, he should maintain a good deal of formality and decorum between himself and the students | −1.77 | < 0.10 |
| 13. Medical students should be represented in curriculum committees. | −0.61 | – |
| *14. If medical students do poorly in medical school it is chiefly because they are intellectually ill-equipped to begin with. | 1.46 | < 0.10 |
| 15. A good teacher concentrates on teaching the latest discoveries in the forefront of medicine, rather than dwelling on basic and general competencies. | −0.67 | – |
| *16. Medical students do their best work when they are told what to do at every step. | −2.09 | < 0.05 |
| *17. Our students are mature enough to set their own goals. | 2.33 | < 0.025 |
| *18. Medical students set high goals for themselves and work hard to achieve them if they are allowed to work on their own. | 1.41 | < 0.10 |
| *19. Medical students do their best work when they assume individual responsibility for their own learning. | 0.36 | – |
| 20. Medical students should be consulted as to the objectives of their curriculum. | 1.15 | – |

Adapted from Joorabchi B., Chawhan AR. Effects of a short educational workshop on attitudes of three groups of medical educators. Br J Med Educ 1975;9:38–41.
*Not significant.

this questionnaire are the following: Should the medical teacher transfer knowledge to students or should he facilitate independent learning? Are medical students able to bear responsibility for their own learning? Eight items that made no sense in the context of the workshop were removed. The remaining 20 are shown in Table 17.1. Inspection of the items reveals that some of them have direct relevance to the goals of the workshop (e.g., items 2, 3, 8, 16, and 17). Other items deal with more general topics (e.g., items 9, 11, and 13). Our hypothesis was that if attitudinal changes took place as a consequence of the workshop, they would be strongest with respect to the category of directly relevant items. This hypothesis was tested in the analysis of the data.

Each item consists of a statement followed by a five-point scale, ranging from "strongly agree," "agree," "neutral," "disagree," to "strongly disagree." Respondents had to circle the alternative of their choice. In order to discourage response sets, some items were phrased negatively and others were phrased positively. The questionnaire was administered twice, before and after the workshop. In order to minimize the possibility that the respondents would mainly give socially desirable answers,[5] they were asked to fill out the questionnaire anonymously and to give honest answers. Respondents had to choose a number known only to them, which permitted us to calculate individual difference scores between pre- and posttest scores.

## Results and Discussion

First, attitudinal changes with respect to the questionnaire as a whole were studied. The answers of the respondents were transformed into scores ranging from 1 to 5. Negatively phrased items were scored in the reverse.

Subsequently, a total score for each individual was obtained by adding the item scores. The differences between pre- and posttest total scores were to be expected, using a $t$-test for correlated samples. The value of $t$-observed was 4.76 ($p < .001$). From this result one can conclude that during the workshop reliable changes in attitude toward aspects of medical education, as measured with the Joorabchi and Chawhan[4] questionnaire, took place. However, because of the specific research design used in this study (a one-group pretest-posttest design) these changes cannot be clearly attributed to the workshop as such. Events between pre- and posttest other than the workshop may have been responsible for the observed changes. In order to rule out this possibility at least one control group should have been used. In this type of study, however, this requirement is rarely fulfilled because one cannot withhold treatment from half of the subjects, and there is generally not enough time available to hold the workshop twice. What can be done is to look for secondary evidence that may or may not support the hypothesis that the observed differences are caused by the workshop. This secondary evidence can be obtained by inspection of attitude changes on individual items.

Table 17.1 contains the main results of this analysis. For each item it shows observed $t$-values, resulting from $t$-tests of correlated samples, and chance probabilities. It was expected that if the workshop was really effective in changing the participants' attitudes the differences between pre- and posttest scores should be greatest on items that were considered directly related to the goals of the workshop. The items in Table 17.1 that are marked by asterisks were considered to be related directly to the workshop objectives. Inspection of these results shows that the differences between pre- and posttest are found mainly on items directly relevant to the objectives of the workshop. Thus it seems to be acceptable to attribute attitude changes among the participants of the workshop to the workshop itself.

## Conclusion

The workshop appears to be effective in bringing about the desired attitudinal changes in the new staff of MF/SCU. This result is encouraging because implementation of educational innovations heavily relies on the willingness of teachers to accept a new philosophy of education and their role in it. An institution that provides education cannot pursue newly defined objectives without the active support of its educators. This result is all the more encouraging because the workshop exerted its greatest influence on ideas of the staff that are vital to the goals of the new medical faculty.

The items on which the staff's attitudes changed most have to do with the extent to which medical students are able to formulate their own learning objectives. The participants switched from a "teacher-oriented" attitude to a "student-oriented view, in which the teacher looks upon himself as a facilitator of learning, acknowledges the needs of the students, and attempts to foster in them independent, self-directed learning habits."[4]

The research presented here is a first step toward a more extensive evaluation of MF/SCU workshops. Attitude changes among medical teachers represent a necessary condition, not a sufficient one, for the implementation of new educational principles. Further research will be focused on the extent to which the new staff is acquiring new professional *skills* necessary to teach in a problem-based, community-oriented educational climate.

## References

1. Nooman Z: The new faculty of medicine at Suez Canal University. Presented at the Meeting of the Network of COmmunity-Oriented Educational Institutions for Health Sciences, Bellagio Study and Conference Center, 1981.
2. Barrows HS, Tambly RM: Problem-Based Learning, An Approach to Medical Education. New York, Springer, 1980.
3. Schmidt JG: Problem-based learning: rationale and description. Med Educ 1983, 17, 11–16.
4. Joorabchi B, Chawhan AR: Effects of a short educational workshop on attitudes of three groups of medical educators. Br J Med Educ 1975;9:38–41.
5. Edwards AL: Techniques of Attitude Scale Construction. New York, Appleton-Century-Crofts, 1957.
6. Cook TD, Campbell DT: Quasi-Experimentation, Design and Analysis to Field Settings. Chicago, Rand McNally, 1979.

# 18
# Training Medical Teachers: Rationale and Outcomes*

## Dan E. Benor and Sophia Mahler

Teacher training is gradually becoming prevalent in medical education. A variety of training methods are used, ranging from independent competency-based modules[1] to systematic didactic courses.[2] The prevailing method, however, which is also most recommended for in-service teacher education is still the short training workshop.[3,4] Some evidence suggests that even a rather short workshop improves the quality of instruction, probably by increasing the teacher's self-confidence.[5] Nevertheless, almost no long-term and wide-range evaluations have been attempted to assess the effectiveness of the various training methods and the duration of their effect. Teacher training thus remains the province of each institution, which develops its own program, often based on beliefs rather than on facts and on contingency rather than on needs.

The following is a description of a multiphasic teaching-training program that has been implemented in the Faculty of Health Sciences, Ben Gurion University (BGU). The program is based on the assumptions that different teachers have different needs and expectations, that no single format can meet all these needs, and that training in didactics and instructional methods should be preceded by attitudinal change. The program acknowledges the great variability in teachers' abilities, competencies, needs, and wishes. The program also reflects the conception that training should be stepwise, gradually progressing toward mastery through repeated reinforcement. The program is evaluated by two independent methods that relate to personal growth on the one hand and faculty development on the other.

## Issues and Responses

Study of current trends and practices in medical education[6,7] reveals several major issues concerning teachers' performance. They may be classified into the following categories: (1) motivational aspects; (2) quality of instruction; (3) personal development of teachers; and (4) faculty development.

---

*Modified from an article, Teacher training and faculty development in medical education, reprinted by permission of the *Iraëli Journal of Medical Science*.

The motivational aspect is by far the most important issue. It includes motivation toward both teaching and participation in planning, program evaluation, course renewal, and other facets of curriculum development.

Among the many reasons for the lack of motivation one can find psychological isolation,[8] lack of reinforcement and reward,[9] and possible profession-role conflict between being a physician and being a teacher.[10] The medical teacher is more service-oriented than his fellow teacher from the general university and further detached from the academic-scholastic environment.

In order to enhance motivation a training program should create personal involvement at the earliest possible phase. The individual faculty member should feel a part of a multidisciplinary team acting together toward a worthwhile goal. The individual should identify with the institutional objectives, philosophy, and educational approaches.[11] Such a process may involve a change of attitudes and thus require appropriate strategies as well as continuity. Certainly it requires information on the institutional history, structure, and objectives, as well as an overview of the entire curriculum and the educational principles that govern it. The teacher may then see his or her own contribution in the proper context. Teachers may end this phase of training with many doubts. They thus must have an appropriate support system to approach with questions, ideas, and grievances for informal off-the-record assistance. Of course, external motivation may be tremendously enhanced by appropriate reward for excellence in teaching. However, such reward cannot replace the internal motivation stemming from identification.

The issue of quality of instruction has been intensively addressed and need not be repeated here. Nevertheless, it may be briefly summarized under four interlocking headings: (1) Orientation toward student rather than teacher, and learning rather than teaching.[12] This category includes the self-learning concept and the inquiry method in education.[13] (2) Systematic approach to curriculum design and to instruction, ranging from the institutional level to the particular course to a single lesson.[14] This category includes the selection of proper methods, materials, and instruments. (3) Cognitive level of instruction, which relates to the development of problem-solving skills.[15] (4) Evaluation of performance, which includes the issues of validity and reliability of measuring instruments.

Teacher training programs should, however, take into account considerable variability among teachers, with or without previous training. They also should consider the specific needs of individual teachers. A basic phase of training may provide the educational language and establish a conceptual framework. It also may increase the teacher's repertoire by additional instructional methodologies.[16] In-depth study of any of the above-mentioned educational issues may be postponed until the following phases, which would be more specific and task-oriented, aimed at defined groups of trainees. It should be stressed, though, that acquisition of basic instructional skills may and should be accompanied by further creation, promotion, and sustenance of motivation. Strategies for attitudinal change may thus still be required. It is suggested that a technical approach to the issue of improving the quality of instruction may be erroneous.

The issue of personal development of teachers, although closely related to the motivational aspect through personal satisfaction, deserves separate consideration. Such personal growth may be regarded as the major safeguard against "faculty fatigue." In its absence the teachers' behavior tends to take the "fidelity" pattern,[17] which means passive acceptance of dictates concerning curriculum and instruction. Such acceptance can never bridge the planned curricular objectives and their actual implementation.[11] On the other hand, personal development may shift the behavior toward the "mutual adaptation" pattern, which means "us" instead of "them," and "let's try it" instead of "do it their way." The common teacher training programs sometimes try too much too early, preventing the feeling of growth. Such feeling may be created by a carefully designed multiphasic program in which opportunities to implement the acquired skills are interwoven with appropriate reinforcement training sessions. Also essential for personal development is the provision of formative evaluation of teachers' performance, including self-assessment tools.

The issue of faculty development is threefold. It implies interdisciplinary and interdepartmental communication. It also involves support of colleagues and professionals to combat the psychological isolation of the individual.[8,9] In addition, it ought to promote the evolution of the educational leadership of tomorrow.

Closely attached to the faculty development issue is the need to protect and maintain educational innovations wherever they have been attempted. In the face of faculty mobility on the one hand and faculty fatigue on the other, only wide dissemination of the new educational approaches together with a constant reinforcement may counteract the tendency to fall back to traditional routines. Furthermore, one can hardly imagine moving away from the biomedical model to the biopsychosocial one[18] without effective channels of communication between disciplines, mutual team effort, skills in systematic curriculum design, and knowledgeable leadership, all included in the term faculty development. It thus becomes apparent that a high level phase of teacher education may be required, supplementing the acquisition of both generic and specific instructional skills.

Thus, teacher training programs should be continuous and multiphasic, involve interdisciplinarity, provide appropriate feedback and support, and consider individual variability of both needs and capabilities.

## Training Program

The BGU Faculty Development Program includes three phases, and a fourth phase is planned for the near future. The first phase aims at enhancing the identification of the individual teacher with the institution, its philosophy, and its educational approaches.[11,19] This phase thus appeals to the attitudinal domain.

The second phase introduces the teacher to the educational language, concepts, and methods. In addition to the acquisition of this generic knowledge, an attempt is made in this phase to develop the participants' self-acceptance as teachers rather than as professionals who are obliged to teach. The second phase thus addresses both the cognitive and attitudinal domains. It does not, however, provide the teacher with specific skills for instruction. These skills are acquired during the third phase, which offers a variety of specific workshops, each designed to improve a specific instructional skill. The third phase thus refers mainly to the psychomotor domain and capitalizes on both the occurrence of attitudinal change and the acquisition of the knowledge base achieved in the former phases.

The fourth phase has not yet started. It will aim at a small, select group of teachers who have been through all previous phases. It will combine all three domains: cognitive, attitudinal, and psychomotor. The teacher will be expected to acquire additional detailed educational knowledge, to further develop their own instructional abilities as well as skills to train other teachers, and to conduct research. As a result teachers may develop a new self-perception as a future educational leader.

The four phases may also be illustrated in a different way: The first phase presents the frame in which the teacher performs. The second phase introduces the teacher to a set of educational "building blocks" and teaches him or her the rules by which these blocks may be interlocked to form constructions. The third phase enables the teacher to use the blocks to construct his own structure within the frame. The fourth phase develops the ability to create frames and to modify them.

A description of the workshops in the program follows. Figure 18.1 summarizes the program and illustrates its multiphasic structure.

## First Phase

The first phase is a 2-day orientation workshop. The participants are 10 to 15 faculty members of varying backgrounds, experience, and seniority from various clinical and scientific disciplines. Most are new to the faculty. The workshop is based on small-group activity. Each group of four to six participants tries to identify health needs and to delineate in rough outlines an ideal medical school that may meet these needs. This imaginary scheme is then confronted with the BGU philosophy, history, structure, and curriculum. Within this framework information is provided on the various facets of the school's life, including open discussions with the dean, senior faculty members, and students. The expected outcome of the workshop is attitudinal change. The teacher discovers that the institutional objectives are not arbitrary and that the curriculum indeed stems from defined objectives and meets real needs. Moreover, the novice teachers discover that many of their own ideas and suggestions are incorporated into the curriculum, and that their further involvement is sincerely welcomed. The educational approach of the school is thus no longer perceived as capricious innovation for its own sake but, rather, as an understandable solution to well defined problems. Participation in this phase is a prerequisite for academic promotion.

## Second Phase

The second phase is an intensive 3-day workshop entitled Basic Instructional Skills. The second phase also hosts a multidisciplinary assemblage of teachers,

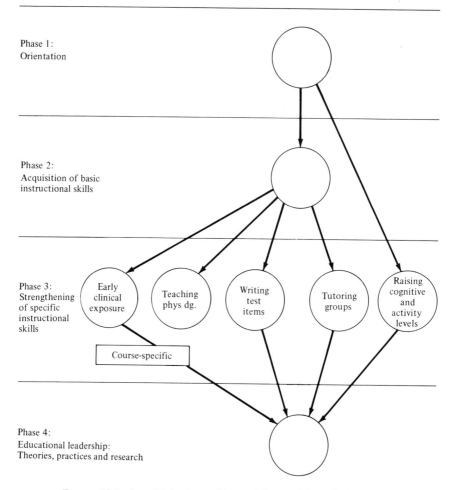

Phase 1:
Orientation

Phase 2:
Acquisition of basic
instructional skills

Phase 3:
Strengthening
of specific
instructional
skills

Early clinical exposure    Teaching phys dg.    Writing test items    Tutoring groups    Raising cognitive and activity levels

Course-specific

Phase 4:
Educational leadership:
Theories, practices and research

FIGURE 18.1. A multiphasic teaching-training model medical school.

working in small groups. The workshop is modularly structured. Each module includes a written or audiovisual simulation related to a single concept. It triggers small-group activity in which participants accomplish a structured task and create their own solution to a problem. The group work is followed by a plenary discussion and is summarized by a short lecture. The concepts covered are setting and formulating instructional objectives, selecting appropriate instructional methods, defining subject matter for learning, and selecting appropriate student evaluation procedures. These modules, when organized in sequence, draw a systematic approach to instruction, both on the macro level of curriculum design and on the micro level of the instructional unit.[14]

The module devoted to instructional objectives may illustrate the process. The group starts by roughly delineating a multidisciplinary course of its choice and elaborates on its objectives. The product is presented to the plenary for feedback and is summarized by a short lecture on purpose, use, and formulation of objectives. On this basis, the group then reformulates a given set of improperly stated objectives that are also scrutinized later in the plenary. A discussion on the interplay between objectives, method, subject matter and evaluation summarizes the module. The rephrased objectives serve the group in the following modules for selecting instructional methods and evaluation measures. At the end of the second phase each teacher is expected at least to be able to identify his or her own needs and interests to be addressed in the third phase.

## Third Phase

The third phase offers five workshops of 3 to 4 days each. The first one is entitled High Level Questioning. It aims to improve instructional behavior in two respects: The first is to replace the traditional lecturing modality by a pattern that elicits students' self-initiated verbalization.[20] The second is to both use and stimulate the students to use the highest possible cognitive level in their verbal exchange.[21] The workshop hosts 8 to 10 participants. During the first day they practice intensively the skills of identifying cognitive levels of given questions using Bloom's taxonomy,[22] raising lower levels to higher ones by reformulating given questions and composing new questions on various levels. During the following 3 days, each participant presents each day a 15-minute lesson to his peers. The teachers are encouraged to use the same content area and the same method they use in their real-life teaching. Upon termination of the presentation, the group provides feedback to the presenter, specifically relating to his or her success in stimulating student discussion by proper questioning. Following this period the presenter leaves the group for 30 minutes of private review of his videotaped performance with an educationalist. On the last day, all three daily performances are reviewed, enabling the teacher to evaluate his progress. This microteaching technique has long been adopted and proved effective in teacher training in general education.[23]

The second workshop in this phase prepares tutors for self-learning problem-based instruction.[24] The expected behavior of a tutor requires a major departure from the traditional teaching patterns. Unlike a teacher, the tutor is neither the source of information nor the leader of the learners.[25] This situation is threatening to many teachers and requires aggressive behavior modification training methods in order to achieve behavioral change in 3 days. For this purpose, both group dynamics and microteaching techniques are used. The 8 to 10 participants, representing varying disciplines, act out in turn all of the following roles: a learner in a group, solving an unknown problem taken from other than his own discipline; a tutor to the peer group that learns a problem; a member in the group that provides feedback to the acting tutor on his performance immediately after the learning session; a moderator of the peer group that provides this feedback, both directing the discussion and protecting the feelings of the acting tutor; and, finally, a personal instructor to the acting tutor, either in private or in front of the group, helping him to gain insight into his performance. Each participant also has an opportunity to discuss his own performance in private with an educationalist while reviewing the videotaped tutorial. It may be noted that the workshop oscillates between "here and now" and "there and then," as well as between the processes of learning new subject matter, learning how to tutor, and training another tutor. This multiple folding considerably increases the vigor of the workshop. It is hoped that the requirement to apply the nondirective, nonimposing mode of instruction to so many situations increases the transferability of the newly acquired skill to real-life educational activities.

The third workshop offered during the third phase develops the skill of writing test items. This 3-day workshop hosts up to 20 teachers, preferably from few disciplines. It is structured in modules, each devoted to a different aspect of evaluation, such as various formats of test items, their cognitive level, and the mental processes that are actually evaluated by the item. Other issues addressed are scoring, item analysis, reliability and validity. Each module includes a short presentation, a group exercise on given material, a plenary discussion, self-composed items, and a summary lecture. Nonconventional evaluation instruments are briefly described, and criteria for selecting a particular instrument are both discussed and practiced.

The third phase also offers a workshop for preceptors instructing first- and second-year students in the early clinical program. This course-specific 4-day workshop is devoted primarily to the teaching of communication skills. The training methods include a number of role-playing sessions followed by group discussions in which the "patient" and the "interviewing student" may reveal their feelings and their expectations from the "preceptor," and the observers may provide objective feedback. Role-playing sessions with real students are interwoven into the workshop. Also, an overview of the entire early clinical program enables each preceptor to regard his or her part in the teaching in a wider context.

Finally, the third phase includes a number of ad hoc miniworkshops of one to two sessions each on specific issues such as teaching physical diagnosis, tutoring students who follow a family, improving communication skills of family practice residents, and others. These miniworkshops are set up in response to an expressed need of a group of teachers. In a sense, those "extracurricular" workshops are "boosters" that reinforce previously acquired skills.

The fourth phase has not yet started and is not discussed here.

## Range of Participation

All workshops are offered several times each year. The attendance is voluntary except for the orientation phase, which is conditional for promotion. Participation is usually self-initiated. However, teachers may be recommended for training by chiefs of services, heads of departments, or course coordinators on the basis of observed need to improve performance. In both cases, the teacher may

TABLE 18.1. Participants in teacher training program.

| | | | | | | | | Participations | | | | |
| | Participants | | | No. of workshops | | | | 1st | 2nd | 3rd | Total | |
| Discipline | Senior | Intermed. | Junior | 1 | 2 | 3 | 4 | Phase | Phase | Phase | Members | Times |
|---|---|---|---|---|---|---|---|---|---|---|---|---|
| Internal | | | | | | | | | | | | |
| medicine | 8 | 21 | 18 | 29 | 14 | 3 | 1 | 17 | 9 | 45 | 47 | 71 |
| Surgery | 5 | 18 | 31 | 31 | 18 | 3 | 2 | 25 | 20 | 39 | 54 | 84 |
| Pediatrics | 2 | 13 | 22 | 32 | 4 | 1 | | 15 | 8 | 20 | 37 | 43 |
| Ob-gyn | | 3 | 17 | 15 | 4 | 1 | | 9 | 7 | 10 | 20 | 26 |
| Psychiatry | 1 | 4 | 21 | 18 | 5 | 3 | | 15 | 15 | 7 | 26 | 37 |
| Family | | | | | | | | | | | | |
| medicine | 2 | 7 | 15 | 11 | 7 | 1 | 5 | 4 | 10 | 35 | 24 | 49 |
| Basic | | | | | | | | | | | | |
| sciences | 4 | 16 | 24 | 17 | 16 | 7 | 4 | 22 | 23 | 42 | 44 | 87 |
| Others | 6 | 11 | 35 | 35 | 15 | 1 | 1 | 15 | 13 | 45 | 52 | 73 |
| Total | 28 | 93 | 183 | 188 | 83 | 20 | 13 | 122 | 105 | 243 | 304 | 470 |

take part in a workshop only if his or her service obligations permit it. In spite of this restriction, 304 faculty members have taken part 470 times in workshops during the 5 academic years between 1980 and 1985. This figure constitutes 62% of the 490 scientists, physicians, and allied professionals who held faculty appointments at any time during this period.

Table 18.1 presents the background of the participants and the attended phases. It reveals a high participation rate in disciplines that are not traditionally found in the front line of medical education. BGU philosophy perhaps accounts for the high involvement of allied professionals (included in Table 18.1 under "Others") and family practitioners. It does not explain, however, the frequent participation of basic science teachers and surgeons. Furthermore, the data indicate higher participation in the voluntary third phase than in the obligatory first one. This phenomenon may indicate a real need, keen interest, and the good reputation of the program.

Table 18.1 shows a small group of teachers who completed all phases of training. They form the nucleus of the future educational leadership of the Health Science Faculty. The fourth phase of the program, mentioned earlier, will begin when their number reaches a "critical mass," hopefully in the near future.

## Evaluation of Training

The earlier mentioned lack of systematic, quantitative assessment of the effectiveness of teacher training programs is caused by several factors. The most important of these is the lack of clear objectives for the training, which stems from lack of criteria for good teaching.[26] Still another hindrance is the large number of confounding variables that arise during a longitudinal follow-up of training, e.g., changes in the teachers' status and seniority or in the curriculum, instructional methods, class size, and the like. Nevertheless, three major evaluation approaches are utilized. It may be noted that these evaluations are in addition to the participants' end-of-workshop questionnaires, which invariably reflect a high degree of satisfaction and can hardly be considered an evaluation. The first approach is a pre/post testing, usually written, before and immediately after the training, sometimes followed by a retest after a period of time.[26,27] Such evaluation may reveal only the cognitive component of the training. It does not disclose actual teacher behavior and says little about his or her attitudes. Pre/post testing is thus used at BGU for training rather than for evaluation purposes, and therefore it is anonymous.

The second approach to evaluation of training is based on students' questionnaires relating to posttraining teacher performance.[28] The strength of this approach is that it relates directly to performance, yet it may bear a price in the teacher–student relationship. It was also shown in BGU that internalization and implementation of nondirective tutoring or questioning skills taught in the workshops sometimes received negative response from students who were not prepared for the abrupt change in the instructional method.[29]

The third approach to evaluating the outcomes of teacher training utilizes direct observations of performance, either live or videotaped.[26,27,30] Different authors, however, recommend different criteria for the observations. The teachers' behavior, which was monitored at BGU for assessment of training, relates to some of the objectives of the training specified earlier, i.e., activation of students and raising the cognitive level of the lesson. The method of observation is described in detail elsewhere.[31,32] It included monitoring of the lesson time spent by teachers' talk compared to the time students spoke and the kind of verbalization (self-initiated, responses to questions, asking questions), as well as its cognitive level. The combination of these parameters indicates the extent of problem-solving activity in the class in contrast to passive acceptance of factual knowledge. The shift in teachers' behavior following the training reflects the achievement of its goals.

The results of such repeated observations on 60 teachers for 500 days reveal a significant change in teachers' performance. The data, which are presented elsewhere,[31,32] show that the activation of students significantly increased and was sustained at the new, high level for the entire 2 academic years of observations, indicating establishment of a new instructional pattern. The cognitive level was also significantly raised, but the new level was maintained for only one year, indicating a need for reinforcement at this time.

The authors suggest an additional, nonconventional approach to assessment of teacher training. It is based on the changes in teachers' educational responsibilities following the training. For this purpose, a role of "educational leader" has been defined by meeting any two of the following three criteria: (1) The teacher is also a coordinator of a major course, providing guidance to a number of other teachers. (2) The teacher has developed an educational innovation that may be an instructional method, evaluation instrument, integrative course, etc. (3) The teacher assumes an active role in and contributes to one of the educational decision-making committees or task forces. This approach thus relates to the outcome of training on an institutional rather than an individual level.

TABLE 18.2. Educational leaders "discovered" in the teacher training workshops.

| Discipline | Position of Educational Leader | | | "Discovered" in workshops | |
|---|---|---|---|---|---|
| | Total | Excluding founders | "Discovered" in workshops | % of total | % of new |
| Internal medicine | 31 | 22 | 6 | 19.4 | 27.3 |
| Surgery | 17 | 13 | 3 | 17.6 | 23.1 |
| Pediatrics | 15 | 13 | 1 | 6.7 | 7.7 |
| Ob-gyn | 7 | 6 | 1 | 14.3 | 16.7 |
| Psychiatry | 7 | 3 | 1 | 14.3 | 33.3 |
| Family medicine | 13 | 10 | 6 | 46.2 | 60.0 |
| Basic sciences | 26 | 10 | 2 | 7.7 | 20.0 |
| Others | 12 | 6 | 1 | 8.3 | 16.7 |
| Total | 128 | 83 | 21 | 16.4 | 25.3 |

Using these criteria, 128 educational leaders were identified during the screened period of 1980 to 1985. Thirty of the 128 assumed their roles during the early, formative years of the school and were defined as the "founding fathers". Fifteen additional teachers were hired specifically for educational tasks, which means that they possessed leadership qualities before joining the faculty. Of the remaining 83, 25.3% (21 teachers) undertook their educational responsibilities shortly after the training. It may be said that they were "discovered" in the workshops. Table 18.2 summarizes the faculty development aspect of teacher training at BGU.

It is not suggested that the training allots leadership qualities to individuals. It is more probable that existing creativity, instructional competencies, and administrative abilities were channeled to educational avenues by the training. Such "discovered" educational leaders were drawn mostly from junior and intermediate ranking staff rather than senior members, suggesting that perhaps junior teachers, including residents, are underestimated in medical education.

## Summary and Conclusions

Many components of the described teacher training program are implemented elsewhere.[2,4,10,19,25] However, two features of the BGU program, when combined, make it unique. One is the timewise hierarchical structure that enables gradual acquisition of instructional skills, progressing from generic to specific[16] and from curricular generalities to particulars of a course and of a lesson. The teacher himself determines the pacing. Opportunities to implement already acquired skills precede the development of additional ones. Moreover, the program acknowledges individual differences and thus offers a variety of themes and training methods to fit personal needs and expectations.

The second feature is the emphasis placed all along the program on the motivational aspects. Indeed, the term "training" becomes alien to the program. Its very essence is to create personal involvement of every trainee on both emotional and practical levels. The individual is guided to become a member in a multidisciplinary team, working together toward an understandable and worthwhile cause. The involvement of the teachers is encouraged and welcomed. When this feeling is combined with the revelation of the educational discipline, a feeling of belonging to both the institution and to the teaching profession arises. Such feelings might well be a prerequisite for any educational innovation.[11] The high proportion of educational leaders who emerged from the program illustrates these two features. Personal growth and institutional development are intertwined.

The BGU training program has been rigorously evaluated and has proved to be effective. However, continuous assessment must be instituted and maintained. Such formative evaluation may also meet the requirement of ongoing on-the-job reinforcement.[26] Nevertheless, BGU cannot yet afford further expansion of the program. It must wait for the graduation of the fourth phase trainees.

Overall, we believe that a responsive teacher training program in medical education should comprise a two-dimensional matrix. One dimension is a time-wise hierarchical structure that enables gradual acquisition of instructional skills. The second dimension is that of mental domains and includes acquisition of conceptual and specific knowledge, opportunities to practice skills, and the establishment of motivation and positive attitudes. Gradual development in each domain is recommended; yet all three must be considered in each phase along the first dimension. Both personal growth and faculty development depend on the careful adjustment of the two dimensions and on their continuity. One may apply in this context the analysis of curriculum orientation in general to the teacher training curriculum. Eisner stated[33]: "Virtually all curricula will reflect different degrees of each of the orientations . . . as a development of cognitive processes, as a technology, as self-actualization, for social reconstruction and relevance, and as academic rationalism."

Nevertheless, it may be concluded that research data on the effectiveness of various training programs are urgently needed to ameliorate the present status of medical education.

## References

1. Cooper JM, Weber WA, Johnson CE: A system approach to program design, in: Competency Based Teacher Education (2). Berkeley, CA, McCutchan, 1973.
2. Schaefer R: Teacher education in the United States, in Yates A (ed): Current Problems of Teacher Education, Hamburg, UNESCO, 1970.
3. Guilbert JJ: Educational Handbook for Health Personnel. Geneva, WHO, 1977.
4. Bland CJ: Faculty Development Through Workshops. Springfield, IL, Charles C Thomas, 1980.
5. Greenberg LW, Goldberg RM, Jewett LS: Teaching in the clinical setting: factors influencing residents' perceptions, confidence and behavior. Med Educ 1984;18:360–365.
6. Maddison DC: What's wrong with medical education? Med Educ 1978;12:97–106.
7. Abrahamson S: Diseases of the curriculum. J Med Educ 1978;53:951–957.
8. Sarason SB: The Culture of the School and the Problem of Change. Boston, Allyn & Bacon, 1971.

9. House ER: The Politics of Educational Innovations. Berkeley, CA, McCutchan, 1974.
10. Bazuin CH, Yonke AM: Improvement of teaching skills in a clinical setting. J Med Educ 1978;53:377–382.
11. Shulmann LS: Research on teaching: the missing link in curriculum implementation, in Tamir P, Bloom A, Hofstein A, Sabar N (eds): Curriculum Implementation and Its Relationship to Curriculum Development in Science. Jerusalem, Hebrew University, 1979.
12. Rogers CR: Freedom to Learn. Columbus, Ohio, Merrill, 1969.
13. Bruner JS: The Process of Education: Cambridge, Harvard University Press, 1960.
14. Segall AJ, Vanderschmidt H, Burglass R, Frostman T: Systematic Course Design. New York, Wiley, 1975.
15. Barrows HS: Problem-Based Learning in Medicine: Rationale and Methods. Educational Monograph 4. Hamilton, Ontario, McMaster University, 1973.
16. Segall AJ: Generic and specific competence in medical education and health care. Med Educ 1980;14(suppl):19–22.
17. Fullan M, Pomfret A: Research on curriculum and instruction implementation. Rev Educ Res 1977;49:335–397.
18. Engel GL: The need for a new medical model: a challenge for biomedicine. Science 1977;196:129–136.
19. Cole CC Jr: Improving Instruction: Issues and Alternatives for Higher Education. American Association of Higher Education, 1982.
20. Flanders NA: Analyzing Teacher Behavior. Reading, MA, Addison-Wesley, 1970.
21. Hunkins PP: Questioning Strategies and Techniques. Boston, Allyn & Bacon, 1972.
22. Bloom BS, et al: Taxonomy of Educational Objectives. New York, McKay, 1956.
23. Allen DW, Ryan K: Microteaching. Palo Alto, Addison-Wesley, 1969.
24. Schmidt HG: Introduction, in Schmidt HG, De Volder ML (eds): Tutorials in Problem-Based Learning. Assen, Van Gorcum, 1984.
25. Barrows HS, Tamblyn R, Jenkins M: Preparing faculty for innovative educational roles. J Med Educ 1976;51:592–594.
26. Rezler AG: Suggested Scheme of Evaluation for Health Personnel Teacher-Training Programmes. Document HMD 73.41. Geneva, WHO, 1973.
27. Sheets KJ, Henry RC: Assessing the impact of faulty development programs in medical education. J Med Educ 1984;59:746–748.
28. Calkins EV, Wakeford R: Perception of instructors and students of instructors' role. J Med Educ 1983;58:967–969.
29. Mahler S: Raising cognitive level of medical school teaching. Doctoral dissertation. Jerusalem, Hebrew University, 1983 [Hebrew].
30. Gall MD, Dunning B, Weathersby R: Higher Cognitive Questioning: Minicourse 9. New York, McMillan Educational Service, 1967.
31. Mahler S, Benor DE: Changes in the rhythm of lessons following a teacher-training workshop in medical education, in Tamir P, Hofstein A, Ben-Peretz M (eds): Pre-service and Inservice Training of Science Teachers. Philadelphia, Balaban International Scientific Services, 1983.
32. Mahler S, Benor DE: Short and long term effects of a teacher-training workshop in medical school. Higher Educ 1984;13:265–273.
33. Eisner EW: Applying the five curricular orientations to man: a course of study, in Eisner EW, Vallance E (eds): Conflicting Conceptions of Curriculum. Berkeley, CA. McCutchan, 1974.

# 19
# Preparing Faculty and Students for Problem-based Learning

JOS H.C. MOUST and HENK G. SCHMIDT

The literature of faculty development pays a great deal of attention to the preparation and training of teachers[1,2] for educational innovation. Less attention, however, is given to the preparation of students, even though both parties involved in the teaching–learning process play an important role in the implementation of new instructional methods.

Dutch universities do not require special qualifications in teaching for the new academic staff entering their faculties. Many faculty members have a rather naive approach to teaching based on their own experiences as a student. Therefore in-service teacher training programs may play an important role in preparing faculty members for the various teaching activities they must perform.

In Dutch medical schools in-service teacher training has a short history. Only since the mid-1960s did a number of Dutch medical faculties create small units for faculty development. Preparation of students for how they can benefit most from what is taught is even more lacking. Some universities have a small center in which students can voluntarily take a study-skills course, but that is all there is. When in 1974 the pioneers of the Faculty of Medicine, University of Limburg, Maastricht, started a problem-based, student-centered medical school, they were confronted with the problem of hiring staff and enrolling students, all of whom lacked basic skills in this new approach.

At the same time, however, these pioneers believed that preparing staff members and students for this new instructional approach was important for the success of this innovation in medical education. During the initial years, when the number of faculty members and students was small, preparation took place on an informal basis. Colleagues informed each other about how they used the various possibilities inherent in problem-based learning. Students underwent a short training program in group dynamics organized by behavioral scientists.

As the number of faculty members and students increased, the preparation of newcomers needed a more structured strategy. A faculty development group was founded to prepare staff and students for the skills necessary for adequate performance in problem-based learning.

In this chapter we describe how students and faculty are prepared for problem-based learning. The preparation of students focuses on the first block period in the first curriculum year. Faculty members are trained in small groups shortly after they join the medical school. Two workshops are obligatory for all those who participate in the education program.

## Training of Students

When students enroll in the medical school they are usually unaware of the possibilities and difficulties of small-group learning as a viable alternative to conventional instruction. Secondary education in The Netherlands can be characterized as highly teacher-centered. Teachers lecture in their own area of competence and do not bother too much with what their colleagues are doing. They direct the learning activities of students to a great extent. They decide on what should be studied and in what way, and leave little room for student initiative. Students being trained in such an educational atmosphere are extremely dependent on their teachers. They come to behave competitively and defensively. Consequently, as these students enter the Maastricht problem-based curriculum, unacquainted with small-group instruction, they are unable to use each other as learning resources. They are unaware of problem-solving strategies. They can hardly plan their own study independent of the directives of a teacher. They are only poorly able to take responsibility for their own learning. In general, they need no less than 6 months to adapt to a learning environment that is alien to their previous experiences.

To support these men and women in their process of adjustment, we offer them a special training program during the first 6 weeks (called a "block") of the first curriculum year. Twelve weeks later a follow-up week emphasizes reflection on the students' actual experiences in the new curriculum. Table 19.1 outlines the first curriculum year.

In order to be able to describe the contents of this training program in some detail, a few general remarks must be made about the problem-based-learning approach to medical education. Usually medical education attempts to achieve three broad objectives.

1. Students must be enabled to acquire a thorough understanding of biological, psychological, and social processes underlying health and disease.

TABLE 19.1. Curriculum of the first year at Rijksuniversiteit Limburg Medical Faculty.

| Block | Topic | Duration (weeks) |
|---|---|---|
| 1 | Introduction to medical study | 6 |
| 2 | Trauma | 6 |
| 3 | Infection and inflammation | 6 |
| 4 | Psychosomatic disorders | 6 |
| 5 | Atherosclerosis | 6 |
| 6 | Tumors | 6 |

2. They must be enabled to acquire a number of manual, cognitive, and social skills.
3. They have to develop a caring attitude toward ill people.

The problem-based approach to instruction tries to meet these objectives, not by lecturing about them but by confronting medical students with assignments called "problems" or "tasks." Groups of eight or nine students, guided by a tutor, "discuss" or "analyze" these problems based on prior knowledge and common sense. This analysis produces a set of learning objectives that are pursued by individual self-directed learning activities. To that end, students screen available handbooks, audiovisual aids, or other learning resources. Subsequently, the knowledge acquired is compared, synthesized, and tested at a follow-up meeting of the group.[3]

In order to fulfill the three objectives stated above, assignments of different types are used. "Explanation tasks" or problems are used as a stimulus for the acquisition of relevant knowledge. Case histories, role playing, and field assignments give students opportunities to learn and practice various cognitive and social skills. For manual skills a skills "laboratory" is available. "Discussion tasks" lend themselves for reflection on attitudes and emotions related to health care. Appendix 1 shows three types of assignments and several examples. Each of these problem types requires its own kind of systematic working procedure, which must be learned by students. As well, students must acquire cooperation skills, e.g., chairing a discussion, explaining difficult concepts, asking clarifying questions, listening to other contributors, summarizing, evaluating a discussion.

## Structure of the Training Program

Learning how to analyze tasks and how to cooperate are closely interwoven during the training. Analyzing the tasks presented, students discover in a natural way which discussion skills are most important. On regular occasions, each group looks back at its own functioning, and shortcomings are diagnosed and remedied. If necessary, special exercises focusing on important discussion skills (e.g., summarizing) are interjected.[4-6] Each week a different type of task is emphasized. The same applies to the training of communication skills. The last 2 weeks of the first block are devoted to a medically relevant theme, influenza. This portion of the block consists in a set of 12 assignments of various types, where the students can integrate and apply the task-analysis and communication skills learned during the weeks before. Table 19.2 outlines the training program in detail.

After 12 weeks there is a second period of training and discussion. During this week of reflection, the following questions are emphasized: To what extent have your skills developed since the introductory training? What problems did you encounter? What do you see as advantages and disadvantages of problem-based, self-directed learning?

Program evaluation indicates that nearly all students (90%) are satisfied with the training approach outlined above. They report that they now are able to distin-

TABLE 19.2. Design of introductory student training.

| Week | Topic | Type of task emphasized | Type of skill emphasized |
|---|---|---|---|
| 1 | Doctor and society | Discussion-task | Summarizing Explaining |
| 2 | Doctor and knowledge | Problems | Brainstorming Asking questions |
| 3 | Doctor and professional practice | Case histories Role play Field experiences | Decision-making Chairing Evaluating Discussing |
| 4/5 | Influenza | All types of tasks | All skills |

guish between different types of assignment and have learned to pursue each type in a systematic fashion. Seventy to eighty percent of the students indicate that they have acquired an understanding of how one could and should cooperate as a tutorial group. However, 62% of the students thought that their acquisition of communication skills needed more practice and further training.

## Preparation of Faculty Members

Up to now teachers working in tertiary education in The Netherlands have not been expected to have had any formal educational training. Many of the new faculty members entering Maastricht Medical Faculty hold idiosyncratic ideas about education in general and about problem-based earning in particular. These prospective teachers were themselves mostly trained in traditional medical schools and were acquainted only with lecture-type instruction. Many have a general approach to teaching derived from rather uncritical modeling of their own teachers.

Entering a medical school where instruction is organized according to the concept of problem-based learning asks for drastic changes in the practice of newcomers with respect to the teaching–learning process, the framework of the curriculum, and the teacher's role. In this educational setting they lose a great deal of autonomy. They have less control over students and their learning. The traditional view that teaching must be in the hands of one teacher is abandoned. The preparation of block books is done by multidisciplinary teams, and the tutorial groups are guided by other staff. Responsibility for the assessment of students' academic progress rests with yet another group of faculty. Also the faculties' relationship with students changes drastically. Because one of the objectives of problem-based learning is to develop a self-directed, self-responsible attitude among students, teachers are not expected to direct and control students over and over again with respect to what and how they have to study. Their task is to facilitate the learning process, not direct it.

Newcomers are not always convinced of the advantages problem-based learning may have for the professional training of medical students. Starting from their own superficial but nevertheless pertinent ideas about teaching, they resist this teaching approach. Misconceptions and concerns come up easily. In order to introduce these faculty members to their new work setting, the faculty development group organizes a workshop several times a year to provide a general overview on principles underlying problem-based learning. In these workshops teachers acquire insight into the different roles teachers are asked to perform. In addition to an introductory workshop they participate in a tutor training in order to get better insight and skills with respect to facilitating and stimulating student learning.

## Framework of Teacher Training

The workshop "Introduction to Problem-Based Learning" is offered four times a year. It lasts 2 days and is obligatory for every faculty member who wishes to play a role in the curriculum. The workshop is set up according to the ideas that are characteristic for problem-based learning: learning in small groups, active participation by group members, and a high degree of self-directedness. The goal of the workshop is threefold.

1. To make new faculty members familiar with educational concepts relevant to problem-based learning
2. To provide insight into the various teaching roles they may fulfill, e.g., that of a tutor, member of a planning group, developer of teacher-independent learning resources, assessor
3. To discuss problems the faculty encounters in implementing the educational philosophy and to invite them to participate in attempts to improve the approach

The participants of the workshop engage in four learning activities: simulations, small discussion groups, short lectures, and live or videotaped demonstrations. For the design of this workshop, see Appendix 2.

The second part of the new faculty training, which is also obligatory, is a 2-day experience in tutoring. This training is also offered four times a year, approximately 3 weeks after each introductory workshop. A small group of nine participants work with a semistructured program. The goal of this training is twofold: to experience personally the impact problem-based learning can have on learning and to learn the basic skills every tutor has to acquire. Participants work on the same tasks with which students are confronted. Sometimes tasks from neighboring Maastricht faculties, e.g., The Faculty of Law, are used, to put the trainee more realistically in the position of a beginning student. Attention is given to the ways in which students can discuss different types of assignment; the aptitudes of group members and discussion leaders; and the skills of the tutor: posing stimulating questions, evaluating a group session, giving feedback to individual students, facilitating the development of the group.

TABLE 19.3. Number of staff participating in faculty development workshops since 1984.

| Year | Introductory workshop | Tutor training |
|------|-----------------------|----------------|
| 1984 | 37 | 62 |
| 1985 | 48 | 59 |
| 1986 | 55 | 65 |
| 1987 | 56 | 47 |
| 1988 | 67 | 93 |
| Total | 263 | 326 |

Each participant takes the role of discussion leader and tutor several times. After each exercise, coparticipants and trainer—the latter being an experienced tutor—provide feedback. Videotapes, handouts, and a handbook specifically written for this purpose[7] provide the necessary background information. The design of this training is shown in Appendix 3.

Faculty members who want to learn more about how to teach adequately in problem-based learning can voluntarily participate in other workshops organized by the faculty development project group. Among those available are "Developing Teacher-Independent Video Materials," a small course for "Study Supervisors," and a workshop "Manufacturing Assignments for Block Books."

Table 19.3 shows how many participants have attended faculty development programs since 1984.

Program evaluation of the workshops "Introduction to Problem-Based Learning" and "Tutor Training" indicates that nearly all participants are satisfied with the way they were introduced to problem-based learning. They believe that they now have a better understanding of the basic ideas underlying this teacher-learning approach, and that they are able to perform as a tutor.

The fact that both programs are obligatory has a great influence on the percentage of participation. Of course, this figure masks the percentage of faculty who are really interested. Hence it is quite surprising that so many participants report that they have become convinced of the possibilities problem-based learning offers for the education of students. In their remarks trainees often write that their initial options have changed, and that even though they have some objections they now are really able to judge the consequences of this instructional method for students and teachers. Faculty members also feel more secure in their tutor role. Changing long-vested ideas about education is not simple. Workshops in which the participants come to know the value of a certain instructional approach for the intellectual development of students can be a first step. The main factor influencing the success or failure of educational innovation, however, is the educational climate. Faculty and students should encourage each other to become more informed and intrinsically interested teachers and learners.

# Appendix 1

*Type of task*

*Problem*: A neutral description of a number of phenomena or events between which there seems to be a certain relation. The students are asked to find explanations for the underlying biological, physiological, and chemical processes or principles, in order to explain the problem.

*Example*

*Sweating*: It is a hot day in August. You are exhausting yourself on the lawn-tennis court in an attempt to be selected by your club for a provincial game. After you have lost from the number 8 player of your club in three sets (4-6,4-6,0-6), you are going to take a shower; your face has turned a deep red, moisture is exuded through every pore, and the muscles of your arms and legs are shaking.

*Dizziness*: You are roaming about an amusement park one evening. You sit in the giant wheel, the octagonal roller-coaster, and the bumping cars, meanwhile eating a spun-sugar candy, a sour-sweet stick, and a few nougat bars. You have tried several times to win a watch in an angling game. By eleven o'clock you are spending your last dollar on a merry-go-round. When you leave this you are dizzy; it seems as if the whole world is whirling around you. You feel a little sick and decide to go home.

*Patient problem*: A neutral description of a case in which a patient has complaints and visits a doctor. Students are asked to imagine, cognitively, what has happened and how (and why) they would handle such a situation. To make the situation more realistic, teachers can design, when possible, a role play.

*Little Eveline*: A girl of 4, who has been listless for a few days and has a cold (runny nose, dry cough), is now becoming really ill and has a fever of 39.2 °C. Her mother first gives her a child's aspirin. However, seeing that the temperature hardly falls, she decides to call the family doctor. The latter thinks that the girl definitely looks ill. The eyes are inflamed. Auscultation of the lungs does not reveal any distinct abnormalities. In her mouth he finds tiny, white spots surrounded by a reddish zone on the mucous membrane. The next day the physician pays her another visit. The girls appears to have meanwhile developed an exanthem: small, dark-red spots behind the ears, on the forehead, and on the chest. Four days later the exanthematous eruption has largely disappeared, and she no longer feels ill.

When you have studied the case and have formed an idea of the possible pathological processes that may be the source of the symptoms here described, you may jointly determine what you would do as a physician during the first and the second visits (on the basis of the knowledge you have so far acquired).

*Discussion task*: A more or less neutral description of a situation in which a doctor can become involved and in which personal values play a role in the way he handles it.

*Blood transfusion for a child of Jehova's witnesses*: A child is admitted to the emergency room of a hospital. She has been knocked down by a motorcar and has lost a substantial amount of blood. The only way to save the child's life in the judgment of the attending physician is a transfusion. However, there is a problem, i.e., that the parents are not likely to give their consent because their creed forbids transmission to their child's body of another person's blood. Should transfusion be given, the parents would repudiate the child.

*Medical examination of the population*: In 1985 the government decides that every 5 years complete physical screening is to take place of all people aged 25 and over. The following methods of diagnosis are to be used: complete physical examination, urinalysis (tests for albumin and glucose), complete blood test (hemoglobin, erythrocyte sedimentation rate, hepatic and renal function tests, glucose), thorax x-ray film, blood smear for cervical carcinoma.
    Are you for or against this examination?

# Appendix 2. Workshop. Introduction to Problem-based Learning

| | Time | Activity | Brief description | Instructional method |
|---|---|---|---|---|
| **First day** | | | | |
| AM | 9:00 | Introduction: goals, working method, acquaintance | | |
| | 9:30 | Some basic concepts of PBL | Background information | Discussion* |
| | 10:30 | Tutorial group | First acquaintance with the tutorial group, role of the tutor | Observation |
| | | | | Discussion |
| | 11:30 | Participation in your own tutorial group | Experience it personally | Simulation |
| | | | | Discussion |
| PM | 13:00 | Lunch | | |
| | 14:00 | Role of teacher-independent learning resources in PBL | | Lecture |
| | | | | Discussion |
| | 15:00 | Visit to the skills laboratory | Simulation: patient contact | Simulations |
| | | | Social skills | Discussions |
| | | | Diagnostic skills | |
| | 17:30 | Wrap-up | | |
| **Second day** | | | | |
| AM | 9:00 | Development of a block book | Distinguishing different types of tasks | Simulations |
| | | | Writing different types of tasks | Discussions |
| | | | Development of problems in a multidisciplinary curriculum | |
| | 12:30 | Lunch | | |
| | 13:30 | Summative assessment: progress test | Development of these tests | Lecture |
| | | Summative and formative assessment: block test | Problems, experiences | Discussion |
| | | | | Simulation |
| | 16:00 | Program evaluation | Student evaluation of the curriculum, teachers, tutorial groups | Lecture |
| | | | | Discussion |
| | 17:00 | Evaluation of workshop | | Verbal and written feedback |
| | 17:30 | Conclusion | | |

PBL = problem-based learning.
**Participants receive written information at home before the workshop starts.

# Appendix 3. Tutor Training*

| | Time | Activity | Brief description | Instructional method |
|---|---|---|---|---|
| **First day** | | | | |
| AM | 9:00 | Introduction: goals, working method, getting acquainted | | |
| | 9:30 | Role of a tutor in PBL: three opinions | Three styles how a tutor can (non) facilitate group learning | Videotape Discussion |
| | 10:15 | Leading a discussion group | Role of the chairman Summarizing | Simulation exercises |
| | | | Task and socioemotional aspects in a study group | Videotape feedback |
| PM | 12:30 | Lunch | | |
| | 13:30 | Role of the tutor | Analyzing different types of tasks: "seven-jump" | Simulations |
| | | | Facilitating learning: posing and simulating questions | Discussions Videotape feedback |
| | 17:00 | Wrap-up | | |
| **Second day** | | | | |
| AM | 9:00 | Role of the tutor | Other methods to analyze different types of tasks | Videotape feedback |
| | | | Group processes | |
| PM | 12:30 | Lunch | | |
| | 13:30 | Role of the tutor | Evaluating interaction in a tutorial group | Videotape feedback |
| | | | Incidents in groups: how to handle them | |
| | | | Giving and receiving feedback | |
| | 17:00 | Evaluation of the training | | Discussion Evaluation sheet |
| | 17:30 | Conclusion | | |

PBL = problem-based learning.
*Participants receive written background information before and during the training.

## References

1. Bergquist WH, Philips SR. A Handbook for Faculty Development. Volumes 1, 2, 3. Berkeley, California, Pacific Soundings Press, 1970, 1976, 1978.
2. Lindquist J (ed). Designing Teaching Improvement Programs. Washington DC, The Council for the Advancement of Small Colleges, 1979.
3. Schmidt HG. Problem-based learning: rationale and description. Med Educ 1983;17:11–16.
4. Schmuck RA, Runkel PJ, Arends JH, Arends RJ. The Second Handbook of Organisation Development in Schools. Palo Alto, Mayfield Publishing Company, 1977.
5. Sharan S, Hare P, Webb CD, Hertz-Lazarowitz R. Cooperation in Education. Provo, Brigham Young University Press, 1980.
6. Sharan S, Sharan Y. Small Group Teaching. Englewood Cliffs, New Jersey, Prentice Hall, 1975.
7. Schmidt HG, Bouhuijs PAJ. Onderwijs in Taakgerichte Groepen. Utrecht, Spectrum, 1980.

# 20
# Introducing Problem-based Learning into a Conventional Curriculum

David Newble

Much of the work on problem-based learning has been undertaken in the innovative medical schools. The exemplar in this regard has been McMaster University where the work of Barrows and his colleagues has been particularly noteworthy.[1] The "McMaster philosophy" propounds a curriculum centered on problem-based learning as an alternative to the conventional content-based and sequentially structured curriculum.[2] Anyone who has had the opportunity to work in one of the innovative schools would find it difficult not to be convinced that the problem-based approach offers an attractive alternative to the traditional approach, even though it has yet to be proved that the outcome is significantly different.

The problem-based approach has been introduced in a substantial way only in the new medical schools, e.g., the University of Newcastle in Australia, Ben Gurion University in Israel, and the University of Limburg in The Netherlands. There have been few reports on the development of problem-based learning activities suitable for use in most medical schools in the world, which have more conventional curricula and are likely to have them for the foreseeable future.

The University of Adelaide has such a curriculum. This chapter describes how problem-based learning activities have been introduced into the fifth-year medicine/surgery teaching program in order to emphasize decision-making and problem-solving in the areas of clinical diagnosis, laboratory investigation, and management.

## Description

The University of Adelaide has a 6-year curriculum that was extensively revised in 1971 to incorporate a topic teaching program during the early clinical years (late third and fourth years).[3] Although a substantial amount of time was allocated to ward-based instruction during topic teaching, the heavy load of theoretical instruction appeared to be distracting the students from the development of clinical skills, a feature common to many traditional medical schools.[4] A concern for this problem led the Departments of Medicine and Surgery to use the 6-week period allocated to these subjects during the fifth year to provide students with additional training in basic clinical skills. This program has been described in detail elsewhere.[5] Therefore this chapter concentrates on the activities that developed to enhance the students' skills in decision-making and problem-solving.

Students rotate through the medicine/surgery program in groups of 9 to 11. Though the course is predominantly preceptor-based, with three or four students allocated to one staff member, the whole group meets together for a variety of other supporting activities dealing with such issues as emergency care, data interpretation, medical imaging, and medical and surgical decision-making. For all of these sessions a problem-based approach is adopted. The focus here is on two examples, one involving the preceptor and the other the whole group.

The staff of the Departments of Medicine and Surgery were convinced several years ago of the value of the problem-oriented medical record (POMR) as a useful adjunct not only to patient care but also to teaching.[6,7] The POMR can be divided into three main components: the data base, the master problem list, and the problem-oriented progress notes. The data base is recorded in the same way as in the conventional record. The master problem list is used to encourage the student to identify and attempt to categorize all the problems presented by the patient. Each problem is then considered separately using a structure (SOAPE) that forces the student into a problem-solving mode. The student must identify from the data base the key subjective (S) and objective (O) data that are relevant to the solution of each problem. However, it is the next section, the assessment (A), that is crucial. The conventional medical record is notoriously lacking in written assessments. Using the structure of the POMR, we challenge the student to write full assessments that contain not only the possible diagnoses but also the justification for their choice. It is very easy for teachers to identify students who are unable to approach this assessment in a rational manner. Having produced the assessment, the student goes on to write a plan (P) for the management and treatment. The students soon recognize that this stage is relatively easy if they have made a clear problem assessment. The consideration of each problem is completed with a statement about education (E) of the patient.

Records of this type are prepared for the preceptor twice per week. They are assessed by the staff member and discussed in detail with the student. Though no formal evaluation has been undertaken, there is little doubt that the students' skills in clinical problem assessment improve dramatically over the 6 weeks of the course.

The second approach to teaching clinical problem-solving using a problem-based approach is illustrated by the medical decision-making session that is held once per week. This session uses a structured format that utilizes some of the principles developed for patient management problems and modified essay questions. At least a week before the session, one or two students are delegated to prepare the case for discussion. Most frequently they choose a case that they themselves have seen, though it is also perfectly permissable to prepare one from a suitable case record. A protocol is prepared along the lines shown in Figure 20.1. It can be seen that the protocol is divided into several sections. The first

Mr. C.                Aged 36 years:  Admitted to emergency service 22/7:  9.00 p.m.

Presenting illness:

Sudden onset of central chest pain while playing squash previous night.
Pain eased after stopping the game.  Pain was gripping in type and
radiated to both shoulders.  Later, pain became localized in the center
of the chest and persisted until the following morning.  However, he
went to work as usual.  At 6.00 p.m., he went to see his general
practitioner, who referred him to hospital.

Significant past history:                    Family history:

Pulmonary embolism 5 years ago               Father alive, 77 years, mild diabetes.
following surgery.                           Mother alive, 76 years, well.
                                             No family members with heart disease.

Examination findings:

Fit-looking young man in no distress.
Pulse 120, regular.  B.P. 135/80.
Heart sounds normal.  No signs of cardiac failure.
Left calf:  37 cm.  Right calf:  35 cm.

Initial investigations:    ECG
                           CXR

Admitted to Coronary Care Unit:  10.30 p.m.

Further investigations:

                Cardiac enzyme studies
                PTTK and TCT (baseline)

Management:

                Monitor
                Heparinize

Seen by consultant 9.00 a.m. 23/7  ECG thought to be within normal limits.

Consultant's plan:

Keep in CCU until enzyme studies available.
Organize lung scan.
Exercise ECG if these normal.

Results (11.30 a.m.):

                CPK 426  (N20 - 110)
                AAT 130 (N  0 -  50)
                LDH 395 (110 - 250)

Assessment:

Myocardial infarct most likely, but not certain.

Consultant's plan:                    Results 24/7:

Defer lung scan.                      Scan suggests small anterior
Organize cardiac scan.                infarction.

FIGURE 20.1. Decision-making session protocol.

contains the presenting data, the information available to the doctor who first saw the patient on arrival in the hospital. At this time some decisions must be made about diagnosis and initial investigations, so a line is drawn across the page and identified as decision point 1. During the whole group session, the students are asked to fold the protocol so that they can read only the information up to this first decision point. The group discusses what decisions they would have made. Once consensus is reached, the next section is revealed. A brief discussion ensues on any differences between the group's decisions and the actual decisions that were made. The process is then repeated at each identified decision point in the patient's management.

Interactive discussion of this type poses problems for some students brought up in a conventional curriculum in which small-group teaching is relatively uncommon. It is particularly so in a session where a rational justification must accompany each contribution. A certain degree of skill is thus required by the tutor to develop a supportive environment. However, once the aims of the exercise are understood, few difficulties arise. Once again, no formal evaluation has been undertaken, but there seems little doubt as to the value of the session in promoting a more critical approach to clinical decision-making.

## Conclusion

Our work has shown that it is possible to introduce problem-based learning activities into a conventional curriculum. It has also been achieved with the support of staff with no particular educational commitment or knowledge of the "cult" of problem-based learning. The fact that the program has been running largely unchanged for more than 10 years, with the continued support of both staff and students, seems to indicate that it is seen as relevant and worthwhile. It also should encourage others in conventional medical schools to introduce similar activities without having to contemplate the need for major curriculum revision.

## References

1. Barrows HS, Tamblyn RM: *Problem-Based Learning: An Approach to Medical Education.* New York, Springer, 1980.
2. Neufield VR, Barrows HS: The "McMaster Philosophy": An Approach to Medical Education. Education Monograph No. 5. Hamilton, Ontario, McMaster University Faculty of Medicine, 1974.
3. Cox LW: New medical course in Adelaide. *Med J Aust* 1971;1:1395–1397.
4. Yonke AM. The art and science of clinical teaching. *Med Educ* 1979;13:86–90.
5. Newble DI: The way we teach basic clinical skills. *Med Teacher* 1982;4:12–15.
6. Weed LL: *Medical Records, Medical Education and Patient Care: The Problem Oriented Record as a Basic Tool.* Cleveland, Case Western Reserve University Press, 1969.
7. Newble DI, Judd SJ, Wangel AG: Quality control of patient care – the practical application of problem oriented medical records. *Aust N Z J Med* 1974;4:23–28.

# Conclusions

Traditional medical schools have been said to emphasize research at the expense of service or teaching. This statement may be true of the balance of prevalent attitudes, a research-and-disease focus is characteristic of faculty views. Medical faculties have deservedly accepted credit for the glories of present-day medicine—the molecular biological revolution, new modes of imaging and diagnosing, and new surgery and drugs. Therefore, faculties must accept their roles in contributing to the presently perceived deficiencies of modern medicine and take part in solving the problems.

The primary criticisms of medicine today are that it is not efficient or equitably distributed. Patients also variously describe alienation from medical practitioners who cannot talk to or with them and hence cannot understand or respond appropriately to the problems patients perceive. In extreme situations such as terminal care or experimental care of untreatable problems, ethical issues and dismaying examples of dehumanization also occur.

More profound—from the intellectual and scholarly viewpoints—are criticisms about the intellectual structure of medical classification of disease and illness and the fact that medicine based on experience in elite referral institutions necessarily biases the learning and approaches of physician-scholars. The result is that patient-care training settings distort the future physicians' expectations. There is an inclination toward extreme cases and dire outcomes and away from an understanding of the common and usual disorders and of health. In this way, medicine fails to train physicians appropriately so that they may become population-based practitioners.

Finally, medical schools are criticized for being inhumane to their students or inefficient with regard to their educational goals. Medical students are often unhappy and have well-documented high rates of serious mental disorder, some of which may be environmentally induced or precipitated, or at least not detected, in the onerous conditions of some programs. Some medical schools attribute the undesirable traits of graduate physicians to their training or acculturation. Not all of this criticism is fair—medicine is not exempt from the ills and errors of mankind. Yet it is thought within the profession that it should be judged by a higher standard than other professions because of its high status and its high stakes in life-and-death issues.

Overall, then, the social, intellectual, and educational criticism suggests that modern medical schools have, in part, failed to produce adequately trained personnel or ones with inappropriate values and intellectual beliefs. Furthermore, modern medical schools have not met community needs nor have they demonstrated sufficient concern for the learning and personal needs of the individual learner. To respond to this line of argument, old and new medical schools are developing innovative educational programs that change the structure of education and alter the place and orientation of its teaching to the population and community. In addition, the argument is based on new theories and new experiments. These efforts are now more than a decade old. Preliminary results and much useful experience have accrued, highlights of which have been presented in this book. In this conclusion, we briefly sketch what we take to be the principal lessons of these cumulative experiences with innovative efforts in medical education.

As the chapters of this volume and their associated references document, problem-based learning and community-oriented medical education have been successfully implemented. Problem-based learning is the better developed in that several schools have adopted it as their primary teaching modality. In addition, faculty development approaches and assessment methods have been created and tested so that it is now possible to adopt problem-based learning without having to start from scratch. However, is it safe to do so, and does it work? Problem-based learning has been documented to work at least as well as traditional approaches. The evaluations seem to suggest that problem-based learning works as well as traditional methods for cognitive learning and retention. Students also seem to be happier during the process. There is, however, no convincing evidence for the claim that students develop better problem-solving skills or that they become more effective lifetime learners. This is partly due to the insufficient time in which to test these claims or the inability to test these matters adequately. At present, traditional educators have not thought these matters through sufficiently to test their students for the final outcome.

It is also evident that problem-based learning is seldom used as the exclusive teaching mode as its proponents assert it might be. Most schools find places for visiting lecturers and symposia in which to use more traditional formats. Lectures, structured laboratories, and canned learning approaches are used even at universities such as McMaster and Maastricht. Ironically, the students at these schools seem to like—and even long for—lectures, normally the bane of students who sit through lectures all day in traditional schools. This does not mean that problem-based learning is simply an equal alternative. The evaluative research findings are clear: problem-based learning produces more satisfied students who do as well or better cognitively on standardized tests.

In contrast, community-oriented medical education is less fully developed and evaluated. The schools at Beer-Sheva, Israel; Ismailia, Egypt; and Gezira, The Sudan for example, are still in the process of making this exciting approach a reality. It is clear that Beer-Sheva has succeeded in interesting more of its graduates in primary care than had been the case for the other schools in Israel. Yet they are now learning that because the rest of the medical establishment (especially the residency training processes and the specialty boards) is traditional, their graduates face a demoralizing experience upon leaving medical school. Thus, for community-oriented medical education to succeed, it may have to have an impact on the entire medical training process and on the boards. Similarly, in Israel, Holland, and elsewhere, the status of primary care is damaged by the scarcity of effectively trained teacher-role models who have intellectual and scholarly status as well as effectiveness as practitioners. Planners must alter this trend with effective faculty if the primary-care career is to become attractive and durable.

It is apparent from the examples described here that it is easier to accomplish these changes when starting a new school than when working in an old one. In such situations, the Dean can choose innovative faculty who are willing to experiment and who do not have as many of the issues of turf, status, and tradition to overcome. However, Harvard's experiment shows that even very traditional settings can move into new formats when there is sufficient drive from the Dean and the President. Already, the New Pathway at Harvard is attracting much attention from other schools in the United States.

In this process of change, the experience of the schools farther along in the process can be extremely useful. To exchange experience is the reason that the Network of Community-oriented Health Care Institutions was developed. As the Appendix shows, there are now about 44 schools in the Network or in Associate status. The complex of committees and the frequent workshops and meetings provide an opportunity to learn about the specifics of the methods and their adoption. The Network also has specific resource materials catalogued and available, including specialized consultants, bibliographies, and the like.

It is an exciting time for medicine. The growth rate of knowledge, the increasing demand and diminished real resources, and the innovations described in this volume come together at a time of intense challenge and opportunity. Along with the technical changes we face—computerization of knowledge systems and availability of new media for instruction—we can see an era of smaller faculties, more innovative and creative students, and superior educational results.

Faculties today face the choice of being part of the solution or part of the problem. It is not an easy choice, but it is one that must be made. We hope that this volume has helped its readers toward a position of improved information and access to sources that help solve the problems facing the medical educator or planner. We also hope that readers will explore the ways in which the experiments described here can be useful. If they do, we will have achieved our goals.

# Appendix A
# The Network

JACOBUS M. GREEP and HENK G. SCHMIDT

The 40 or so medical schools that form the Network of Community-oriented Educational Institutions for Health Sciences are dedicated to the health needs of the populations they serve. They place special emphasis on primary health care in their education, research and health care activities. The Network is an independent organization governed by an Executive Committee chosen by the medical schools, and has its headquarters at the University of Limburg in Maastricht, the Netherlands. Half the schools are in developing countries and the other half in developed countries.

In the 1970s, a growing interest developed in the relationship between educational programs for the health professions and the actual practice of health care. In the developing world, the concern for an optimum use of scarce resources led to a questioning of the traditional approaches to medical education. WHO sponsored an international Network in support of this critical attitude, and encouraged the search for new solutions. In the industrialized world, concern over the rapidly increasing cost of health care triggered off a search for new solutions for the delivery of health care. A close relationship between the universities and the development of health services in the region which they serve seemed to be an important condition of success. The Organization for Economic Cooperation and Development (OECD) convened a series of meetings of all the partners in a series of promising experiments in community-oriented education.

In this way contacts developed between certain Schools of Medicine and Schools of Health Sciences that had several characteristics in common:

- A focus on health problems across the broad spectrum from primary health care (community) to secondary and tertiary health care (institutions), and a focus on factors influencing human health (a population-health perspective);
- Emphasis on *health* research, rather than on a more narrow biomedical approach, so that it includes research concerned with the factors influencing population health and the provision of effective and efficient health care;
- Facilities for educating health care personnel where the health science centers are based, and recognition that those centers should work with the health care services in the region and not be excluded from them;

- Educational programs that are based not only on the institutional care services (hospitals) but also on primary health care settings in the community;
- Flexible curricula with emphasis on health problems in the community, on more effective teaching/learning methods, and on more reliable evaluation procedures.

In 1979, WHO – and, more specifically, members of the Division of Health Manpower Development, Dr. Tamas Fülöp and Dr. Fred Katz – took the initiative in bringing together 20 of these "innovative" schools at a conference in Kingston, Jamaica. They felt that not enough educational institutions provide students with adequate learning experiences of community health care and at the same time prepare their students for lifelong learning, using a problem-solving approach. Those institutions dedicated to providing their students with orientation on community-health care and using teaching/learning methods which are problem-based rather than discipline-centered encounter considerable opposition because their very existence challenges the status quo. At the same time, the experimental nature of the program makes heavy demands on finite resources. Further, they have to prove their worth in contrast to the established institutions and programmes.

So the 1979 meeting explored the possibility of getting those responsible for these programs to provide mutual assistance, in a variety of ways, through the formation of a Network of cooperating institutions. It sought some preliminary answers to the following questions: What are the principal characteristics of the programs? What are the existing constraints and what constraints are likely to arise in the future? What are the possible ways of tackling these obstacles? What collaborative actions could mutually benefit the programme represented? And lastly, what action might be taken to enhance the potential success of other programs with similar objectives?

Two follow-up meetings took place in 1981 in Bellagio, Italy, and in 1983 in Havana, Cuba, to monitor progress. Both were sponsored by WHO and the Rockefeller Foundation.

In 1979, the Network set the following objectives:

- Strengthening of member institutions in their realization of both community orientation and problem-based learning;
- Strengthening of individual faculty capacities related to community-orientation and problem-based learning;
- Development of technologies, approaches, methodologies and tools appropriate to a community-oriented and problem-based educational system;
- Promoting and coordinating the population-based concepts in the health services system and the educational program;
- Assisting institutions in countries that have made a political decision to introduce innovations in the training of health personnel, with the ultimate goal of improving health care and contributing to the commitment to Health for All by the year 2000.

In 1983, additional specifications were thought necessary and were formulated as follows. The Network facilitates the development of education programs which help students to become competent in solving health problems of communities as well as of individuals and family in a community context. Problem-based learning is seen as a powerful educational strategy to maximize students' achievement of relevant knowledge, skills and attitudes. Specific considerations include the following:

- The systematic selection of problem- and population-based concepts which represent health needs of the community. This will require a balanced understanding of scientific technological advances and social systems;
- The definition of relevant skills, including skills in problem-solving, independent learning, critical appraisal of evidence and teamwork;
- The strengthening of teaching staff capacities related to community-orientation and problem-based learning;
- The development of curriculum design methods and learning tools appropriate to a community-oriented and problem-based educational system;
- A system of selecting health professional students, if feasible;
- The design of procedures and tools for assessing student and graduate performance;
- The evaluation of innovative programs including their contribution to the development of effective, efficient and human health care, and the commitment to Health for all.

The Network attempts to establish health research programs that include basic, applied and operational research that is relevant to health and health care problems in the community served. And it attempts to establish the relationships with all the health care services and with health care delivery. This linkage will promote coordination between health services and health manpower development, and will encourage health care systems based on the primary health care approach.

## Community-oriented Education

A good example of community-oriented education is taking place at the University of Ilorin, in mid-Western Nigeria, to which a Faculty of Health Sciences was assigned in 1978. A regular exodus of students and staff into the rural areas takes place twice a year. Small groups of students, each accompanied by two staff-members, settle in a village for a month. Here they study disease patterns in the natural environment, make epidemiological surveys and contribute to the local health care by direct communication with residents. At the end of the 6-year period of study, the students have been exposed to community experiences for almost a year, and are fully sensitized to the primary health needs of the community. They should be capable of seeing diseases in their social, economic and cultural contexts. They should be able to participate actively in efforts made to improve the community's health. And in principle they should have full competence to deliver health care.

The Network considers that learning experiences like this are of the utmost importance for medical students. It forces them to see the real health needs of the population they will be caring for in later years, helps them to perceive individual problems in a social context, sensitizes them to the importance of joint preventive and curative measures, and provides them with the skills necessary to deal with these problems.

Workshops on various topics, information exchanges, bilateral contacts, consultation activities and publications all form part of the Network's activities. The workshops try to practice what the Network preaches. Lectures are avoided; active participation is fostered. A newsletter, sent out twice a year, keeps members informed about workshops, new developments, and the agenda of forthcoming events. A good example of the bilateral contacts that are stimulated and supported is the collaboration between the medical school of the Gezira University in the Sudan and the Suez Canal University Medical Faculty in Egypt. These two innovative schools now jointly run regional workshops for schools in the Arab countries on such topics as small-group tutorials, problem-based learning, and community-oriented education.

Most of the faculties feel that their educational programs stimulate the two concepts of self-learning and self-evaluation. The students are taught how to read scientific articles and how to evaluate their contents critically. Lectures are kept to a minimum as teaching devices and small-group discussions are preferred. There is a continuous mixture of theory and practice, and the students will practice in the community as much as possible.

The students and the faculty and administrative staff—without exception—demonstrate a commitment to the innovative approach. There have been many obstacles but they have overcome most hurdles successfully. Nevertheless, it will be many years before the goal of educating community-oriented physicians, rooted in primary health care, will be achieved all over the world. In many countries, planning for health manpower has no relation to plans for educating physicians and other health professionals. And that should be a matter of great concern.

There are now approximately 40 schools that are members of the Network, and they are scattered throughout all regions of the world, in both developing and developed countries. Some have already graduated several cohorts of students and some are only beginning their activities. There is only space here to name a few of these schools which will serve as examples: Xochimilco (Mexico) and MacMaster (Canada) in the Americas; Ilorin (Nigeria) in Africa; Gezira (Sudan), Ismailia (Egypt) and Beer Sheva (Israel) in the Eastern Mediterranean Region; Maastricht (Holland) in Europe; Newcastle (Australia) and Tacloban (Philippines) in the Western Pacific; and Khon Kaen (Thailand) in the South-East Asia Region.

---

*Used with permission of *World Health*, April 1984, pp 18–21.

# Appendix B
# Network Member Institutions

## Full Members

1. Alausa, Dr. O.K.
   Faculty of Medicine
   Bayero University Kano
   P.M.B. 3011
   Kano
   Nigeria

2. Barrows, Prof. Howard S.
   Assistant Dean for Educational
     Affairs
   School of Medicine
   Southern Illinois University
   P.O. Box 19230
   Springfield, Illinois 62794–93230
   U.S.A.

3. Bjurulf, Dr. Per
   Dean, Faculty of Medicine
   Health University
   581 83 Linköping
   Sweden

4. Boon, Dr. Louis
   Dean, Faculty of Health Sciences
   University of Limburg
   P.O. Box 616
   6200 MD Maastricht
   The Netherlands

5. Bureau, Dr. Michel A.
   Dean, Faculty of Medicine
   University of Sherbrooke
   3001, 12th Avenue, Fleurimont
   Sherbrooke, Quebec
   Canada J1H 5N4

6. Carlevaro, Dr. Pablo V.
   Dean, Facultad de Medicina
   Universidad de la República
   Avda. General Flores 2125
   Montevideo, Uruguay

7. De Benedictis, Dr. Giuseppe
   President, Medical School of
     Bari
   University of Bari
   Policlinico, Department of
     Pathology
   Piazza G. Cesare, 11
   70124 Bari
   Italy

8. Ezzat, Dr. Esmat
   Dean, Faculty of Medicine
   Suez Canal University
   Ismailia
   Egypt

9. Gebert, Dr. Ronald A.
   Dean, Facultad de Medicina
   Universidad de la Frontera
   P.O. Box 54-D
   Temuco
   Chile

10. Glick, Dr. S.
    Dean, Faculty of Health Sciences
    Ben Gurion University of the
       Negev
    P.O. Box 653
    Beer Sheva 84105
    Israel

11. Greer, Dr. David
    Dean, Faculty of Medicine
    Brown University
    97 Waterman Street, Arnold Lab
    Providence, Rhode Island 02912
    U.S.A.

12. Al-Hamer, Dr. Faisal Y.
    Dean, College of Health Sciences
    Ministry of Health
    P.O. Box 12
    Bahrain
    Arabian Gulf

13. Hamilton, Dr. John
    Dean, Faculty of Medicine
    The University of Newcastle
    Rankin Drive
    Newcastle N.S.W. 2308
    Australia

14. Johnson, Dr. Tom M.
    Ass. Dean, College of Human
       Medicine
    Michigan State University
    Office of the Dean
    East Fee Hall
    East Lansing, Michigan
       48824-1316
    U.S.A.

15. Kaufman, Dr. Arthur
    Director Primary Care
       Curriculum
    School of Medicine
    University of New Mexico
    Albuquerque, New Mexico 87131
    U.S.A.

16. Khalidi, Dr. Usama Al
    Acting Dean
    College of Medicine and Medical
       Sciences
    Arabian Gulf University
    P.O. Box 22979
    Manama
    Bahrain

17. Lythcotte, Dr. D.
    Dean, New York Medical School
    The City University of New York
    Convent Ave. and 138th St.
    New York, N.Y. 10031
    U.S.A.

18. Macleod, Dr. Stuart M.
    Dean, Faculty of Health Sciences
    McMaster University
    1200 Main Street West
    Hamilton, Ontario L8N 3Z5
    Canada

19. Martey, Dr. J.O.
    Dean, School of Medical
       Sciences
    University of Science and Tech-
       nology
    University Post Office
    Kumasi
    Ghana, West Africa

20. Mora-Carrasco, Dr. Fernando
    Division Director, Faculty of
       Health Sciences
    Universidad Autónoma
       Metropolitana Xochimilco
    Calz. del Hueso no. 1100, Col.
       Villa Quietud, Del. Coyoacan
    04960 Mexico, D.F.

21. Odesanmi, Dr. W.O.
    Dean, Faculty of Health Sciences
    Obaferni Awolowo University
    Ile-Ife
    Nigeria

22. Ogunbode, Dr. O.
    Dean, Faculty of Health Sciences
    University of Ilorin
    P.M.B. 1515
    Ilorin
    Nigeria

23. Ordonez, Dr. Cosme
    Representative
    Ministry of Public Health
    Higher Institute of Medical
       Sciences
    Ermita 248, esq. a San Pedro
    Havana
    Cuba

24. Owor, Dr. Raphael
    Dean, Faculty of Medicine
    Makerere Unviersity
    P.O. Box 7072
    Kampala
    Uganda

25. Pasternack, Dr. Amos
    Dean, Medical Faculty
    University of Tampere
    Box 607
    33101 Tampere
    Finland

26. Prasai, Dr. Bhishma Raj
    Dean, Institute of Medicine
    Tribhuvan University
    P.O. Box 1524
    Kathmandu
    Nepal

27. Radjiman, Dr.
    Dean, School of Medicine
    Gadjah Mada University—Sekip
    Yogyakarta
    Indonesia

28. Reyes, Dr. Marita V.T.
    Dean, College of Medicine
    University of the Philippines
    547 Pedro Gil St., Ermita
    P.O. Box 593
    Manila
    The Philippines

29. Roslani, Dr. Mohammed
    Dean, School of Medical
       Sciences
    University Sains Malaysia
    Minden, Penang 11800
    Malaysia

30. Salafsky, Dr. B.
    Director, College of Medicine at
       Rockford
    The University of Illinois
    1601 Parkview Avenue
    Rockford, Illinois 61107-1897
    U.S.A.

31. Sanpitak, Dr. Pisit
    Dean, Faculty of Medicine
    Khon Kaen University
    Friendship Highway
    Khon Kaen 40002
    Thailand

32. Skelton, Dr. W. Douglas
    Dean, School of Medicine
    Mercer University
    1400 Coleman Avenue
    Macon, Georgia 31207
    U.S.A.

33. Sturmans, Dr. F.
    Dean, Faculty of Medicine
    University of Limburg
    P.O. Box 616
    6200 MD Maastricht
    The Netherlands

34. Suwanwela, Dr. Charas
    Rector
    Chulalongkorn University
    Bangkok 10500
    Thailand

35. Taha, Dr. Salah
    Dean, School of Medicine
    University of Gezira
    P.O. Box 20
    Wad Medani
    Democratic Republic of the
      Sudan

36. Vasanthakumar, Dr. M. Boosha-
      nam
    Principal, Christian Medical Col-
      lege
    Vellore-632002
    Tamil Nadu
    S. India

37. Vasinanukorn, Dr. Mayuree
    Ass. Dean of Academic Affairs
    Faculty of Medicine
    Prince of Songkla University
    P.O. Box 4
    Hat-Yai, Songkla 90110
    Thailand

## Associate Members

1. Alam, Dr. S. Mahmood
   Baqai Medical College/Baqai
     Foundation
   III-B, 1/7, Nazimabad
   Super Highway/Toll Tax Plaza
   P.O. Box 2407
   Karachi – 18
   Pakistan

2. Alkafajei, Dr. Ahmed M.B.
   College of Medicine
   Department of Community Medi-
     cine
   University of Mosul
   Mosul, Baghdad
   Iraq

3. Al Qirbi, Dr. Abobackr
   Dean, Faculty of Medicine and
     Health Sciences

Sana'a University
P.O. Box 1247
Sana'a Yemenaraq Republic

4. Aristizabal A., Dr. Gerardo
   Dean, Faculty of Medicine
   Escuela Colombiana de Medicin
   Calle 134 No. 13-81
   Bogotá
   Colombia, S.A.

5. Baggio, Dr. Adelar Francisco
   President, Fidene
   Rua Sao Francisco
   501 Caixa Postal 560
   98.700 Ijui RS
   Brasil

6. Bhachu, Dr. Sem Singh
   Course Coordinator, AMREF
     Training Centre
   Diploma in Community Health
   Wilson Airport
   P.O. Box 30125
   Nairobi
   Kenya

7. Bolanos, Dr. Oscar
   Dean, Medical Faculty
   Universidad del Valle
   Apartado Aereo 2188
   Cali
   Colombia

8. Camp, Dr. Martha G.
   Assistant Director, Office of
     Educational Research and
     Services
   The Bowman Grey School of
     Medicine
   Wake Forest University
   300 South Hawthorne Road
   Winston Salem, North Carolina
     27103
   U.S.A.

9. Carabeo, Dr. Joseph M.
   Executive Officer

Philippine Youth Health Program
Room 703, Manufacturer's Build-
ing
Plaza Santa Cruz
Santa Cruz, Manila
The Philippines

10. Chawla, Dr. Livtar Singh
Professor and Head of Depart-
ment of Medicine
Dayanand Medical College
Ludhiana 141001 (Punjab)
India

11. Cox, Dr. K.R.
Head of the School of Medical
Education
University of New South Wales
P.O. Box 1, Kensington
New South Wales, Sydney
Australia 2033

12. Day, Prof.dr. Stacey B., M.D.,
Ph.D., D.Sc.
Professor of International Health
and Director
World Health Organization Col-
laborating Center
6 Lomond Avenue
New York, New York 10977
U.S.A.

13. Donhuijsen, Dr. H.W.A.
Asst. Dean I, School of Medicine
Padjadjaran University
Jalan Pasirkaliki 190
Bandung 40161
Indonesia

14. Al-Faleh, Dr. Faleh Z.
Dean, College of Medicine
King Saud University
P.O. Box 2248
Riyadh
The Kingdom of Saudi Arabia

15. Farah, Dr. Abdi Ahmed
(Pakistan)
Dean, Faculty of Medicine
National University
P.O. Box 933
Mogadishu
Somalia

16. Flores-Medina, Dr. Octavio A.
Dean, Facultad de Medicina
Universidad Autónoma de
Zacatecas
Carretera a la Bufa s/n
Zacatecas
México

17. Garcia-Barbero, Mrs. Milagros
Head of the Unit of Medical Edu-
cation
Medical School
University of Alicante
Apdo 99
Alicante 03690
Spain

18. George, Dr. C.F.
Dean, Faculty of Medicine
University of Southampton
Centre Block, General Hospital
Tremona Road
Southampton SO9 4XY
United Kingdom

19. Greenblatt, Dr. Charles L.
School Director, Hadassah Medi-
cal School
Hebrew University
P.O. Box 1172
Jerusalem 91010
Israel

20. Gwavava, Dr. N.J.T.
Dean, School of Medicine
University of Zimbabwe
P.O. Box A178
Avondale, Mt. Pleasant
Harare
Zimbabwe

21. Hamad, Dr. Bashir
    Dean, Faculty of Medicine &
        Health Sciences/
    The United Arab Emirates
        University
    P.O. Box 15551
    Al Ain
    The United Arab Emirates

22. Hassan, Dr. Mohamed A.
    Dean, Faculty of Medicine
    University of Khartoum
    P.O. Box 102
    Khartoum
    Democratic Republic of the
        Sudan

23. Hilton, Dr. David
    Assistant Director, World Coun-
        cil of Churches
    Christian Medical Commission
    150, route de Ferney
    1211 Geneva 20
    Switzerland

24. Hoenigmann, Alexander C.
    c/o Austrian Medical Students
        Association (AMSA)
    Liechtensteinstrasse 13
    1090 Wien
    Austria

25. Hori, Dr. Motokazu
    Dean, School of Medicine
    University of Tsukuba
    Tsukuba City, Ibaraki-ken 305
    Japan

26. Isacsson, Dr. Sven-Olof
    Faculty of Medicine
    Office of Medical Education
    Lund University
    Box 117
    22100 Lund
    Sweden

27. Islam, Dr. Nurul
    Coordinator
    Institute of Applied Health
        Sciences
    University of Chittagong
    63 Central Road, Dhanmondi
        R.A.
    Dhaka−5
    Bangladesh

28. Jain, Dr. P.S.
    Dr. B.C. Roy Foundation
    Medical Education Centre
    Medical Council of India
    Kotla Road, Temple Lane
    New Delhi−11002
    India

29. Kelsey Fry, Dr. I.
    Dean, Medical College of St.
        Bartholomew's Hospital
    University of London
    West Smithfield, London EC1A
        7BE

30. Macadam, Dr. Douglas
    Head, Department of Community
        Practice
    The Community Health Research
        & Training Unit
    University of Western Australia
    328 Stirling Highway
    Claremont, WA 6010
    Australia

31. Magen, Dr. Myron S.
    Dean, College of Osteopathic
        Medicine
    Michigan State University
    A308 East Fee Hall
    East Lansing, Michigan
        48824-1316
    U.S.A.

32. Mazzuchi, Dr. Daniel S.
    Assistant Dean
    The Upper Peninsula Health Education Corporation
    A-118 East Fee Hall
    East Lansing, Michigan
    48824-1316
    U.S.A.

33. Monterosa Rogel, Dr. Rafael A.
    Dean, Medical School
    Universidad Nacional de El Salvador (UES)
    San Salvador
    El Salvador, C.A.

34. Mukelabai, Prof. K.
    Dean, School of Medicine
    University of Zambia
    P.O. Box 50110
    Lusaka
    Zambia

35. Orrenius, Dr. Sten
    Dean, College of Medicine
    Karolinska Institute
    P.O. Box 60400
    10401 Stockholm
    Sweden

36. Padonu, Dr. Michael K.O.
    Department of Community Medicine
    College of Medical Sciences
    University of Maiduguri
    P.M.B. 1069
    Maiduguri, Borno State
    Nigeria

37. Parry, Dr. E.H.O.
    Director, The Wellcome Tropical Institute
    200 Euston Road
    London NW1 2BQ
    United Kingdom

38. Pauli, Dr. Hannes G.
    Director, Institute for Research in Education and Evaluation
    Faculty of Medicine
    University of Bern
    Inselspital 14c
    3010 Bern
    Switzerland

39. Pesigan, Dr. Arturo M.
    Executive Director, Community Medicine Development Foundation, Inc.
    c/o Department of Community Health
    College of Public Health
    University of the Philippines
    Manila
    P.O. Box EA79, Ermita 1000
    Metro Manila
    The Philippines

40. Philalithis, Dr. A.
    Assistant Professor in Social Medicine
    School of Health Sciences, Div. of Medicine
    University of Crete
    71409 Iraklion, Crete
    Greece

41. Richards, Dr. Ronald W.
    Professor and Director
    University of Illinois at Chicago
    Center for Educational Development, Health Sciences Center
    808 S. Wood Street, Room 986
    Chicago, Illinois 60612
    U.S.A.

42. Rodezno, Dr. Rafael Amador
    Coordinador Facultativo Estudio Trabajo U.N.A.N.
    Dept. Medicina Preventiva y Salud Pública
    Hospital Esc. Oscar D. Rosales A.
    Leon
    Nicaragua

43. Seraphin, Dr. Bararengana
    Dean, Faculty of Medicine
    National University of Rwanda
    B.P. 30, Butare
    Rwanda

44. Shahabudin, Dr. Sharifah Hapsah
    Asso. Prof., Medical Education
        Unit
    Faculty of Medicine
    Universiti Kebangsaan Malaysia
        (UKM)
    Jalan Raja Muda
    50300 Kuala Lumpur
    Malaysia

45. Shaker-Shubair, Dr. Kandil
    Director
    Center for Educational Develop-
        ment for Health Personnel
    University of Jordan
    Amman
    Jordan

46. Small, Ms. Elaine D.
    Dean, Faculty of Health Sciences
    University of Guyana
    Turkeyen Campus, Box 841
    Georgetown
    Guyana

47. Tajasen, Dr. Tejatat
    Assistant Prof. and Dean, Faculty
        of Medicine
    Chiangmai University
    110 Intavaroras Road
    Maung, Chiangmai 50000
    Thailand

48. Torrado, Dr. A.
    Clinical Director
    Medical Faculty
    Paediatric Hospital
    3000 Coimbra
    Portugal

49. Ulmer, Dr. David D.
    Dean, Faculty of Health Sciences
    The Aga Khan University
    Stadium Road
    P.O. Box 3500
    Karachi-5
    Pakistan

50. Wiedersheim, Dr. Robert
    Dean, Medical Faculty
    University Witten/Herdecke
    Beckweg 4
    5804 Herdecke
    Federal Republic of Germany

51. Wray, Dr. Samuel R.
    Dean, Faculty of Medicine
    University of the West Indies
    Mona, Kingston 7
    Jamaica

52. Zachariah, Dr. A.
    Dean, Christian Medical School
    Ludhiana 141008
    Punjab
    India

53. Zapeta, Dr.
    Dean, Faculty of Medicine
    Universidad Nacional Autónoma
        de Nicaragua
    Aptdo Postal 663
    Managua J.R.
    Nicaragua

54. Zein, Dr. Zein Ahmed
    Dean
    Gondar College of Medical
        Sciences
    P.O. Box 196
    Gondar Ethiopia

55. Zilhao, Dr. Aurelio A.
    Dean, Faculty of Medicine
    Universidade Eduardo Mondlane
    P.O. Box 257
    Maputo
    República Popular de Mozam-
        bique

56. Zwi, Dr. Anthony
    Lecturer in Community Medicine
    University College and Middle-
        sex School of Medicine
    66-72 Gower Street
    London WC1E 6EA
    United Kingdom

57. Jeffers, Mr. Wayne S.
    Student
    International Community-
        Oriented Medical Students
        Ass.
    c/o The University of New Mex-
        ico
    2400 Tucker Avenue
    Albuquerque, New Mexico 87131
    U.S.A.

58. Shalby, Miss Sherein Abd-El
        Hamed
    Chairman, The Standing Com-
        mittee of E.M.S.A.
    Egyptian Medical Students
        Association
    c/o Suez Canal University
    Faculty of Medicine
    P.O. Box 41522
    Ismailia
    Egypt

59. Gur-Aryeh, Mr. Itay
    Chairman, Tel Aviv Medical Stu-
        dents Organization
    IMSF, Sackler School of Medi-
        cine
    University of Tel Aviv
    Ramat Aviv 69978, Tel Aviv
    Israel

60. Ormos, Kleopatra
    Secretary General IFMSA
    Liechtensteinstrasse 13
    1090 Vienna
    Austria

## Corresponding Members

1. Abel, Dr. Rajaratnam
   Head, RUHSA Department
   Rural Unit Health & Social
       Affairs
   Ruhsa P.O. 632 209
   North Arcot Dits., Tamil Nadu
   India

2. Alger, Dr. Elizabeth A.
   Associate Dean
   UMDNJ-New Jersey Medical
       School
   Office of Education
   185 South Orange Avenue
   Newark, New Jersey 07103-2757
   U.S.A.

3. Bamgbose, Dr. Jones Koleade
   Faculty of Health Sciences
   Obafemi Awolowo University
   P.O. Box 1392
   Ile-Ife 040 State
   Nigeria

4. Bicknell, Dr. William J.
   Professor of Public Health
   Office of Special Projects Health
       Policy Institute
   Boston University
   53 Bay State Road
   Boston, Massachusetts 00000
   U.S.A.

5. Boikhan, Dr. M.S.
   Director
   Plot ST/1
   Pakistan Medico International
   Sect. no. 4 Orangi Town
   Karachi–41
   Pakistan

6. Cardona, Dr. Jorge Osorio
   Professor, National School of
       Public Health
   Universidad de Antioquia
   A.A. 66425 Medellin
   Colombia

7. Clarke, Dr. W.D.
   Director, Blithe Centre for
     Health and Medical Education
   BMA House
   Tavistock Square
   Blithe Center for Health and
     Medical Education
   London WC1H 9JP
   United Kingdom

8. Grande, Dr. Nuno Rodrigues
   Professor and Chairman
   Largo do Prof. Abel Salazar, 2
   Instituto de Ciencins Biomedicas
     Abel Salazar
   Universidade do Porto
   4000 Porto
   Portugal

9. Hart, Dr. Julian Tudor
   The Queens
   Glyncorrwg
   West Glamorgan
   Wales SA13 3BL
   United Kingdom

10. Hidajat, Dr. Achmad
    Dean, Faculty of Medicine
    Brawyaya University
    J.L.M.T. Haryono 171 Malang
    East Java
    Indonesia

11. Kumpusalo, Dr. Esko
    University of Kuopio
    Department of Community
      Health
    P.O. Box 6
    70211 Kuopio
    Finland

12. Mangla, Dr. Bhupesh
    General Secretary
    Azad Medicos' Association
    Gole Market
    16/5 Doctor's Lane
    New Delhi – 110 001
    India

13. Montoya, Dr. Carlos A.
    Hospital Infantil Universitario
    Carrera 25, Numero 49-48
    Manizales-Caldos
    Colombia

14. Moss, Dr. John
    Lecturer, Department of Commu-
      nity Medicine
    The University of Adelaide
    3rd Floor, Bice Building
    Royal Adelaide Hospital
    Adelaide
    South Australia 5000

15. Musgrove, Dr. John
    Professor of Family & Commu-
      nity Health
    College of Medicine
    Sultan Qaboos University
    P.O. Box 32-485, Al-Khod
    Sultanat of Oman

16. Petit, Dr. P.L.
    Consultant Public Health, Con-
      sultant for Management of
      Development Programmes
      (C.D.P.)
    Johannes Worpstraat 5-III
    1076 BC Amsterdam
    The Netherlands

17. Reid, Dr. Una V.
    WHO/Pan American Health
      Organization
    Box 508
    Bridgetown
    Barbados, W.I.

18. Seager, Dr. Charles Philip
    Psychiatric Unit
    Herries Road
    Northern General Hospital
    Sheffield S5 7AU
    United Kingdom

19. White, Dr. Donald K.
    Senior Lecturer, Health Services
      Management Centre

Edgbaston
19, Greville Drive
Birmingham B15 2UU
United Kingdom

20. Xing, Dr. Chen Zhi
Vice Director of Shanghai Ninth
People's Hospital
Shanghai Second Medical
University
639 Zhi Zao Ju Road
Shanghai
People's Republic of China

## Honorary Members

1. Fülop, Dr. Tamas
Former Director
Division of Health Manpower
Development
World Health Organization
Geneva
Switzerland

2. Guilbert, Dr. Jean-Jacques
Former Chief Medical Officer for
Education Planning, Methodol-
ogy and Evaluation
Division of Health Manpower
Development
World Health Organization
Geneva
Switzerland

3. Herrera, Dr. Florentino Jr.
In life Dean and Chancellor
College of Medicine
University of the Philippines
Manila
The Philippines

4. Katz, Dr. Frederick M.
In life Chief Scientist for Educa-
tional Evaluation
World Health Organization
Health Manpower Development

Geneva
Switzerland

5. Maddison, Dr. David C.
In life Foundation Dean
Faculty of Medicine
University of Newcastle
New South Wales
Australia

6. Odonez, Dr. Cosme
Representative Ministry of Public
Health
Higher Institute of Medical
Sciences
Havana
Cuba

7. Prywes, Dr. Moshe
Chairman, Center for Medical
Education
Ben Gurion University of the
Negev
Beer Sheva 84105
Israel

8. Sibley, Dr. Jack C.
In life Associate Dean, Education
Faculty of Health Sciences
McMaster University
Hamilton, Ontario
Canada

9. Tiddens, Dr. Harmen
Professor of Health Care Organi-
zation
University of Brabant
Tilburg
The Netherlands

10. Villareal, Dr. Ramón
In life Dean, Faculty of Health
Sciences
Universidad Autónoma
Metropolitana
Xochimilco
Mexico City
Mexico

# Index

Activation of prior knowledge, 105–106
  requirements for, 110
Allocation of resources, 5, 49, 202–203
Appropriate medical care, as term, 137

Ben Gurion University (BGU), Faculty of
  Health Sciences. *See* Training
  Medical Teachers
BGU. *See* Ben Gurion University, Faculty
  of Health Sciences
Brainstorming, 107

Case study method, 103
CBMES. *See* Community-based Medical
  Education and Service Program
Clinical epidemiology, 49
Clinical instruction, reform in, 35–37
COBES (Community-based experience
  and service) educational program
  in Nigeria
  design and objectives of, 79–80
  direct confrontation with health
    problems, 83
  documentation of learning as reflected
    in students' statements, 84
  evaluating program, 86
  evaluating students' performance, 85
  health and disease in relation to
    environment, 84
  limited objectives of, 91
  sixth-year student's impression of,
    91–92
  student reports, 80–83

defining and learning about commu-
  nity, 80–81
guinea worm infestation in Dekala,
  82–83
nutritional status of children, 81–82
student's reflections on, 88–90
terminal objectives of, 91
Collaborative projects, 204
Community-based activities, 69
Community-based curriculum. *See*
  Community-oriented curriculum
Community-based education. *See*
  Community-oriented medical
  education
Community-based experience and service
  educational program in Nigeria.
  *See* COBES
Community-based Medical Education and
  Service (CBMES) Program,
  98–99
Community-based medical education in
  Nigeria (Bayero University), 93–99
  CBMES program, 98–99
  criteria for selection of areas for, 97
  curriculum, 95–96
  educational objectives, 96
  first community-based medical posting,
    98
  institutional objectives of Bayero
    University Medical School, 94–96
  major disease entities in Nigeria, 94
Community health, concept of, 52
Community Health Committees, 96
Community medicine, taught by problem-
  solving, 152–153

Community orientation, in health care,
6, 7
Community-oriented curriculum, 67–76
at Bayero University, 95–96
community-based activity versus, 69
issues in curriculum design, 71–72
new role for teachers, 75–76
task of implementing, 66–67
Community-oriented medical education
basic principles and ingredients of, 68
characteristics of, 56–60
community basis, 53–54
community involvement, 71
conceptual formation in student, 57
coordination between educational institution and health services, 70–71
in current use, 47–50
defining, 51, 67–68
evaluating, 11–12
experiments in, 7
future of, 14–15
health orientation, 52–53
humanistic challenge of student, 57–58
institutional commitment to, 56
institutional involvement in delivery of health care to community, 57
integration across disciplines, 58–60
leadership in, 70
life cycle, 55–56
management and organization, 76
"natural history of disease" model,
54–55
network of, for health sciences, 12–14.
See also Network of Community-oriented Educational Institutions for Health Sciences (The Network)
primary goal of, 11
problem-based learning and, 10–11,
72–73
problem-solving, 60
reasons for, 4–7
selection of students, 60–61
self-learning, 60
sites of learning, 74–75
social and behavioral sciences in, 58
spiral model, 59–60
summary of features of curriculum in,
61–63
three-dimensional model, 63–64

Comparative studies, of innovative institutions, 203–204
Conventional medical education,
problems of, 112–115
Critical appraisal of data/evidence, 160,
172
Curriculum. *See also* Community-oriented curriculum
structure of, in problem-based learning at Newcastle, 119–121
systematic development of, at Newcastle, 115–117

Diagnostic errors, 28
Discipline-based learning, 8
Discovery-learning approach, 103
Disease
"natural history of disease" model,
54–55
psychological and social factors in, 26

Elaboration of knowledge, 106
Encoding specificity, 103, 106
Environment, health and, 6
Ethics, 25
Evaluation of health sciences education programs
evaluation of student performance,
169–173
critical thinking ability, 170
knowledge, 170
methods of student evaluation, 171
patient management problems,
171–173
personal characteristics, 170
principles of evaluation, 169
problem-solving, 169–170
self-directed learning, 170–171
specific evaluation strategies, 171
program evaluation, 173–174
program evaluation at McMaster,
175–179
data bank outcome studies, 176
external evaluation and accreditation,
176
ongoing evaluation by students,
175–176

studies on graduates, 176–179
programs, 165–179
selection of students, 167–169
ultimate effectiveness of, 165–166
Evaluation system at Maastricht Medical
School, 180–194. *See also* Maastricht Medical School

Faculty development, 239–241. *See also*
Training medical teachers
beliefs held among teachers, 239
instructional qualities necessary for
problem-based, community-
oriented curricula, 239
teacher-training programs, 240
Financial costs of medicine, 5, 18–19,
26, 30–31, 48

Health
defining, 52
person-centered/population-based
model of, 4
psychological and behavioral factors in,
23–24
Hospital-based model of medical education, 93

Iatrogenesis, 4
Immune system, psychological and social
factors and, 26
Information processing approach to learning, 105–106
Innovative institutions: Assessment, 203–
205
collaborative projects, 204
comparative studies, 203
Innovative medical education, 157–163
evaluation procedures and curriculum,
157–163
objectives of, 157
protecting and maintaining, 250

Laboratory tests, use and costs of, 30
Lancaster Approaches to Studying Inventory, 226

MAAS. *See* Maastricht Historytaking and
Advice Checklist
Maastricht Historytaking and Advice
Checklist (MAAS/MHAC),
161–162, 206
categories of questions in, 209–210
construction of, 208–210
description of, 210–211
evaluating undergraduate students with,
213
growth in interviewing skills, 213–217
patients' contribution to interview,
211–212
protocol and psychometric properties
of, 212–213
Maastricht Medical School, 206–218
achievements, 234–235
clinical ratings, 189
dropout rates and performance,
234–235
education counseling and graduation,
193–194
evaluation program, 182–188
block tests, 183
progress tests, 183–186
skills tests, 186–188
graduation and dropouts, 233–234
outline of curriculum, 181
overview of medical curriculum,
230–231
positive and negative evaluations of
curriculum by students, 232
problem-based learning, 180–182
problem-based learning training programs, 240
Progress Test Review Committee
(PTRC), 184–185
progress tests at, 221
self-assessment units, 189–193
Modified Essay Questions (MEQ),
191
Patient Management Problems
(PMP), 190–191
Portable Patient Problem Pack
(P4-Deck), 192
Problem Boxes (PB), 191–192
Simulated Patient Encounters (SPE),
188
Structured Orals (SO), 188

Maastricht Medical School (*cont.*)
  study load, 233
  teaching program in medical interview-
    ing, 206–208
  triple jump exercise (TJE), 193
  tutorials, student response to, 232
McMaster Medical School curriculum,
    147–156
  achievement of graduates, 222
  benefits of problem-based learning,
    149–150
  case 1, Mary Cornell: typical problem,
    154
  case 2, lazarus problem: phase II
    problem, 154–155
  case 3, Sally Moutarde: phase II
    problem, 155–156
  clinical competence and internship per-
    formance, 223
  community medicine taught by,
    152–153
  curricular objectives, 148–149
  faculty use of problem-solving, 153
  integration of knowledge through
    problem-solving, 151–152
  phase I, 147
  phase II, 148
  phase III, 148
  phase IV, 148
  problem selection, 150–151
    faculty use of, 153
    in large classes, 153
  science education, 150
  summary of objectives, 167
  tutors, 158
"McMaster philosophy," 272
Medicaid, 18
Medical care
  costs of, 5, 18–19, 26, 30–31, 48
  public's expectations of, 6
Medical education, 3–16
  community-oriented, 4–7
  criticisms of, 47
  objectives of, 166
  obstacles to change in, 22–24
  post World War II revolution in medi-
    cine, 19–22
  problem-based learning, 7–10
  reason for teaching science in, 33

reform in, 28–37
  stress factors in, 19–20
Medical environment, new forces in,
    24–28
Medical interviewing. *See also* Maas-
    tricht Historytaking and Advice
    Checklist (MAAS/MHAC)
  design of Maastricht interview training
    program, 206–208
  importance of, 206
  principles for designing teaching pro-
    grams in, 206–207
Medical schools
  entrance requirements for, 31–32
  established schools, challenges in, 69
  first two years of, 20
  nonscientific side of medicine
    presented in, 21–22
  problems of, 21
  reform in, 29
  status of teachers, 22
Medical teachers. *See also* Faculty
    development, Training medical
    teachers
  attitude changes in, 243–247. *See also*
    Suez Canal University
  preparation of, 263–264
Medicare, 18
  post World War II, 17–19, 47–48
  psychological and behavioral factors in,
    25
  specialization in, 48–49
MHAC. *See* Maastricht Historytaking and
    Advice Checklist
Modern medicine, critiques of, 4–5


Network of Community-oriented Educa-
    tional Institutions for Health
    Sciences (The Network), 12–14,
    275–278
  achievement of graduates, 222
  community-oriented education,
    277–278
  member institutions, 279–289
  objectives, 276
Organization for Economic Coopera-
    tion and Development (OECD),
    275

"Newcastle experiment," 39–46. *See also*
    Problem-based medical education:
    Newcastle approach
  basic philosophy for medical education,
    39–40
  development of objectives, 41–42
  education program and its assessment,
    43–46
  faculty of medicine with University of
    Newcastle, 40–41
  selection of students, 43

Organization for Economic Cooperation
    and Development (OECD), 275

Patient Satisfaction with Communication
    Checklist (PSCC), 212
Physicians
  ethical dilemmas faced by, 25
  number and distribution of, 29
  performance expectations or compe-
    tence of, 165–166
  relations with patient, 178
  role of, 26–28
  specialists, 48–49
  use of quantitative data by, 24–25
POMR. *See* Problem-oriented medical
    record
Population-based medicine, 6
Preclinical education, 32–35
Premedical education, 31–32
Preventive medicine, 29–30
  "natural history of disease" model,
    54–55
  in pediatrics, 49
Primary care, choosing careers in,
    223–224
Primary care orientation, 158
"Priority" problems, 104, 136–137
Problem-based, community-oriented cur-
    ricula, 220–228
  academic achievement, 220–222
  career preference and career choice,
    223–224
  clinical competence and internship per-
    formance, 222–223
  learning styles, 225–226

perceptions of students regarding cur-
    riculum, 224–225
  problems of comparing educational
    approaches, 226–227
Problem-based learning, 7–10, 101–104
  benefits of, 149–150
  cognitive and motivational effects of,
    230–238
  community-oriented medical education
    and, 10–11, 72–74
  comparisons of medical knowledge
    achievement scores, 236
  conditions that facilitate, 105–106
  description of, 101–102, 106–109, 231
  design of introductory student training,
    263
  evaluating, 11–12
  future of, 14–15
  graduation and dropouts, 233–234
  historical perspective on, 102–103
  introducing, into conventional curricu-
    lum, 272–275
  learning objectives in, 102
  at Maastricht Medical School, 180–181
  McMaster approach to, 9–10
  as means of instruction from first day
    to last, 9–10
  model for, 122–124
  objectives of, 261–262
  positive motivational effects of,
    233–234
  preparation of faculty members for,
    263–264
  problem-solving performance, 235–236
  rationale behind, 105–111
  reordering of priorities in, 122
  staff for, 130
  student attitudes toward instruction,
    231–233
  study load, 233
  teacher training, framework of, 264–265
  as term, 122
  training program for, structure of,
    262–263
  training students for, 261–262
  tutor training, 269
  utility of, 9
  workshop: Introduction to problem-
    based learning, 268

Problem-based learning activities, 130
Problem-based medical education: New-
    castle approach, 112–144
  anticipated advantages, 117–118
  assessment, 138–140
  continuing management decision,
    128–129
  curricular structure, 119–121
  diagnostic decision, 127–128
  educational model, 127–129
  education structure, 141–142
  evaluation, 144
  functional organization, 142–143
  general organization, 140–141
  learning environment, 130–131
  learning process skills, 124
  learning resources, 131
  Mark 1 curriculum, 124–125
  Mark 1 problem materials, 131–133
  Mark 2 curriculum, 125–127
  Mark 2 problem materials, 133–136
  matrix, 143–144
  objectives, 118–119
  organization and management of
    resources, 140–144
  problem selection, 136–137
  problems of conventional medical edu-
    cation, 112–115
  staff for, 130
  systematic development of curriculum,
    115–117
  tutors, role and activities of, 127
  using problems for learning, 122–140
Problem-oriented medical record
    (POMR), 273
Problem-solving, 60
  community medicine taught by,
    152–153
  integration of knowledge through,
    151–152
  for large classes, 153
  as term, 122
Program evaluation, 199–203
  allocation of resources, 202–203
  clarification of aims, 199–200
  definition of outcomes, 200–201
  design of research projects, 201–202
  reasons for evaluation, 200

PSCC. *See* Patient Satisfaction with
    Communication Checklist
Psychological and behavioral factors, in
    medicine, 25

Quantitative data, physicians' use of,
    24–25

Resource allocation. *See* Allocation of
    resources

Self-directed study, at McMaster, 178
Self-learning, 60
Social progress and public health, 4–5
Socratic teaching method, 8
Student assessment, 196–199
  assessment and independent learning,
    196–197
  designing appropriate assessment tools,
    198–199
  "steering effect" of assessment,
    197–198
Suez Canal University
  institutional goals toward development
    of new medical schools, 243
  items measuring attitude toward aspects
    of medical education, 245
  new curricula, 243
  workshop, 244
    evaluation of, 244–246

Teachers in community-based education,
    role of, 75–76
Training medical teachers
  educational leaders "discovered" in
    teacher training workshops, 257
  evaluation of training, 255–257
  faculty development, 250
  framework of training, 264–265
  motivational aspects, 249, 257–258
  multiphasic teaching-training model,
    252
  personal development of teachers, 250
  phase I: orientation workshop, 251

phase II: Building Instructional Skills
workshop, 251–253
phase III: four workshops, 253–254
protecting and maintaining educational
innovations, 250
quality of instruction, 249
range of participation, 254–255
role of "educational leader," 256
timewise hierarchical structure, 257
training program, 250–251
two-dimensional matrix, 258
Triple-jump exercises (TJE), 172, 193,
198, 199
Tuberculosis, drops in rates of, 5
Tutors
difficulties of adapting to problem-
based medical education, 130

in problem-based learning at McMaster
Medical School, 150
role of problem-based learning tutor,
130–131

University of Adelaide, problem-based
learning at, 272–275

WHO. See World Health Organization
World Health Organization (WHO), 275,
276
community-oriented educational
programmes, 12–13
definition of health, 52
on public health care, 6

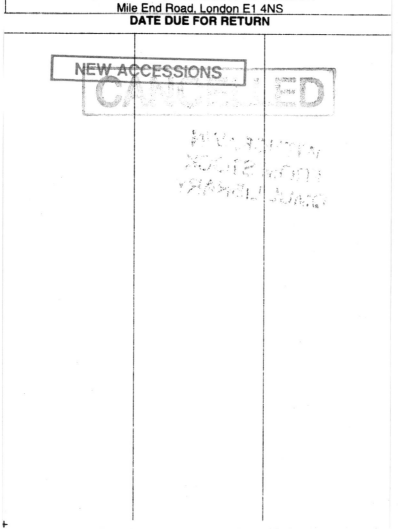

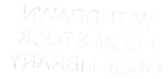

IICRC implements projects to develop and promote international cooperation in the fields of science, technology and culture. The organisation is jointly formed by the United Nations University (UNU), the Ishikawa Prefecture Government in Japan, and the City of Kanazawa in Japan. IICRC was established on 3 October 1996 with the aim of providing local input into UNU efforts on sustainable development and international cooperation. In this context, IICRC acts as a programme office for UNU-IAS.

Website: http://www.ias.unu.edu/iicrc

The United Nations University Institute of Advanced Studies (UNU-IAS) is a global think tank whose mission is "advancing knowledge and promoting learning for policymaking to meet the challenges of sustainable development". UNU-IAS undertakes research and postgraduate education to identify and address strategic issues of concern for all humankind, for governments and decision makers and, particularly, for developing countries. The Institute convenes expertise from disciplines such as economics, law, and social and natural sciences to better understand and contribute creative solutions to pressing global concerns, with research focused on Urban Studies, Biodiplomacy, Sustainable Development Governance, Science Policy and Education for Sustainable Development, and Ecosystems and People.

Website: http://www.ias.unu.edu

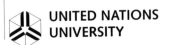

**UNITED NATIONS**
**UNIVERSITY**

**UNU-IAS**
Institute of Advanced Studies

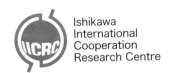

Ishikawa
International
Cooperation
Research Centre